A Progress in Cardiovascular Diseases Reprint
May/June and July/August 1975

POSTOPERATIVE CONGENITAL HEART DISEASE

Edited by
Amnon Rosenthal, M.D.
Senior Associate in Cardiology
The Children's Hospital Medical Center
Boston, Massachusetts
Edmund H. Sonnenblick, M.D.
Professor of Medicine, and
Chief, Division of Cardiology
Albert Einstein College of Medicine
Bronx, New York
Michael Lesch, M.D.
Director, S.A. Levine Cardiac Center
Peter Bent Brigham Hospital
Associate Professor of Medicine
Harvard Medical School
Boston, Massachusetts

GRUNE & STRATTON
A Subsidiary of Harcourt Brace Jovanovich, Publishers
New York San Francisco London

The chapters of this book appeared originally in the May/June and July/August 1975 issues (Vol. XVII, No. 6 and Vol. XVIII, No. 1) of *Progress in Cardiovascular Diseases,* a bi-monthly journal published by Grune & Stratton, Inc., and edited by Edmund H. Sonnenblick, M.D., and Michael Lesch, M.D. Amnon Rosenthal, M.D. was guest editor for these issues.

Grune & Stratton, Inc.
111 Fifth Avenue
New York, New York 10003

Library of Congress Catalog Card Number 75-37081
International Standard Book Number 0-8089-0934-7

Printed in the United States of America

Contents

To

Prudence, Jonathan, Eben and Nathaniel

FOREWORD

THE BENEFICIAL EFFECTS of surgical treatment of congenital heart disease are unquestionable. Overall mortality for infants critically ill with heart disease has been halved, at least. For selected diagnoses, like D-transposition of the great arteries with intact ventricular septum, survivors increased from 10 to 90%. Significant prolongation of life, through surgery, for those remaining asymptomatic beyond the first year of life is less well documented, but seems increasingly likely as clinical course studies, with and without operation, are being completed. The improvement in the quality of life, a hackneyed phrase of the past decade, cannot be doubted by anybody who has ever witnessed the dramatic postoperative changes in a skinny, blue, irritable, squatting youngster with tetralogy of Fallot, or examine the steep rise in the growth curve, after successful closure of a large ventricular septal defect. This is heady stuff; the surgeon and his cardiologist colleague cannot help but feel elated as they see themselves, much larger than life, reflected in the eyes of the grateful parents. With the help of the large supply of rose colored glasses, standard equipment in all cardiac and cardiac surgical departments, loud residual murmurs become faint, heart blocks are referred to as A-V dissociations, and persistent radiograhic changes are often disregarded.

The present volume, a very important one, evaluates the long term survivors. The papers originate from major centers of excellence on the East Coast, the South, and the Middle West. The principal authors of five of the nine chapters are present or former members of the Cardiology Department of the Children's Hospital. Review, thus, is bound to be somewhat slanted but is, at least, harmonious. None of the senior authors are surgeons, although our two surgical colleagues appear as co-authors; this should guarantee a degree of objectivity. The material is approached first from the point of view of various diagnostic tools (X-rays, ECG, VCG, Echo, Radionuclide angiocardiography, Ear Oximetry). Next, specific aspects of the post-operative state (myocardial performance, pulmonary vascular obstruction, growth and development and the fate of valve prostheses) and finally the general, long term, post-operative evaluation of the patients is addressed.

This excellent volume presents a hopeful but somewhat sobering view. The majority of the survivors are competitive products of surgical and medical skills. Still, many, even most, carry residual, albeit minor sequelae of congenital heart disease. These facts should not make the cardiologist any less positive in his attitude towards these patients, or the cardiovascular surgeon any less aggressive in his approach. Familiarity with the information so beautifully presented should make us, however, a little more cautious in discussing the future with the parents preoperatively, and somewhat more critical when discharging the child from the hospital. Postoperative hemodynamic evaluation is mandatory for all but the simplest defects, at set time intervals. Only a minority should be discharged completely from clinical supervision although the check-ups may be limited from two to five year intervals in those with excellent postoperative results.

Finally, the attentive reader of this volume will feel a bit less lonesome when he discovers an unexpected complication in one of his postoperative patients. It happens to the best of us.

Alexander S. Nadas, M.D.
Professor of Pediatrics at
Children's Hospital,
Harvard Medical School;
Chief, Department of Cardiology
Children's Hospital Medical
Center

The Patient With Congenital Heart Disease After Surgical Repair: An Overview

Amnon Rosenthal

THE ERA of surgical treatment of congenital cardiovascular disease was ushered in when Dr. Robert Gross successfully ligated a patent ductus arteriosus in 1938. During the subsequent two decades, corrective surgery was performed on patients with relatively simple cardiovascular malformations; such as coarctation of the aorta, atrial septal defect or pulmonary stenosis, and palliative surgery in patients with more complex lesions such as tetralogy of Fallot or complete transposition of the great arteries. In the last decade, the surgeons ingenuity and improved techniques have resulted in successful repair of the most complex malformations. Transposition of the great arteries, tricuspid atresia, and complete atrioventricular canal, for example, have become amenable to surgical repair. Recently, the most profound and far reaching changes have been the introduction of one stage surgical correction in infants instead of palliation followed by correction in childhood. Malformations such as ventricular septal defect, tetralogy of Fallot, and transposition of the great arteries can now be corrected in infancy utilizing deep hypothermic circulatory arrest. Corrective surgery in the neonate and infant has significantly altered the pattern of care and quality of life.

Survival and relief of symptoms are the immediate goal of surgery. The long term objective of surgical and medical treatment for infants and children with cardiovascular malformations remains to provide optimal physical, intellectual, and emotional growth that will enable them to be healthy adults.

Many of the children who have undergone surgical correction or palliation have reached adulthood. They present new and challenging clinical and laboratory findings with which the internist or the adult cardiologist may not be familiar. For example, pulmonary regurgitation is commonly present in postoperative patients with tetralogy of Fallot and right bundle branch block is nearly a uniform electrocardiographic pattern in patients who have had a right ventriculotomy for correction of tetralogy of Fallot or ventricular septal defect. Awareness of the cardiac and extracardiac complications, sequelae, and residua that follow surgery will permit the physician to assess the significance of the clinical findings and laboratory studies observed. Evaluation of the cardiovascular status in the postoperative patient may require exercise testing, electrophysiologic, or myocardial function studies by cardiac catheterization in addition to the customary examination, chest x-ray, and electrocardiogram.

Management may differ considerably from the nonoperated patient with congenital heart disease. The majority of postoperative patients can lead a normal family life. However, with few exceptions, they require closer medical supervision than other young adults. Susceptibility to infective endocarditis persists in most postoperative patients. They also should be given recommendations regarding recreational and occupational activities and may require genetic counseling. Women who have reached childbearing age may be expected to have an increased frequency of offspring with congenital cardiac malformations. How well these patients would tolerate hypertensive or coronary artery disease remains unknown. I would suspect that these may have a more adverse effect on the postoperative patient with congenital heart disease because of the frequent presence of conduction or rhythm abnormalities, poorer myocardial function, or injury associated with previous prolonged volume or pressure overload, chronic hypoxemia, or residual pulmonary vascular obstructive changes.

The purpose of this symposium is to provide the internist and cardiologist with up-to-date information on the clinical and laboratory findings, course, management, and prognosis of the postoperative patient with congenital heart disease. The individual manuscripts review problems common to many postoperative patients, the diagnostic tools utilized and, when appropriate, include an in depth discus-

From the Departments of Cardiology and Pediatrics, The Children's Hospital Medical Center, Harvard Medical School, Boston, Mass.

Reprint requests should be addressed to Amnon Rosenthal, M.D., Senior Associate in Cardiology, The Children's Hospital Medical Center, 300 Longwood Ave., Boston, Mass. 02115.

sion of specific problems associated with the common cardiac lesions. In many instances, particularly with regard to the long-term prognosis of the very complex cardiac lesions, only scant information is available and further recommendations must await more clinical research.

Residua, Sequelae, and Complications of Surgery for Congenital Heart Disease

Jill H. Morriss and Dan G. McNamara

IN THE 36 yr since patent ductus arteriosus was first repaired by operation, almost all of the congenital malformations of the heart and great vessels have been surgically "attacked." The range of success of these operative attempts varies from total cure in some to only temporary relief of symptoms in others. Current methods of surgical treatment, properly applied, can benefit about 80% of all patients with congenital heart disease. The undisputed value of surgery in the management of patients is well enough established that the remaining limitations can be discussed with candor.

The intent in presenting an outspoken review of the long-term residuae, sequelae, and complications of congenital heart operations is twofold. First, this review is meant to aid the physician who is concerned infrequently with congenital heart disease, but who will nevertheless be called upon from time-to-time to refer children for surgical treatment. Secondly, it should provide a reminder to those who are daily concerned with these patients that not all of the problems in congenital cardiovascular surgery are solved.

It is the patient's privilege and the physician's responsibility to know in advance of surgery both the likelihood of operative success and what "success" means in terms of the physical, social, educational, and vocational activities of the patient. Reasonable and pertinent questions include: (1) what is the extent of disability that might remain in spite of "successful" surgery, (2) what new problems might arise as a result of the operation, and (3) will cardiac or extracardiac developments appear later despite a technically successful operation?

For common cardiac defects which have been managed surgically for the past 20 yr or more, the answers are becoming available but for rare defects and for those first operated upon in recent years, the answer to many of these questions awaits longer follow-up.

DEFINITION OF TERMS

There might be differences of opinion among cardiologists and cardiovascular surgeons whether an abnormality identified after heart surgery constitutes a residual defect, a sequela of the operation, or a complication of the repair. Thus, the usage of these terms in this article requires definition.

Residua

The term postoperative *residua* refers to any of the remaining anatomic and hemodynamic abnormalities which existed as part of the congenital malformation or those which developed or could develop as a consequence of the defect. The residua in some instances might eventually be preventable in future patients by improvement in diagnostic or surgical techniques or by closer attention to those techniques currently available. In other instances, the nature of the malformation is such that a residual abnormality either could not be corrected or correction was not worth the added risk to the patient. It may be the case that the residua was located away from the area of primary operative exposure and no attempt was made to approach the additional defect surgically. The likelihood of certain defects remaining after surgery is unpredictable, while the chance that others will persist despite an otherwise successful operation can be anticipated quite accurately.

Sequelae

The term *sequelae* will be used to refer to those anatomic and hemodynamic consequences of the operative procedure which are apparently unavoidable in our current state of knowledge. However, once the method of avoiding an important sequela has been developed, its continued occurrence constitutes a *complication* as defined in the following section. Some sequelae, whether clinically obvious or not, are inconsequential, while

---

From the Section of Cardiology, Department of Pediatrics, Baylor College of Medicine, Houston, Tex., and the Texas Children's Hospital, Houston, Tex.

Supported in part by USPH NIH grant HL-5756, and by USPH NIH grant RR-00188 from the General Clinical Research Branch.

Reprint requests should be addressed to Jill H. Morriss, M.D., 6621 Fannin, Houston, Tex. 77025.

others lead to manifest or potential problems. A few of the sequelae may be more devastating than the original circulatory problem for which surgery was performed.

Complications

Complications are unexpected events related to the surgery though their occurrence is not always without precedent. Complications do not necessarily imply a mistake in judgment or performance on the part of the cardiologist, anesthesiologist, nurse, or surgeon, but certainly errors, however excusable, do sometimes result in complications. Some of the complications to be discussed are currently unpreventable.

CARDIOVASCULAR DYSFUNCTION IN CONGENITAL HEART DISEASE

Some of the manifestations of cardiovascular dysfunction and the potential consequences resulting from congenital heart disease are listed in Table 1.

Enlightened recommendation for operation is based on the extent to which surgery may remove or diminish the manifestations or prevent the potential consequences of the specific defect.

Table 1. Cardiovascular Dysfunction in Congenital Heart Disease

Manifestations
1. Cardiac enlargement (including hypertrophy and dilatation)
2. Pulmonary hypertension secondary to a structural anomaly
3. Arterial oxygen desaturation
4. Pulmonary edema
5. Myocardial insufficiency
6. Dysrhythmias
7. Airway obstruction
8. Systemic arterial hypertension
9. Exercise intolerance
10. Growth failure
Potential Consequences
1. Predisposition to infective endocarditis
2. Tendency to pulmonary infection
3. Pulmonary vascular obstructive disease
4. Central nervous system complications
5. Personality, psychologic, and intellectual consequences
6. Chance of sudden death

THE SPECIFIC MALFORMATIONS

This review concerns the eight most common malformations among those which are treated by operations usually considered "corrective" or definitive, as opposed to palliative.

Ductus Arteriosus

Any residuum or important sequela from surgery for simple ductus arteriosus would be unexpected by anyone with even a layman's knowledge of the operation, since the procedure reputedly is the simplest, safest, and most successful heart operation yet devised.

Simple Ductus Arteriosus

A simple ductus is one which is: (1) unassociated with elevated pulmonary artery pressure, (2) has sufficient length to permit occlusion without interference with flow through the adjacent aorta or pulmonary artery, (3) is unassociated with sclerotic changes in the wall of the ductus, pulmonary artery, or aorta, and (4) is unassociated with other cardiovascular defects.

Residua

Persistent patency or recanalization. Mere ligation rather than division and suture of the ductus may result in either incomplete closure or recanalization of the lumen. Thus ligation, while technically simpler, is rarely performed. As an exception, ligation may be preferable in the infant with a large ductus, especially when the diagnosis is uncertain or when the ductus is associated with large ventricular septal defect; then, banding of the pulmonary artery may be required. Under these conditions, the anterior approach required for exploration of the outflow tract or banding of the pulmonary artery prohibits the exposure needed for division of the ductus.

Susceptibility to infective endocarditis. The usual site of vegetations in subacute bacterial endocarditis (SBE) in patients with ductus is on the pulmonary artery opposite the orifice of the ductus at the site of a "jet" lesion. Once the "jet" lesion has formed (and there is no means of knowing when this occurs short of direct observation), the susceptibility to SBE is established. The older the patient, the more likely is the presence of the "jet" lesion. Thus, a residual tendency to SBE after successful ductus repair is theoretically possible, though we do not know of reported cases.

Persistent abnormalities. After surgical obliteration of the simple ductus, all indices of cardiac enlargement return to normal within a few weeks to a few months postoperatively. In those cases in which there is preoperative left axis deviation of the QRS complex on the frontal plane of the electrocardiogram (ECG), there will be no change postoperatively since left axis deviation does not result from left ventricular hypertrophy per se, but rather represents an additional anomaly of the conduction system. This ECG abnormality is of no functional consequence, however, and can be ignored in the follow-up of the patient.

Any persisting exercise intolerance, growth failure, or tendency to pulmonary infections after successful repair of simple ductus can be assumed to have another basis.

In most centers children who have had successful repair of simple ductus are dismissed from follow-up in a cardiac clinic and the use of prophylactic penicillin for dental procedures is discontinued. The acceptability for life insurance coverage without increased premium by most companies is further reassurance to the patient of his complete normalcy.

Sequelae

There is no sequela resulting from surgery for simple ductus even though some of the complications listed below may have been considered the unavoidable result of surgery a number of years ago.

Complications

Recurrent laryngeal nerve injury. Unfavorable operating conditions during dissection to reach the ductus may result in trauma to the recurrent laryngeal nerve. Paralysis of the larynx may interfere not only with the voice but also with patency of the airway in the early postoperative period.

Phrenic nerve injury. Injury to the phrenic nerve during any thoracic operation requiring mediastinal dissection may occur despite skillful technique. The diaphragmatic paralysis usually subsides within 3 mo after surgery. While the injury may be clinically silent in the patient with unimpaired lung function, it can seriously interfere with ventilation in the patient who has existing respiratory insufficiency (Fig. 1).

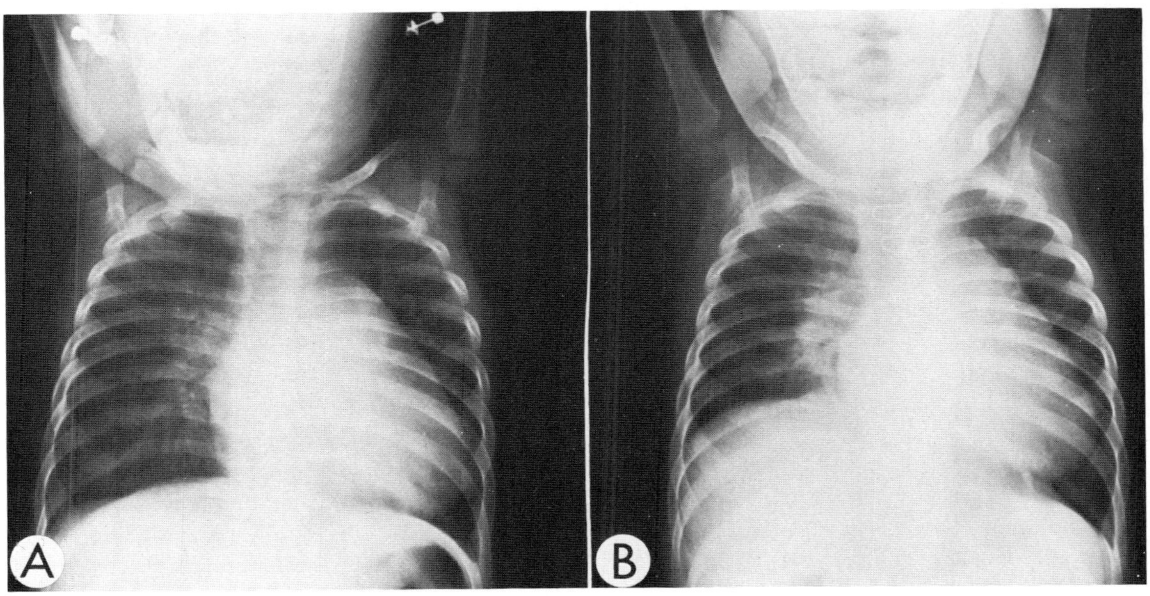

Fig. 1. (A) Preoperative chest film in a patient with left-to-right shunt demonstrating cardiomegaly and increased pulmonary vascularity. (B) Postoperative chest film with elevation of the right hemidiaphragm resulting from intraoperative phrenic nerve injury.

False aneurysm. False aneurysm may result from inadvertent separation of the layers of the pulmonary artery wall during dissection or during suturing of the ductus with the resultant formation of a hematoma in the pulmonary artery wall. This complication may not become clinically obvious until several weeks after operation when the patient develops unexplained fever and the radiographic appearance of a mass in the mediastinum. False aneurysm is more likely to complicate surgery for a large ductus with elevated pulmonary artery pressure associated with degenerative changes in the arterial wall.

Large Ductus Arteriosus with Elevated Pulmonary Artery Pressure

Usually a medium-sized ductus (internal diameter of ductus about $\frac{1}{3}$ to $\frac{1}{2}$ that of the aortic isthmus) produces a left-to-right shunt with a calculated pulmonary-to-systemic flow ratio of about 2-to-1. The pulmonary circulation accepts this flow without a resulting elevation of pulmonary artery pressure even though left ventricular enlargement and a wide pulse pressure ensue. However, when the internal diameter of the ductus measures over three-fourths that of the aorta, the pulmonary artery pressure is usually elevated as a consequence of the large flow and direct transmission of systemic pressure. Provided there are no other congenital or acquired abnormalities of the circulation, the pulmonary artery pressure can return to normal after obliteration of the ductus.

What are the possible explanations when pulmonary artery pressure remains elevated after operation?

Pulmonary Artery Branch Stenosis

The murmur of ductus arteriosus may obscure that of pulmonary artery branch stenosis. Unless cardiac catheterization and angiography are performed preoperatively, this anomaly, which is difficult to recognize at the time of surgery, may go undetected.

Pulmonary Vascular Obstructive Disease (PVOD)

This abnormality of the small muscular pulmonary arteries is not so common with ductus as it is with ventricular septal defect; however, the vascular phenomenon probably accounts for most cases of persistent pulmonary hypertension after ductus surgery.

Anatomic Obstruction of the Return of Pulmonary Venous Blood

When ductus arteriosus is associated with an obstructive lesion of the left side of the heart, some elevation of pulmonary artery pressure is likely to remain after obliteration of the ductus. These obstructive anomalies, often overlooked preoperatively, include stenosis of the individual pulmonary veins or of the common pulmonary vein (cor triatriatum), and mitral stenosis. In addition, restriction of flow into the left ventricle may result from either underdevelopment of the left ventricle or left ventricular failure due to other causes.

SELECTION OF THE PATIENT FOR PDA SURGERY

When ductus arteriosus is not a simple one or when surgery is required in infancy, or if the operation is performed by anyone other than an experienced surgeon, the usual encouraging and optimistic outlook cannot be given to the patient or to his family. Surgery for simple ductus is usually recommended in early childhood whether or not there are symptoms or manifestations of cardiovascular dysfunction.

Atrial Septal Defect (ASD)

There are five types of atrial septal defect, each correctable by a different operative technique. For each of them the result of surgery may differ. They are: (1) ostium secundum defect, (2) ostium primum defect, (3) fenestrated valve of the foramen ovale, (4) sinus venosus defect, (5) single atrium.

Because the secundum defect is the most common it will be reviewed in more detail than the others.

"Simple" ostium secundum defect. A simple ASD is one which is unassociated with other congenital cardiac defects or elevated pulmonary artery pressure and anatomically is of a size which allows direct suture closure rather than the use of a prosthetic patch. A simple ASD secundum is one which is far enough removed from the atrioventricular valves that neither the valve ring nor the atrioventricular conduction system is traumatized in the repair. It is also far enough removed from the sinoatrial node that atrial arrhythmias will not result from repair.

It is usually assumed that any right-to-left shunting with ASD constitutes a complicated defect and precludes surgical repair. This is indeed true if the cause of the right-to-left shunt is high pulmonary artery pressure and resistance. However, one of the uncommon defects associated with an otherwise simple ASD is a persistent functioning Eustachian valve diverting the flow of inferior vena caval blood directly into the left atrium as in the fetal circulation. For these patients, surgical closure can be accomplished with the same good outlook as otherwise simple ASD.

Next to ductus arteriosus, a simple ASD secundum has the best outlook for complete surgical cure. Within a year of operation performed in childhood the heart size is normal by physical, radiographic, and electrocardiographic examination and the great majority of patients are asymptomatic.

Most of the postoperative patients have been allowed to participate in sports and to plan a normal family life including parenthood. Some clinics have dismissed the patient from further follow-up and have discontinued the use of antibiotic prophylaxis for dental work. Even when a prosthetic patch has been used to close the defect, a number of major life insurance companies have granted policies to patients 5 yr after surgery without an increase in premium.

Residua

Persistent atrial communication. It has not been our policy to routinely recatheterize all of the patients after clinically successful repair of simple ASD. Small clinically insignificant persistent communications have been reported in patients submitted to routine postoperative catheterization, but these minute defects should not alter the good outlook with operation.

Cardiac enlargement. Persistent cardiac enlargement has not been noted in the children operated upon at this institution for simple ASD. However, Young[1] reported unexplainable radiographic and/or electrocardiographic signs of persistent cardiac enlargement in 17 of 66 postoperative patients. In an additional five patients with cardiac enlargement, there was either an arrhythmia or persistent shunt.

Pulmonary valve and branch pressure gradients. The systolic murmur of ASD is related to the systolic pressure gradient between the right ventricle and the main pulmonary artery. Commonly the gradient at heart catheterization is 10–20 mm Hg, but rarely it may measure as high as 50 mm Hg in patients with a very large left-to-right shunt. It can be generally assumed that this pressure gradient will disappear after closure of the defect, although the cardiologist usually looks for angiographic evidence of anatomic obstruction of the pulmonary valve when the gradient is found to be quite high.

Likewise, a small gradient of 5–10 mm Hg may develop between the main pulmonary artery and the right and/or left main branch in patients with a large pulmonary blood flow, despite lack of anatomic stenosis of the pulmonary artery branches. One can anticipate that this gradient will likewise disappear after operation.

Mitral valve anomaly unsuspected preoperatively. One of the anomalies associated with ASD is billowing of the mitral valve,[2] however, preoperative recognition may be difficult. While this defect characteristically produces a mid-systolic click and late systolic murmur at the mitral area, these auscultatory events may not be consistently heard at each examination and may not appear at all until late childhood or adult life. This late appearance of the murmur occurs whether the anomaly is associated with ASD or occurs as an isolated defect. Thus, the patient with an apparent simple

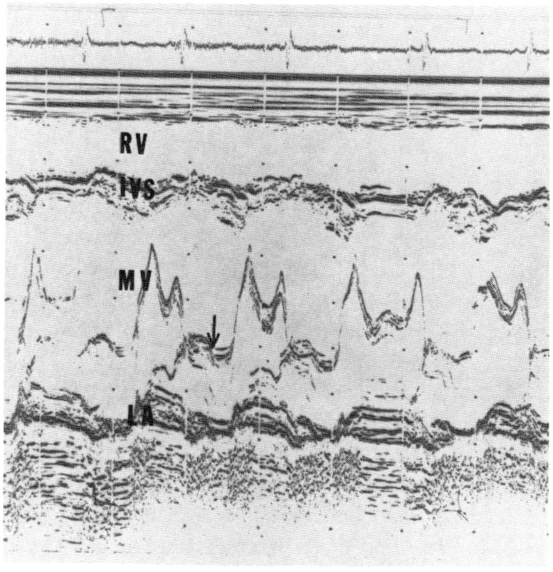

Fig. 2. Echocardiogram in 5-yr-old child with mitral valve prolapse. RV—right ventricular cavity, IVS—interventricular septum, MV—mitral valve, LA—left atrial wall. Arrow denotes point at which there is abrupt posterior movement of both leaflets of the mitral valve during late systole.

ASD may also have a clinically silent anomaly of the mitral valve. The abnormality can be demonstrated by a left ventricular angiogram, but can also be identified more simply by an echocardiogram (Fig. 2). While the mitral insufficiency which results from billowing is usually functionally benign, recognition of the anomaly is important because of the susceptibility it produces to bacterial endocarditis.

Allen et al.[3] reported a series of 62 patients with billowing of the mitral valve. During a 9–22 yr observation period, five of these patients developed SBE related to the mitral valve abnormality. In 46 patients with coexisting ASD and mitral insufficiency (representing 6% of all patients with ASD) Hynes et al.[4] found mitral valve prolapse in eight of them.

Sequelae

There is no sequela peculiar to simple ASD closure but two troublesome aftereffects occur which also may be associated with repair of other congenital cardiac defects.

Postpericardiotomy syndrome. This phenomenon is for some reason common after repair of secundum ASD. In the first year after operation and rarely in the second or third postoperative year, the patient who has recovered uneventfully from surgery may develop chest pain, neck and shoulder pain associated with fever lasting for three to ten days. The ECG findings may be confined to a change in the direction of the T waves. There may or may not be an audible pericardial friction rub.

Aspirin in large doses administered for the duration of the illness partially relieves the pain and fever. While corticosteroids also relieve the manifestations of the pericarditis, use of these drugs are rarely justified for a problem which has few permanent residual complications.

In our experience the syndrome was associated with an important degree of pericardial effusion in three children. In these patients, needle aspiration was performed in two and steroid therapy was used in a third because of signs of cardiac tamponade. In one postoperative patient (not one with ASD) who had several recurrences of postpericardiotomy syndrome, constrictive pericarditis developed approximately one year after operation and required surgical relief.

Arrhythmias. To our knowledge, persistent and important arrhythmias have occurred in only 2 of all the patients operated upon for ASD at this institution. The arrhythmia which appeared abruptly several years after operation in both instances consisted of the so-called "sick sinus syndrome"[5] with intermittent episodes of atrial flutter alternating with sinus bradycardia and prolonged pacemaker recovery time after atrial pacing (Fig. 3). This rare occurrence, presumably a sequelae of the operation, should be kept in mind in the postoperative follow-up of patients.

Complications

There is no complication peculiar to simple ASD closure but there are rare potential problems which might arise from total cardiopulmonary bypass such as air emboli to the coronary, or cerebral circulation, blood incompatability, or serum hepatitis. Other complications are those which could theoretically arise from any major operation such as unexpected idiosyncrasy to anesthesia, uncontrollable hemorrhage, infections, or postoperative changes in the personality of the patient who is susceptible to such.

Ostium primum defect. The primum defect belongs to the group of anomalies known as endocardial cushion defects. The mitral valve abnormalities associated with the ostium primum ASD persist after successful closure of the atrial communication. Residual abnormalities are a cleft of the posterior leaflet and anomalous attachment of the chordae to the anterior leaflet of the ventricular septum rather than to the anterior papillary muscle. In some patients the mitral valve deformity is of minor functional significance; (Fig. 4) in other patients, it results in mitral insufficiency which is so severe that there is no clinical improvement from surgical closure of the ASD alone. Patients require postoperative follow-up since they remain at risk for development of SBE.

Formerly, the major sequela of surgery for this defect was complete atrioventricular heart block related to hapless placement of sutures too close to the atrioventricular node. Now that the anatomic location of the conduction system is better understood, the occurrence of atrioventricular block during surgery for ostium primum ASD is a rare complication.

Fenestrated valve of the foramen ovale. Fenestrated valve of the foramen ovale produces clinical and hemodynamic findings similar to ostium secundum ASD. Usually the specific anatomy of this communication is recognized first by the sur-

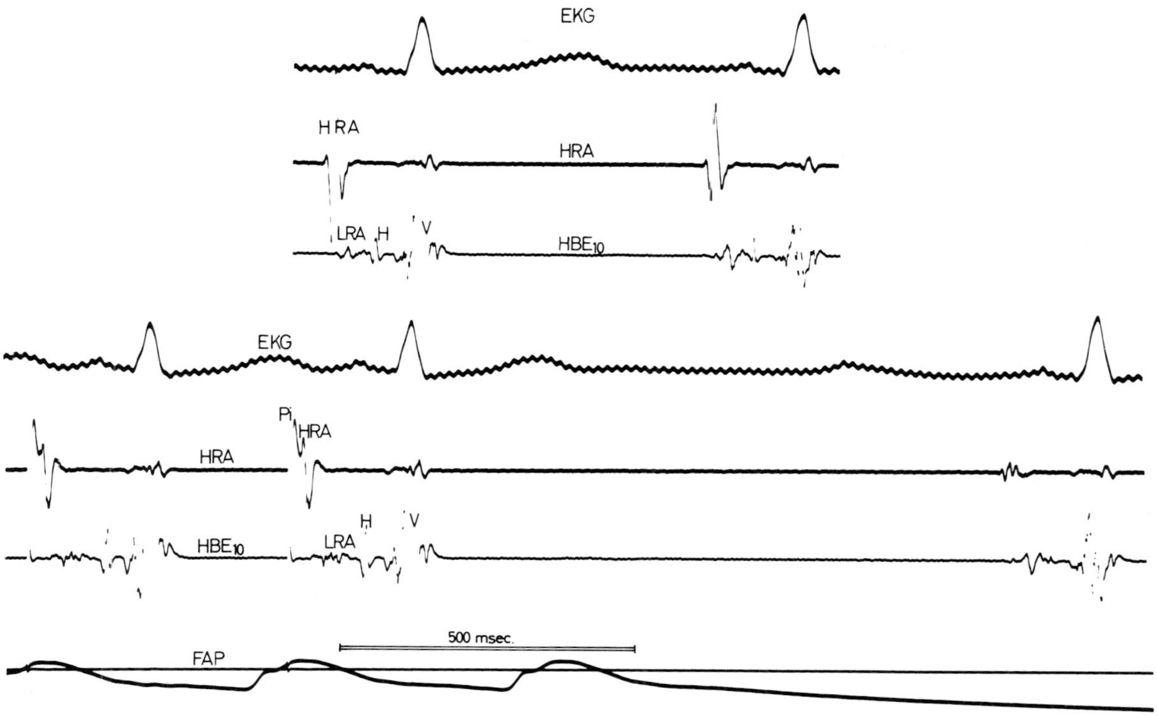

Fig. 3. His bundle electrograms in 18-yr-old female who had atrial septal defect repair at 5 yr of age demonstrating prolonged sinus node recovery time. Top panel shows resting surface ECG (lead II), high right atrial electrogram (HRA) and His bundle electrogram (HBE). Bottom panel demonstrates prolonged sinus node recovery time after cessation of atrial pacing. Low right atrial depolarization (LRA), His bundle potential (H), ventricular depolarization (V), pacemaker impulse (Pi), femoral artery pressure (FAP).

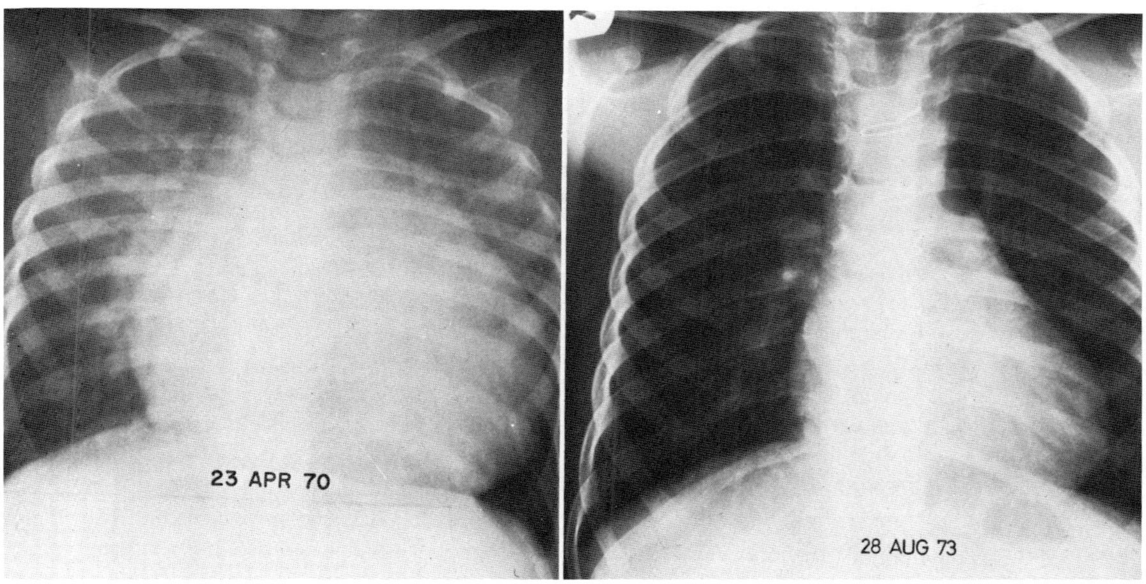

Fig. 4. Decrease in heart size following repair of ostium primum ASD and cleft mitral valve. (A) Preoperative film at 2 yr of age. (B) Film showing decrease in heart size 3 yr after surgery.

geon at the time of operation. The "Swiss cheese" like membrane may have to be excised leaving a single large opening which can then be directly sutured. Attempts to close each of the small defects separately may result in a persistent shunt. The result of a properly performed correction is as good as that for ordinary secundum ASD.

Sinus venosus defect (SVD). Repair of a sinus venosus defect situated high in the atrial septum near the orifice of the superior vena cava necessitates suturing in the region of the sinoatrial node, thus it is no surprise that arrhythmias often develop after the operation. Furthermore, SVD usually occurs in association with a single anomalous pulmonary vein draining to the superior vena cava. If this pulmonary vein opening is situated high on the superior vena cava, its ostium cannot be incorporated under the patch used to close the atrial defect and the surgeon usually leaves the vein to drain anomalously. The resulting left-to-right shunt is small and does not appear to produce any enlargement of the heart or clinical symptoms. The only other choice the surgeon has for management of this single anomalous vein is lobectomy.

Single atrium. While single atrium is a correctable anomaly, it creates an ominous clinical picture with bidirectional shunting of blood, marked cardiac enlargement and elevated pulmonary artery pressure. Its surgical closure requires a large prosthetic patch which must be placed precariously close to the atrioventricular node and to the atrioventricular valves predisposing the patient to AV node dysrhythmias and/or tricuspid insufficiency.

SELECTION OF THE PATIENT FOR ASD SURGERY

Considering the possible residua, sequelae and complications of operation for ASD, it is sometimes difficult for the physician to recommend operation and for the parents to accept it, especially in a child with a simple secundum ASD who has no symptoms. Experience has shown, however, that the natural course of ASD is one of progressive deterioration with cardiac enlargement, arrhythmias and congestive heart failure. This degree of disability usually does not appear until adult life when the risk of surgery is higher and the chance for improvement less likely than in childhood. Therefore, if the patient has an ASD resulting in pulmonary blood flow which is approximately twice systemic flow, or if there is any degree of cardiac enlargement, operation in midchildhood (5–10 years of age) is indicated even in the asymptomatic patient.

Ventricular Septal Defect (VSD)

VSD Without Elevation of Pulmonary Artery Pressure

The VSD of small to moderate size (diameter less than half the diameter of the aortic annulus) allows a variable left-to-right shunt depending on the size of the defect but causes little or no elevation of right ventricular or pulmonary artery pressure. With a small shunt, producing a pulmonary to systemic flow ratio of 1.5-to-1.0, there is no enlargement of the heart and the only threat to the patient is the risk of SBE. A larger shunt resulting from VSD of moderate size leads to slight left ventricular enlargement apparent on radiographic and electrocardiographic examination. Symptoms of exercise intolerance are usually lacking in these patients although some athletically inclined teenagers may complain of an inability to keep up with their peers.

Residua

Persistent left-to-right shunt. A residual shunt may be present despite careful direct suture or closure of the VSD with a Dacron patch. It is difficult to say whether this incomplete closure is caused by sutures pulling out from strong myocardial contractions or technical problems accompanying the repair. Postoperative heart catheterization in 140 patients studied by Allen et al.[6] revealed a residual left-to-right shunt in 29% of patients; in five patients the shunt was large. In a few patients with persistent left-to-right shunting after VSD closure, an additional VSD has been identified as the reason for the residual defect. The coexistence of two separate VSD's may be missed by the cardiologist at the time of heart catheterization as well as by the surgeon at the time of operation. Defects located in the lower anterior muscular septum are especially difficult to see and approach at operation since large papillary muscles in a relaxed empty heart overlap and obscure the defect from view. Considering the care taken by the surgeon to avoid suturing near the conduction bundle, located near the inferior rim of the defect, it is not surprising that a small area of persistent shunt often remains.

Persistent susceptibility to infective endocarditis. One of the stated justifications for surgical closure of a small VSD is prevention of infective endocarditis. It is not yet known whether successful closure of the defect guarantees protection against this complication. In our one patient who developed SBE after VSD surgery, the infection occurred during the early postoperative period; this patient had been on long-term daily prophylactic antibiotics before operation (prescribed "elsewhere") which may have favored growth of a resistant strain of the organism. None of our long-term postoperative patients has yet developed SBE. Certainly this infection could occur at the site of an incompletely closed VSD. Theoretically, SBE could develop on a "jet" lesion which developed before operation. Most cardiologists continue to administer SBE prophylaxis for dental manipulations despite successful repair of VSD. Allen et al[6] report the development of SBE in three patients in their group of 240 survivors of VSD surgery. In 2 of these patients there was a persistent VSD. The VSD was completely closed in a third patient who died four months postoperatively with infection considered by the authors to be related to the operation.

Sequelae

Ventriculotomy scar. In a few patients the ventriculotomy incision heals with excessive fibrous tissue formation which may predispose to ventricular ectopic beats and, rarely, may interfere with right ventricular contractility. This problem theoretically is more likely to result if ventriculotomy significantly compromises coronary supply to this portion of the right ventricle.

Complete right bundle branch block (RBBB). Right bundle branch block usually develops after repair of VSD. By direct monitoring of the ECG during operation, it appears that the conduction abnormality develops most commonly at the time of the ventriculotomy incision; less commonly it occurs with suturing of the patch at the edges of the VSD. Right bundle branch block is troublesome to the clinician because it renders the ECG difficult to interpret in determining if hypertrophy is present, but the conduction delay does not appear to influence the function of the right ventricle. Whether RBBB predisposes to complete atrioventricular block, especially in those cases with left anterior hemiblock is still under investigation. Allen et al.[6] reported a death 14 yr postoperatively in a child who had ECG evidence of RBBB and left axis deviation; they attributed this death to a Stokes-Adams attack.

Complications

Complete atrioventricular block. Suturing in the region of the His bundle near the inferior margin of the VSD is likely to produce complete AV block. Mortality is high with this complication and usually, a pacemaker is required to maintain compensation. In some instances, the AV block is transient and thus permanent pacemaker implantation usually is withheld for a week or so after operation. During this period of observation, the heart rate is maintained with an external pacemaker connected to epicardial wires. Allen et al.[6] reported that 35 of the 341 patients in their series developed complete AV block. In 21 of the 35 patients the block was transient and did not recur during the ten year follow-up. Among the 14 patients with persistent block, there were eight deaths including three patients who had pacemaker implantation.

Aortic insufficiency. The VSD lies near the aortic valve leaflet especially in the type of defect located superior to the crista supraventricularis. Sutures placed to close the VSD may catch the aortic leaflet and produce aortic insufficiency. The murmur of aortic insufficiency may be obscured by respirator noises in the postoperative period and the pulse pressure often does not widen until several weeks after surgery.

Tricuspid insufficiency. A plateau murmur heard following closure of VSD may prove to result from tricuspid insufficiency rather than persistent VSD. Since the most common location for VSD is near the septal leaflet of the tricuspid valve, suture of the defect may unavoidably include the leaflet or the chordae of the septal leaflet of the tricuspid valve. The tricuspid insufficiency does not usually produce serious hemodynamic difficulty as long as the right ventricular pressure remains normal.

VSD With Elevated Pulmonary Artery Pressure

Residua

Persistent elevation of pulmonary artery pressure. In patients who have pulmonary vascular obstructive disease, the right ventricular and pulmonary artery pressure may either remain elevated or fall only slightly after surgical closure of the VSD. Persistent pulmonary hypertension may be well tolerated in the early postoperative period and not suspected until demonstrated by postoperative cardiac catheterization. The process, however, is a progressive one and the patient is likely to develop a further increase in pulmonary artery pressure with right heart failure. After several years the pulmonary pressure may rise in excess of systemic pressure despite complete closure of the defect. Allen et al.[6] reviewed the effect of preoperative pulmonary hypertension on surgical therapy and concluded that: (1) total pulmonary resistance tended to be higher in patients over 3 yr of age both pre and postoperatively, (2) the occasional decrease in pulmonary vascular resistance after surgery in younger patients reflects that there may be greater reversibility in arteriolar changes than in older patients, (3) some patients over 5 yr of age had a further increase in total pulmonary resistance after successful VSD closure demonstrating the progressive nature of pulmonary vascular obstructive disease.

SELECTION OF THE PATIENT FOR VSD SURGERY

Operation for VSD in childhood usually is more acceptable to the patient's family than is operation for ASD, probably because the murmur is loud enough that the startled parents are able to hear it themselves with the ear placed on the child's chest. Furthermore, the intensity of the murmur is alarming to the clinician if he only rarely encounters congenital heart defects and he may unwittingly transmit this concern to the parents. Considering the unavoidable residua, sequelae and complications of VSD closure, operation preferably should be performed for the patient who has cardiac enlargement or a significant left-to-right shunt. Closure of the small hemodynamically insignificant VSD solely to prevent bacterial endocarditis may not be justified.[7]

Coarctation of the Aorta

Coarctation is usually regarded as a malformation which can be "cured" by operation, a claim that this review will not attempt to discredit, but rather to qualify for certain types of coarctation and for operations performed under less than ideal conditions. The term coarctation in this review will be confined to the "curtain" lesion of the thoracic aorta characterized by Edwards.[8] We shall exclude "infantile" coarctation, the misnomer for diffuse hypoplasia of the isthmus which *results* from rather than *causes* reversed flow through a ductus.

In the properly selected patient, complete relief of stenosis can be achieved and a well-performed anastomosis can remain widely patent for an indefinite period of time (Fig. 5). This is especially true when the operation is performed after early childhood yet before the third decade of life to avoid degenerative changes near the coarctation.

Residua

Persistent pressure gradient between arm and leg. A significant pressure gradient which persists after coarctation repair is likely to result from one of several possible factors: (1) surgery performed during infancy or early childhood, (2) technical faults in the repair—use of continuous rather than interrupted sutures for example, (3) the presence of a long narrow segment of aorta between left subclavian artery and coarctation site, and (4) the presence of additional areas of stenosis in the aorta, such as in the descending thoracic or abdominal aorta.

In the early postoperative period, a poor result can be predicted if the femoral pulses are not of good bounding quality. Systemic hypertension may persist for 2 or 3 wk postoperatively and the blood pressure may measure even higher than preoperative values for a few days, however, no pressure gradient should be detectable in the immediate postoperative period.

Simon and Zloto[9] reviewed the late follow-up of 187 patients who survived surgery for coarctation. In 18 patients there was a residual gradient across the coarctation site of 10 mm Hg or more; in only eight of these patients was the gradient $>$ 20 mm Hg. Reoperation was performed in seven of these eight patients.

Degenerative changes in the aortic wall distal to coarctation. Intimal plaques and medial necrosis occur in the aorta *distal* rather than proximal to the coarctation; this process progresses with age so that operation performed in adult life may be unsuccessful due to these changes. When it is necessary to resect a long segment of this unhealthy tissue, approximation of the ends for direct anastomosis is impossible and a graft is required. When the repair includes the degenerative tissue, aneurysm formation may result. An aneurysm distal to the coarctation repair occurred in five of the 187 patients followed by Simon and Zloto.[9]

Persistent hypertension despite relief of the pressure gradient. Long standing systemic hypertension from the coarctation may sometimes produce changes in the systemic arterioles which result in

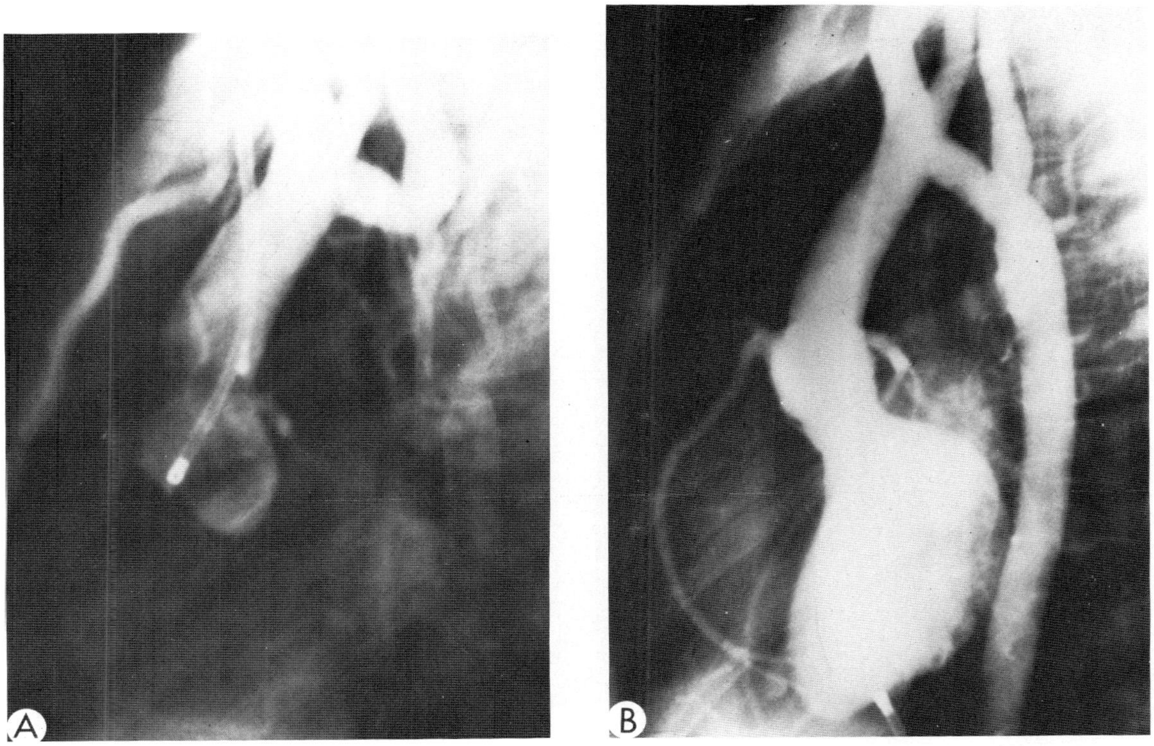

Fig. 5. Coarctation of the aorta. (A) Preoperative aortogram at age 4 yr demonstrating site of coarctation distal to left subclavian artery. (B) Left ventricular angiogram $2\frac{1}{2}$ yr after resection of coarctation demonstrating virtually normal diameter at anastamotic site.

persistent hypertension despite adequate relief of the coarctation. Persistent hypertension on this basis is more common if operation is delayed until late teenage or adult life. In Simon's review only 9% (16/187) of the patients had persistent hypertension of undetermined cause. Four of these patients were less than 15 yr of age at operation. Simon did not feel, however, that the incidence of persistent hypertension was greater than that in the general population.

Bicuspid aortic valve. It has been estimated that 85% of patients with coarctation of the aorta have a bicuspid aortic valve. There are two known consequences of this anomalous valve; the valve may be the site of infective endocarditis or valvulitis and, secondly, there is a propensity for calcific changes to develop in the valve resulting in aortic stenosis in adult life. Sometimes both stenosis and insufficiency may result from a bicuspid aortic valve which is neither infected nor calcified. Simon[9] says that 27% (20/74) of their patients with an abnormal valve had a bicuspid valve without aortic stenosis or insufficiency. A bicuspid valve was found in their series in 43% of the patients who had aortic stenosis and in 24% of the patients who had aortic insufficiency associated with the coarctation.

Cerebral vascular malformations. Aneurysms in the cerebral arteries are known to occur with coarctation and are theoretically more prone to rupture in preoperative patients who have significant systemic hypertension. However, among the five postoperative patients in Simon's series[9] who developed cerebrovascular accidents none had hypertension.

Mitral valve disease. Mitral stenosis or insufficiency may coexist with coarctation as a congenital malformation or mitral insufficiency may occur secondary to papillary muscle necrosis acquired in infancy with severe coarctation and congestive heart failure. Usually the valvular dysfunction is mild but occasionally severe mitral insufficiency results requiring additional surgical treatment. Freed et al.[10] reported a 2% incidence of mitral insufficiency in 861 patients with coarctation. Simon[9] reported a 6% incidence of mitral insufficiency and a 4% incidence of mitral stenosis in his series.

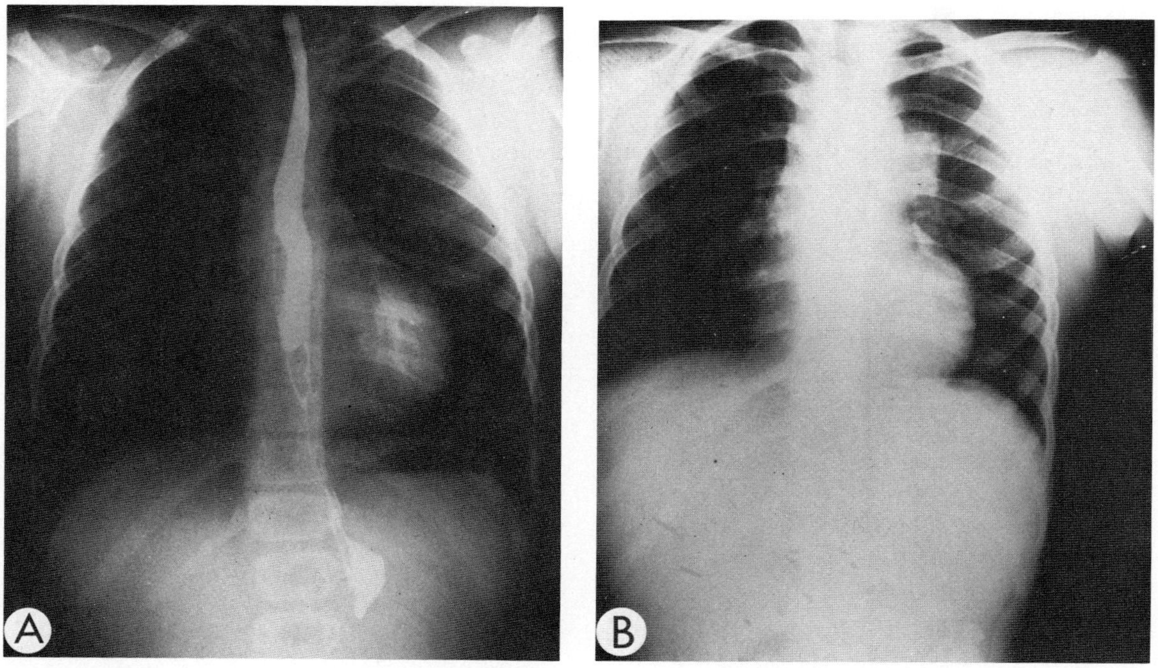

Fig. 6. Mycotic aneurysm at anastamotic site 12 yr after coarctation repair. (A) Chest film obtained 6 mo before that in (B). (B) Bulge which has appeared in left superior mediastinum proved to be a mycotic aneurysm at site of end-to-end anastamosis after coarctation resection.

Susceptibility to infective endocarditis. The patient with successful repair of coarctation remains prone to development of SBE. The infection may occur at the site of the repair, on the bicuspid aortic valve or on an anomalous mitral valve. Three of our patients developed SBE postoperatively with the lesions on a stenotic aortic valve in one patient and on the anastomotic site in the other two patients (Fig. 6). One patient developed the infection within a few weeks of surgery and the other five years postoperatively.

Persistent left ventricular hypertrophy (LVH). Among the 163 patients who had a late postoperative electrocardiogram in Simon's series,[9] 45 had persistent LVH. This finding was more common in patients operated upon after 30 yr of age (36%), than in patients who had surgery before 15 yr of age (14%). Radiographic evidence of LVH was found in 77 of 155 patients who had a late postoperative chest roentgenogram. A persistent hemodynamic lesion was considered to be responsible for the persistent LVH in 69% of these patients.

Sequelae

Stenosis of the left subclavian artery. When the origin of the left subclavian artery lies close to the anastomotic site the pressure pulse in the left subclavian artery may become damped. If the degree of stenosis is severe, the patient may experience pain or fatigue in that arm with exercise. In fact, the stenosis of the subclavian artery may be severe enough that exercise of the arm evokes subclavian steal syndrome through the ipsilateral vertebral artery.

Restenosis of the coarctation site. After initial successful relief of the gradient, the area of resection of the coarctation may again become stenotic. If so, the patient again develops systemic hypertension in the upper extremities, loss of palpable femoral pulses and the reappearance of collateral circulation to the lower extremities. The restenosis may be severe enough to warrant reoperation although this presents a more formidable task than the initial operation. Restenosis does not imply that the initial operation was done incorrectly. Frequently operation performed in a young infant results in excessive scar tissue and leads to restenosis. Diffuse narrowing of the aorta proximal to the coarctation repair may also contribute to restenosis. The use of continuous sutures rather than interrupted sutures predisposes to restenosis. Restenosis becomes functionally significant if the cross sectional area of the anastomosis is narrowed to less than 25%–30% of that of a normal aorta.[11]

Complications

Paraplegia. This complication occurred spontaneously in one patient three years after operation in the series reported by Simon.[9] While this complication has been observed immediately after surgery, its occurrence in the late postoperative period was unexplainable.

Aortic Valve Stenosis

While valvulotomy for aortic valve stenosis should be considered palliative rather than curative surgery, the relief of a dangerously high pressure gradient between left ventricle and aorta can be very effective. As with many other malformations, symptoms of exercise intolerance in the child or other signs of distress which would be obvious to the parents may be absent in spite of a severe degree of obstruction. The ECG does not reliably reflect left ventricular pressure and the radiographic appearance of the heart is usually normal in the child with either severe or mild stenosis. Thus, in the patient with clinic signs of aortic stenosis, cardiac catheterization must be performed to assess accurately the degree of severity. The same clinical limitations in predicting the degree of stenosis apply to the postoperative patient.

Residua

Pressure gradient. Among 19 patients who had aortic valvulotomy in childhood in our institution, the preoperative gradient ranging from 50 to 120 mm Hg was reduced postoperatively to a range of 0–45 mm Hg. There were seven patients in this group who had preoperative pressure gradients >85 mm Hg; two of these had postoperative gradients of <10 mm Hg (Fig. 7).

Tendency to SBE. While none of our post-

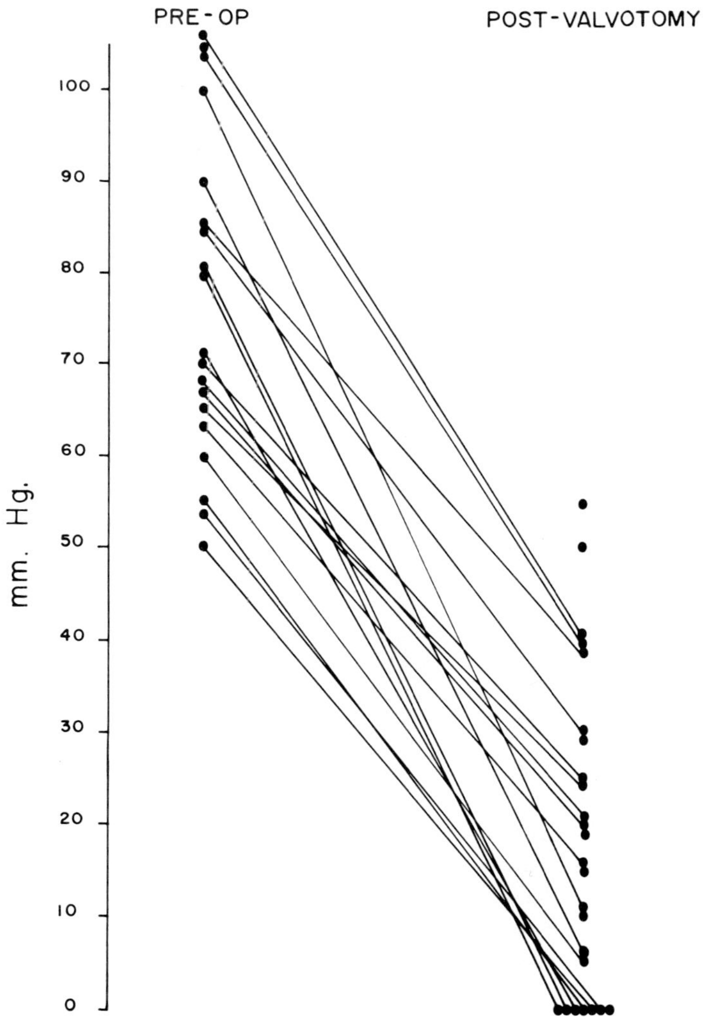

Fig. 7. Comparison of preoperative and postoperative aortic valve gradients among 19 patients recatheterized after aortic valvotomy in childhood.

operative patients has developed SBE, the susceptibility to this infection is theoretically as high after surgery as it was before. Because of this, we have exerted special efforts to caution the patients about the need for continued prophylaxis against SBE.

Susceptibility of the valve to develop calcific changes after valvulotomy. Calcification of the stenotic aortic valve appears to develop first in adult life; when encountered in the patient undergoing surgery for the first time, calcification necessitates aortic valve replacement. Greater than 90% of adults who have surgery for aortic valve stenosis require valve replacement. It is not yet known whether operation in childhood prevents calcification of the valve but none of our patients reaching adult life who had valvulotomy in childhood has developed valve calcification by x-ray.

Unsuitability for competitive sports. In spite of a good postoperative result, competitive sports are not recommended. Strenuous exercise exaggerates aortic insufficiency and there is still the chance of exercise induced arrhythmias.

Sequelae

Aortic insufficiency. In a group of 27 patients operated upon in our institution and followed for an average of 6 yr, 13 patients have moderately severe or severe aortic insufficiency, and in these patients valve replacement is anticipated.[12] Aortic insufficiency is more severe and more frequent in those patients operated upon in early infancy but these operations were done as emergency lifesaving procedures to relieve congestive heart failure.

Aneurysm of the aortotomy site in the ascending aorta. In one child with congenital rubella syndrome an aneurysm with calcific changes developed at the site of aortotomy. Reoperation for removal of the aneurysm was performed.

Complications

Except for complications due to total cardiopulmonary bypass, there is no complication peculiar to surgery for aortic valve stenosis.

Tetralogy of Fallot

Intracardiac repair of tetralogy of Fallot has proved effective in relieving symptoms of cyanosis and intolerance to ordinary activity in the majority of patients. The operation sometimes results in nearly normal resting right heart pressures. However, to call the operation curative may be an overstatement even under the best of circumstances. It is unlikely that the patient with even an "excellent" result can be dismissed entirely from follow-up in a cardiac clinic or that he can be allowed to participate in all competitive sports.

Residua

Residual right ventricular-pulmonary artery pressure gradient. Among the 221 postoperative patients who were recatheterized in our laboratory only 43% (95/221) had a right ventricular-pulmonary artery pressure gradient of < 20 mm Hg at postoperative catheterization.[13] However, the majority of patients with less satisfactory relief of the pressure gradient had no symptoms, while some of the patients with excellent relief of the obstruction had disabling symptoms for other reasons. Persistent stenosis postoperatively was found to be related to the type of preoperative anatomical obstruction. In those patients in whom only infundibulectomy was necessary, 65% had a gradient of < 20 mm Hg. In those who required pulmonary valvulotomy as well, only 43% had an equally favorable pressure response to operation. For patients who required a combination of right ventricular outflow tract prosthesis, valvulotomy and infundibulectomy, only 35% had an excellent result with respect to relief of the stenosis.

Persistent ventricular septal defect. At postoperative catheterization a persistent VSD was noted in 20% (44/221) of all patients recatheterized.[13] Again, the more severe the defect, the more likely was persistence of the VSD. The incidence of persistent VSD ranged from 7% among the patients who required simple infundibular resection to 23% of those who required a right ventricular outflow prosthesis, pulmonary valvulotomy and infundibular resection. However, the persistent defect now resulted in a left-to-right rather than right-to-left shunt. The shunt was large (> 1.5 to 1.0) in only eight of the 44 patients with a persistent VSD.

Donahoo et al.[14] reported the need for a second operation to close a "recurrent" VSD in nine patients among 343 patients who underwent repair of tetralogy of Fallot, but their incidence of well-tolerated "recurrent" VSD is not known. In 1966 Malm[15] reported a 14% incidence of persistent VSD prior to 1965. Kirklin[16] reported an 8% incidence of persistent VSD prior to 1965 but reports none after that time.

The identification of a VSD after repair of tetralogy of Fallot raises the question of need for additional operation. It creates conditions for continued susceptibility to infective endocarditis, and the persistent obvious murmur is a constant reminder to the patient's physician of an unsuccessful operation. However, reports such as the one by Donahoo et al.[14] are helpful in approaching this problem. They state that the persistent VSD in their nine patients who required reoperation was at the anterosuperior margin of the defect between the annulus of the aortic valve and the crista supraventricularis. Sutures had torn through the myocardium rather than through the patch. The authors state that a patch which is too small can predispose to recurrence. They also point out that placement of sutures at the anterosuperior aspect of the VSD is difficult because of poor visualization of the area and the great care taken to avoid injury to the tricuspid valve and the noncoronary cusp of the aortic valve. In their nine patients who required another operation to close a persistent VSD, all survived and all had successful closure.

Obstruction to pulmonary blood flow distal to pulmonary valve. Prior to operative repair of severe tetralogy of Fallot, several different types of obstructive lesions in the pulmonary circulation or in the left side of the heart may be present but are masked by the more proximal obstruction of the right ventricular outflow tract. After surgical relief of the infundibular stenosis, the effect of the more distal obstructive process on the pulmonary circulation becomes manifest by elevated pulmonary artery pressure. In tetralogy of Fallot, five different pathologic mechanisms may produce this phenomenon: (1) obstruction of small arteries by the presence of multiple thrombi which have accumulated from long-standing polycythemia and reduced pulmonary blood flow, (2) obstructive disease of the small muscular pulmonary arteries involving the media and the intima, as a result of a large systemic-to-pulmonary artery anastomosis, especially the Potts anastomosis. Four of the 221 patients recatheterized after surgical repair at our institution had pulmonary hypertension presumably resulting from a large palliative shunt, (3) congenital stenosis of the secondary or tertiary branches of the pulmonary arteries. Pulmonary branch stenosis and large branches of the pulmonary artery may be easily seen on the preoperative angiogram but multiple small stenoses may be difficult to detect preoperatively. Two of the 221 patients recatheterized after intracardiac repair at our institution had elevation of main pulmonary artery pressure because of multiple congenital stenoses of distal pulmonary artery branches, (4) acquired stenosis of the right pulmonary artery resulting from closure of the ascending aorta-to-right pulmonary artery anastomosis at the time of definitive repair. In a study from this institution five of 14 patients had elevated pulmonary artery pressure, ranging from 50 to 100 mm Hg, despite an otherwise good repair due to stenosis at the site of the previous ascending aorta anastomosis.[17] Occasionally ligation of the Potts anastomosis has resulted in stenosis of the left pulmonary artery, (5) lesions obstructing the return of pulmonary venous blood. If obstruction to left heart filling is associated with tetralogy of Fallot, the obstructive nature of the left heart anomaly may not become manifest until after intracardiac repair when the total systemic venous return then flows through the lungs.

Sequelae

Right bundle branch block (RBBB). This sequela to operation for tetralogy of Fallot is listed first because it is undoubtedly the most common, although it is probably functionally benign. As discussed under VSD repair, RBBB may occur with the ventriculotomy incision, or with placement of the sutures in the VSD, or more rarely not at all. It has been postulated that the combination of RBBB with left anterior hemiblock predisposes the patient to subsequent development of complete AV block.[18] However, none of our patients with this combination of ECG abnormalities after tetralogy of Fallot surgery has developed complete AV block.

Pulmonary insufficiency (PI). The murmur of PI is easily audible in 75% of all patients after intracardiac repair of tetralogy of Fallot. The murmur occurred in only 9.5% (4/42) of patients in whom repair of the obstruction was accomplished by mere infundibular resection. However, the murmur was present in 94% of the 104 patients who required an outflow tract prosthesis in addition to valvulotomy and infundibular resection. It is surprising that among the patients who required valvulotomy in addition to infundibulectomy only 70% developed a murmur of pulmonary insufficiency postoperatively.

In contrast to PI associated with pulmonary hypertension in which the insufficiency murmur is of high frequency, the PI murmur heard in the

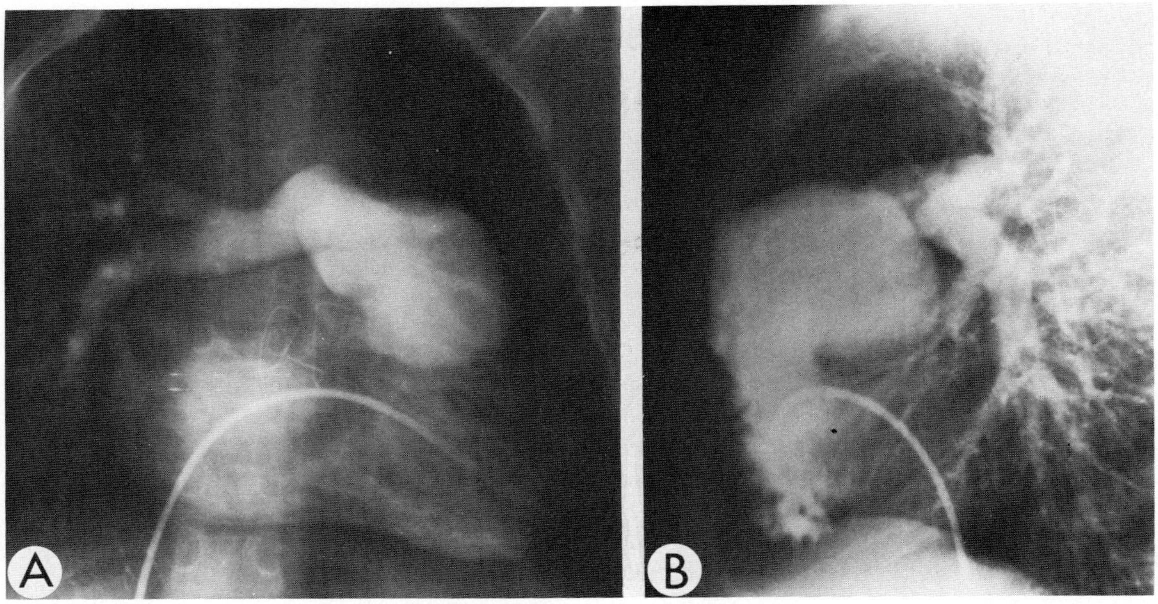

Fig. 8. An aneurysm of the pericardial outflow patch which developed after definitive repair of tetralogy of Fallot is seen in the AP (A) and lateral (B) projections. The aneurysm was resected 18 mo after the original operation.

postoperative tetralogy of Fallot patient is usually a low frequency murmur.

Pulmonary insufficiency in the absence of other residual defects may prove to be a functionally unimportant lesion, but it is bothersome since it may cause a slight elevation of right ventricular end-diastolic and right atrial pressures which may be exaggerated with stress. Following exercise in these patients one can usually see a prominent A wave in the jugular venous pulse. It is not yet known if these pressure effects will lead to eventual right ventricular and right atrial enlargement.

Right ventriculotomy scar. Extensive fibrosis around the right ventriculotomy scar was noted in a patient who died 16 yr after tetralogy of Fallot repair. His death resulted from an episode of uncontrollable ventricular tachycardia occurring a year after the onset of repeated episodes of multiple ventricular ectopic beats. This arrhythmia had been resistant to the usual antiarrhythmic drugs. This sequel to right ventriculotomy is uncommon.

Aneurysmal dilatation of the right ventricular outflow tract patch. In 10% of our cases in which an outflow tract prosthesis was necessary aneurysmal bulging of the patch was noted either by chest radiogram or by angiogram at the time of postoperative catheterization (Fig. 8). Aneurysms occurred more often when the patch material was pericardium rather than Dacron®, and were more common when there was persistent obstruction to flow distal to the outflow patch. Dilatation usually occurred within 6 mo of surgery and remained stable thereafter. Three patients have required reoperation to relieve the aneurysm formation and the distal obstruction.

Complications

Complete atrioventricular (AV) block. During the development of surgery for tetralogy of Fallot, placement of sutures to close the VSD frequently produced complete AV block, Now that surgeons know the precise location of the conduction bundle, AV block is a rare occurrence. The technique of intracavitary mapping for location of the conduction system is now used by several centers to give added assurance in localizing the conduction bundle.

There is no frequent complication related solely to the repair of tetralogy of Fallot.

SEQUELAE FROM PREVIOUS SYSTEMIC TO PULMONARY ARTERY ANASTOMOSIS

In the patient who has had a palliative shunt operation, there are several potential problems to be faced at the time of intracardiac repair. Because of such problems, surgeons are attempting to perform repair rather than palliative operations for the symptomatic infant with tetralogy of Fallot.

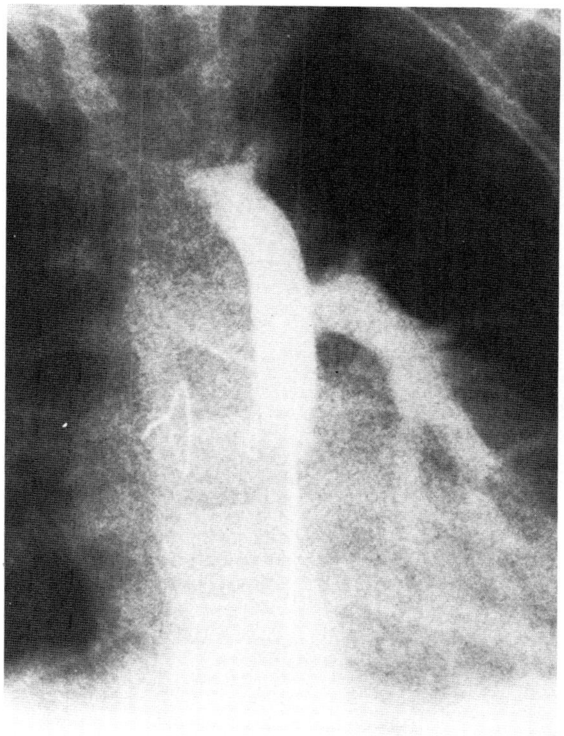

Fig. 9. A persistently patent Potts anastomosis is functioning as demonstrated on this postoperative aortogram after Mustard operation for transposition of the great arteries and attempt at Potts closure.

The Potts anastomosis is technically difficult to close. In 22% of patients in our series who had closure of the Potts anastomosis at the time of intracardiac repair, the anastomosis was found to be partially patent at the time of postoperative catheterization (Fig. 9). The left-to-right shunt in each instance was small and did not produce a hemodynamic problem, but provided a potential site for development of SBE.

Stenosis of the right pulmonary artery may result from the ascending aorta-to-right pulmonary artery anastomosis, relief of which may require special reconstruction of the pulmonary artery at the time of repair (Fig. 10).

The subclavian artery-to-pulmonary artery anastomosis is more easily closed than other palliative shunts. We have, however, encountered several instances of subclavian steal syndrome from this anastomosis. Also, the growth of the arm on the side of the subclavian anastomosis is minimally impaired, but usually the patient is unaware of this and denies any symptoms from ligation of the subclavian artery.

The development of pulmonary vascular obstructive disease after an anastomosis is a rare sequel, usually the result of a very large Potts anastomosis. A very large shunt may also predispose to left ventricular failure which may persist after obliteration of the shunt and repair of the tetralogy of Fallot.

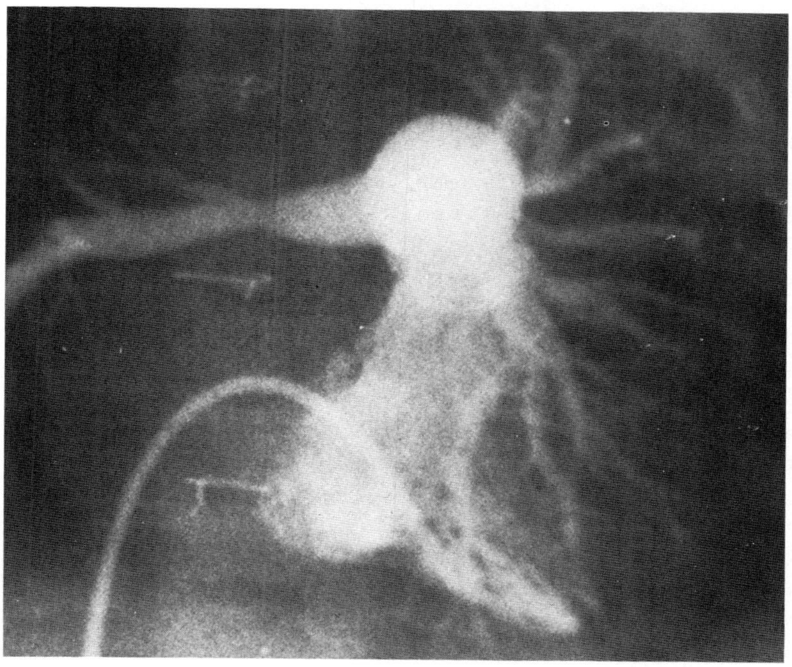

Fig. 10. Stenosis of right pulmonary artery at site of previous ascending aorta-to-pulmonary artery anastamosis producing a gradient of 20 mm Hg on postoperative cardiac catheterization.

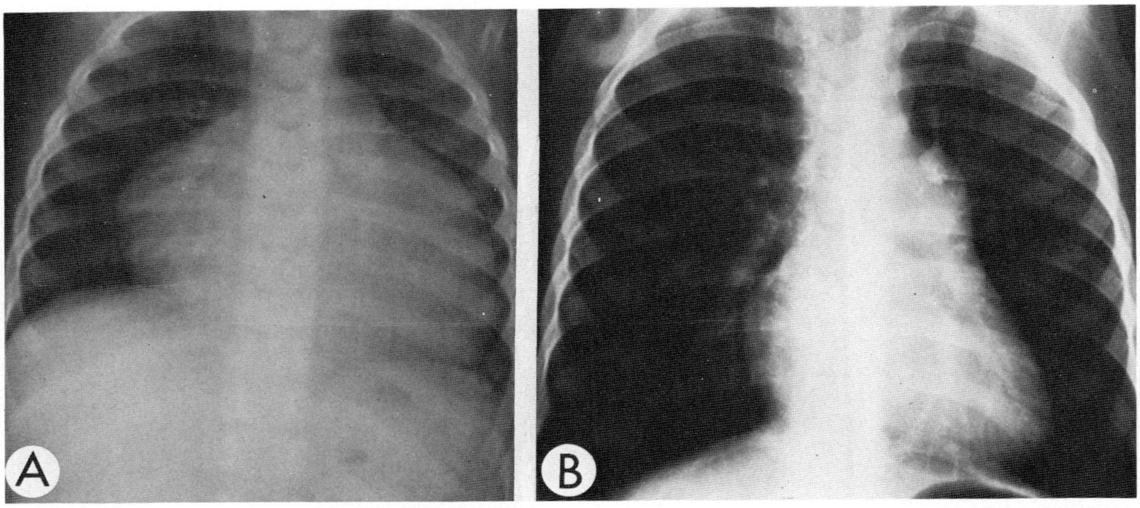

Fig. 11. Change in heart size following successful valvulotomy (Brock procedure). (A) Preoperative film at initial visit at 19 mo of age. Right ventricle (RV) pressure 184/0-16, left ventricle (LV) 100/0-8, pulmonary artery (PA) not entered. (B) Film obtained 2 yr after successful valvulotomy. RV pressure 25/0, PA 20/4, right femoral artery 100/56.

The severe disability associated with tetralogy of Fallot and the high incidence of complications and sudden death without surgical treatment leave little doubt that repair of the defect is indicated in all patients. There is no benign form of tetralogy of Fallot although symptoms may appear in late childhood in some patients, and in rare instances, untreated patients survive into adult life. Review of the many residual defects and surgical sequelae which may be encountered after intracardiac repair is not intended to discourage operation for this anomaly, but individuals with a personal interest in the subject should be made aware of the possible results of corrective surgery.

Pulmonary Valve Stenosis (PVS)

Valvulotomy for pulmonary stenosis, first introduced by Brock in 1949, has gained a reputation for being one of the most successful operations for congenital heart disease with respect to surgical mortality and postoperative clinical improvement (Fig. 11).

Difficulties in recommending operation for the child with PVS exist because the growth of the child from infancy is usually normal and few of the patients have symptoms. However, postoperative studies have demonstrated that a high right ventricular pressure after many years leads to myocardial fibrosis which may interfere with ventricular function even after otherwise successful valvulotomy. Furthermore, long-standing right ventricular hypertension resulting from PVS produces secondary hypertrophy of the infundibulum and may prevent complete relief of the pressure gradient by valvulotomy alone.

Until recently, surgery for PVS was not considered justified unless resting right ventricular peak systolic pressure was elevated to at least 80–90 mm Hg. Now, a lower level of right ventricular pressure, in the range of 50–60 mm Hg, may determine surgical candidacy.

Residua

Right ventricular-to-pulmonary artery peak systolic pressure gradient. Ideally the residual peak systolic pressure gradient after operation does not exceed 20 mm Hg. When there is a significantly high pressure gradient remaining after an expertly performed valvulotomy, it usually reflects an additional area of obstruction, either in the infundibulum or at a small pulmonary valve annulus.

Among 30 patients who underwent valvulotomy and postoperative catheterization at this institution, only five had a residual right ventricular-to-pulmonary artery pressure gradient of >20 mm Hg.

Elevated right ventricular pressure. One of the parameters used in judging postoperative success has been measurement of right ventricular pressures at rest and with exercise. In the report by Tandon et al.[19] only four of 22 patients recatheterized postoperatively had an unsatisfactory result with residual elevation of resting right ventricular pressures of >60 mm Hg (liberally defined!). Stone et al.[20] recatheterized 20 patients after pulmonary valvulotomy and found that two patients in their series had resting systolic right ventricular pressure above 60 mm Hg. This same group also evaluated the effect of exercise on right ventricular pressure. Eight patients with normal right ventricular pressures at rest had elevations to more than 60 mm Hg with exercise. It was striking that the two patients who had resting right ventricular pressures of > 60 mm Hg had elevations to 90 and 115 mm Hg after exercise.

Elevated right ventricular end-diastolic pressure (RVEDP). Stone et al.[20] studied RVEDP at rest and with exercise in 20 patients pre and postoperatively. The average preoperative rise with exercise was 9.6–12.3 mm Hg. Postoperatively, no patient had a rise in RVEDP with exercise.

Impaired stroke index. In the 20 patients studied by Stone et al.,[20] referred to in the preceding section, six patients had a preoperative exercise induced decrease in stroke index. No patient showed this change postoperatively.

All of the patients studied by Stone were children. The age factor influences the outcome of operation since hemodynamic studies in adults after pulmonary valvulotomy have demonstrated impaired cardiac function.[21]

Atrial communication. Right-to-left shunting at the atrial level may occur in association with PVS if a foramen ovale is present and if right atrial pressures are elevated. In less severe cases, when right atrial pressure is normal right-to-left shunting through a foramen ovale does not occur.

When an atrial communication is recognized preoperatively, it should be closed at the time of valvulotomy. An atrial communication which persists after successful valvulotomy may result in a small right-to-left shunt (perhaps detectable only by indicator dilution curves) but can be the route for paradoxical emboli to the systemic circulation. In two of our patients who had successful valvulotomy by the Brock technique (which precludes inspection of the atrial septum) transient hemiparesis developed 5 yr and 8 yr, postoperatively. These patients had normal right ventricular peak systolic pressures. Pulmonary insufficiency reflected by an increase in right ventricular end-diastolic and right atrial pressures may have predisposed to this complication in each of them.

Sequelae

Pulmonary insufficiency (PI). The only frequent sequela to surgery for PVS is the murmur of pulmonary insufficiency. Pulmonary insufficiency after pulmonary valvulotomy appears to be less of a hemodynamic problem than PI after tetralogy of Fallot repair, perhaps because the patient with tetralogy of Fallot repair has had a wide ventriculotomy and is more likely to have residual obstruction.

In a postoperative evaluation of 95 patients by Tandon et al.,[19] 55 of them had the diastolic murmur of PI. In our experience, a PI murmur is heard in almost all of the postoperative patients but may be missed unless the patient is exercised or placed in the supine position for auscultation. The PI murmur after pulmonary valvulotomy is low-pitched in contrast to the high-pitched Graham Steel murmur of PI associated with pulmonary hypertension.

Complications

Operative morbidity and mortality. Pulmonary valvulotomy is associated with a low risk when performed by an experienced team. Specific complications related to this operation are rare.

Transposition of the Great Arteries (TGA)

The Mustard operation currently is the only procedure used for correction of TGA. It consists of the placement of an intratrial baffle made of pericardium or of prosthetic material so as to transpose the return of systemic venous blood to the left side of the heart, and that of the pulmonary venous blood to the right side of the heart. The operation is especially successful in those cases without other associated defects which would require treatment or consideration, i.e., no ventricular septal defect, no pulmonary stenosis and no pulmonary hypertension.

For the treatment of a malformation which has a mortality in the first year of life of about 90% in untreated patients, the operative mortality of the Mustard operation ranging from 10%–20% is encouraging. Furthermore, after successful operation, cyanosis disappears and patients have clear improvement in exercise tolerance. Pulmonary vascular obstructive disease develops very early in infancy, usually by 3 mo of age, when TGA is associated with a large VSD or with a large ductus arteriosus. Once the vascular changes have developed, elevated pulmonary artery pressure is likely to persist postoperatively, jeopardizing survival from the operative procedure.

Sequelae

The Mustard operation is still so new that many of the problems occurring after operation and

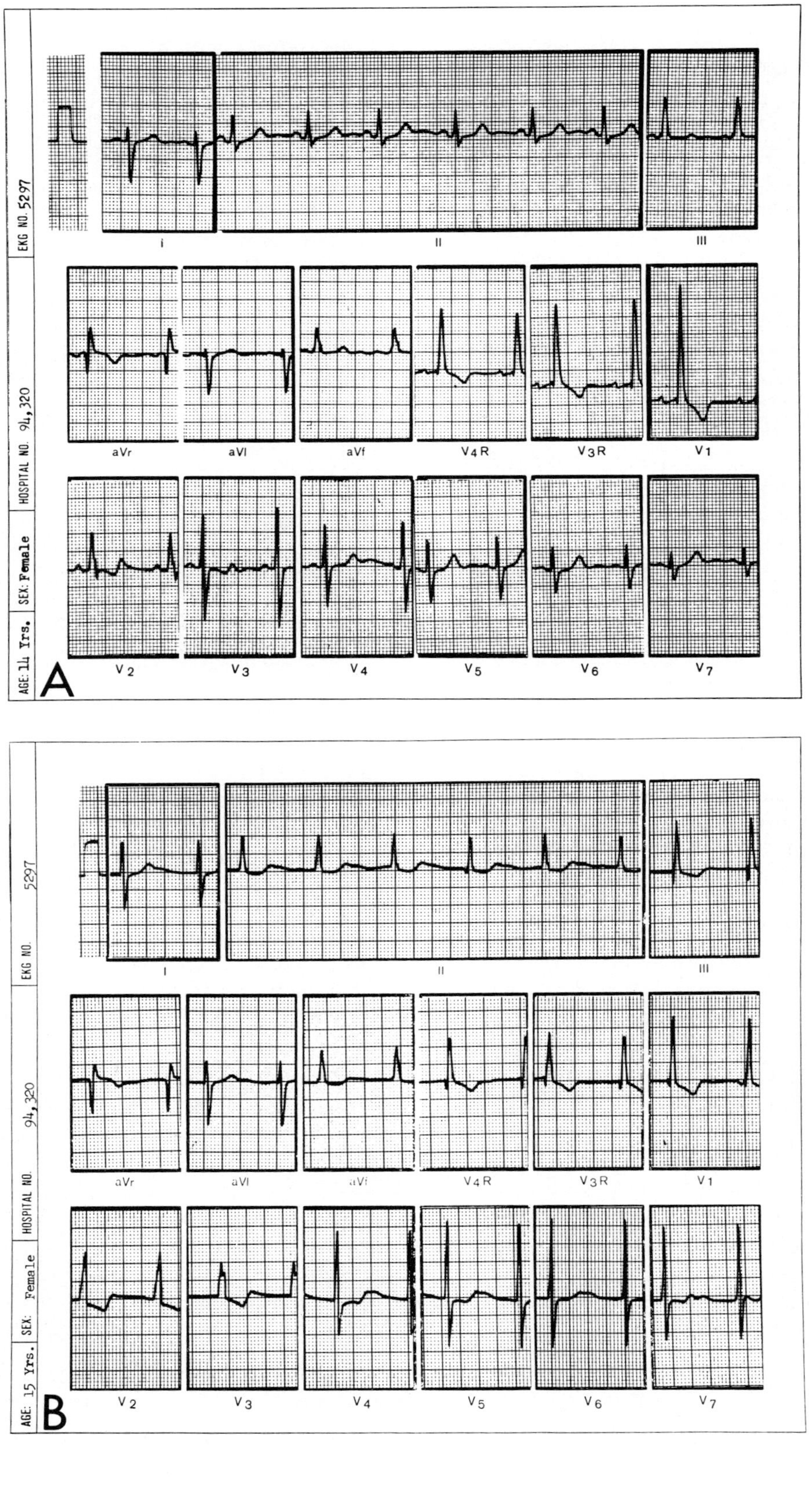
AGE: 14 Yrs.
SEX: Female
HOSPITAL NO. 94,320
EKG NO. 5297
I
II
III
aVr
aVl
aVf
V4R
V3R
V1
V2
V3
V4
V5
V6
V7
A
AGE: 15 Yrs.
SEX: Female
HOSPITAL NO. 94,320
EKG NO. 5297
I
II
III
aVr
aVl
aVf
V4R
V3R
V1
V2
V3
V4
V5
V6
V7
B

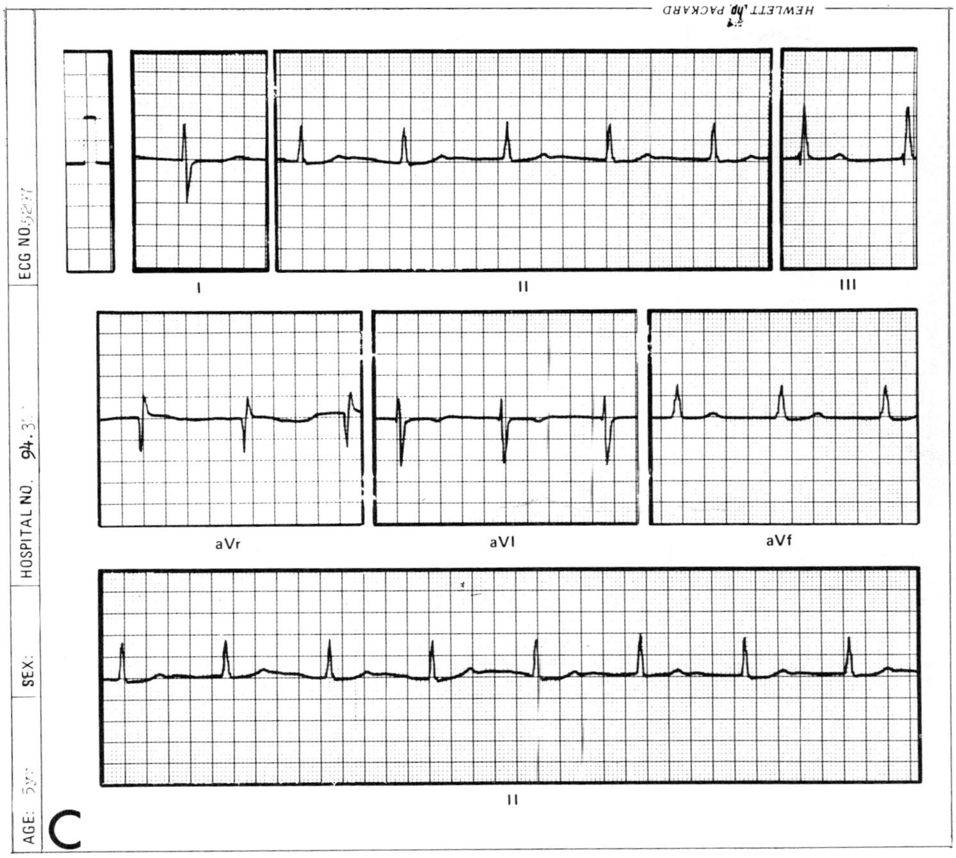

Fig. 12. Change in electrocardiogram from intratrial baffle procedure in 14-yr-old patient (Mustard repair). (A) Preoperative tracing—sinus rhythm at a rate of 80/min with right axis deviation and right ventricular hypertrophy. (B) Tracing on 2nd postoperative day after Mustard procedure with nodal rhythm and AV dissociation. (C) Limb leads and rhythm strip 6 days after Mustard procedure with junction rhythm.

designated as sequelae may well be considered complications within a short time as investigators in the field are learning ways to avoid them.

Arrhythmias. In the first patients operated upon at this institution from January 1964 to March 1971, there was a 90% incidence of some type of arrhythmia either in the early postoperative period or in the follow-up period. Not all of the arrhythmias in this group caused functional difficulties but there were five late deaths attributed to persistent uncontrollable arrhythmias. Improvement in operative technique which avoids suturing in the region of the sinoatrial node has reduced, but not eliminated, the appearance of arrhythmias. Arrhythmias after Mustard repair may occur at anytime during the follow-up period and may be progressive. Among the patients in our series who had a 3-yr follow-up, 30% had sinus rhythm in the early postop period but only 10% had sinus rhythm at the end of a 3-yr follow-up period (Fig. 12).

Obstruction of the superior vena cava (SVC) or inferior vena cava (IVC). Diversion of systemic venous return to a new right atrium has resulted in late postoperative stenosis of the channel between the vena cavae and the atrium (Fig. 13). In our experience this problem has not required reoperation but may account for distended cutaneous veins in the upper or lower extremities. In an early series reported by Stark et al.,[22] SVC obstruction occurred in four of their 113 survivors of the Mustard operation and was attributed to shrinkage of the pericardial baffle. In a later series reported by Stark et al.[23] the incidence of SVC and IVC obstruction was more common when Dacron®, rather than pericardium, was used for the baffle. Ten of 28 survivors of the Mustard procedure who had Dacron® intratrial baffles in their series

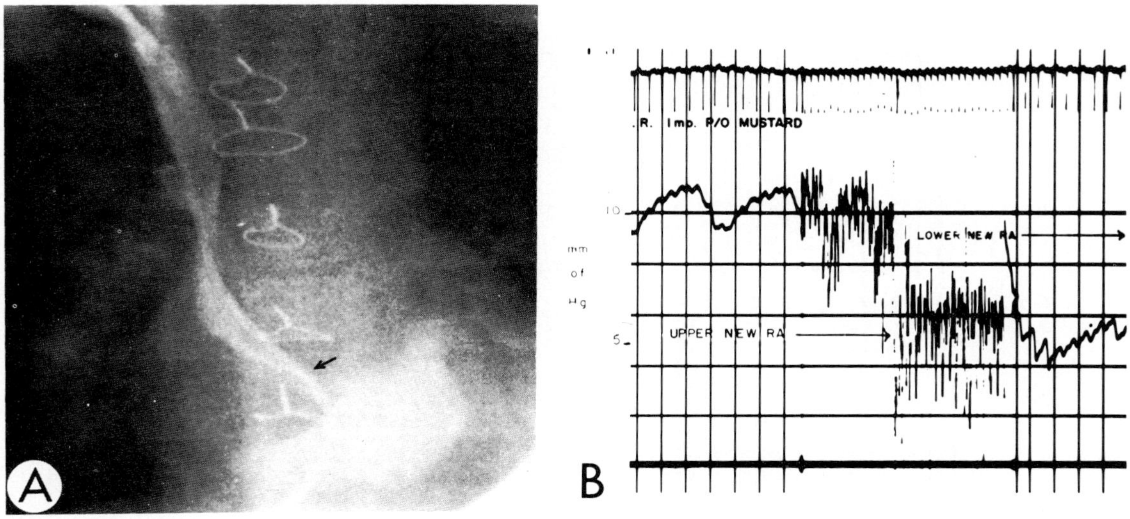

Fig. 13. Superior vena caval obstruction after Mustard procedure with use of pericardium for baffle material. (A) Catheter course from inferior vena cava to new right atrium (RA) to superior vena cava (SVC). (B) Pressure tracing pullback from SVC to new RA with a gradient demonstrated at SVC-RA junction (at site of arrow).

developed obstruction to systemic venous return and nine of these patients required reoperation for this problem.

Tricuspid insufficiency. Late contraction of the intratrial baffle with tension of the tricuspid annulus has been blamed for the appearance of tricuspid insufficiency developing several months or a year after operation. The problem of tricuspid incompetence after the Mustard operation was reviewed by Tynan et al.[24] They related the tricuspid incompetence to pre-existing inadequacy of the tricuspid valve and showed some correlation of this problem with postoperative arrhythmias. Some surgeons suggested that the use of a Dacron® baffle

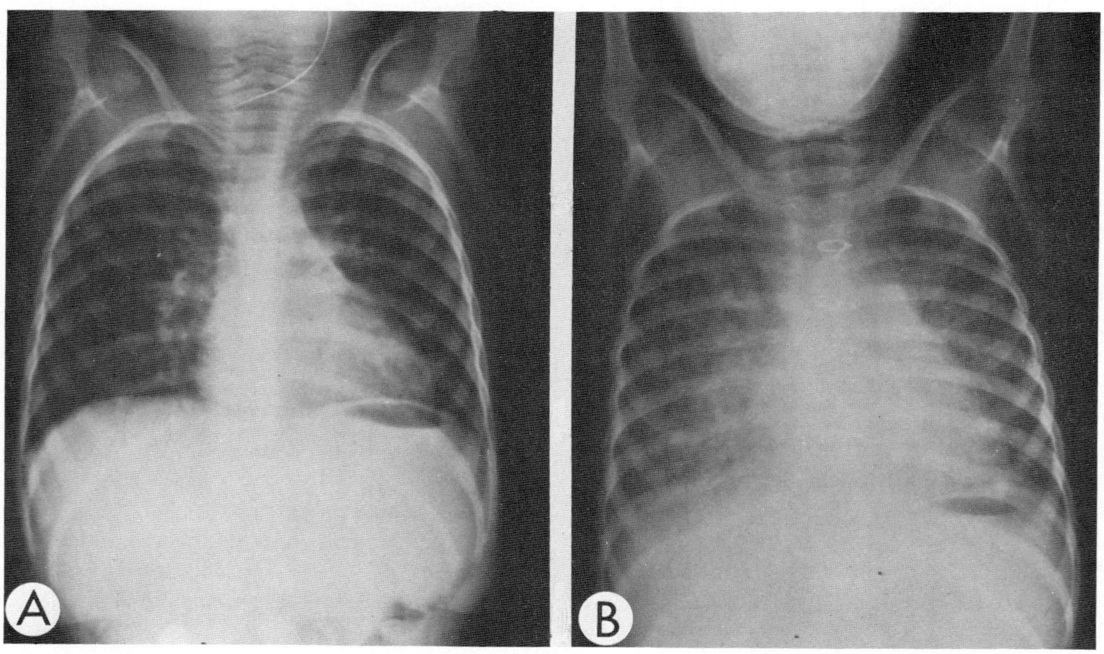

Fig. 14. Pulmonary venous obstruction developing after Mustard procedure with use of Dacron® for the baffle material. (A) Preoperative chest film before Mustard procedure. (B) Film 23 mo after Mustard procedure before reoperation to enlarge the pulmonary venous atrium; pulmonary edema is evident.

might decrease the incidence of this problem; however, this material appeared to be responsible for an even more serious sequel to be mentioned next.

Obstruction to pulmonary venous return. A high incidence of pulmonary venous obstruction developing several weeks after operation was noted in several instances with the use of Dacron® for the intratrial baffle. This problem should be considered as the most likely reason for the development of pulmonary edema appearing after an initial good response to operation (Fig. 14). This problem is technically correctable and if diagnosis is made, reoperation should follow promptly. In our institution a group of 32 patients had Dacron® used as the material for an intratrial baffle over a 15-mo period. Seven of the 24 survivors of this procedure required reoperation 6-23 mo following the original operation because of pulmonary venous obstruction. Reoperation consisted of enlargement of the pulmonary venous atrium with a patch graft. Now pericardium is recommended by most surgeons as the preferred material for intratrial baffle construction, If Dacron® must be utilized because of the unavailability of pericardium, the pulmonary venous atrium should be enlarged at the time of the initial surgery.

Complications

It is to be expected that many of the sequelae will soon be classified as complications as is the case when any new operative procedure is being developed (Fig. 15). Unfortunately, patients with TGA usually cannot await improvement in techniques. Delaying operation provides little hope for the patient who may not survive without definitive treatment. Palliative treatment may sustain some of the patients until the first or second year of life but delaying surgery may allow the complications from the natural history of the disease.

SUMMARY

Definitive, if not curative surgery is available for the eight most common congenital cardiac defects —ductus arteriosus, ASD, VSD, coarctation, pulmonary valve stenosis, aortic valve stenosis, tetralogy of Fallot, and transposition.

The results of surgery for uncomplicated cases of DA, ASD, VSD, and coarctation usually can be determined by clinical means (including chest radiogram and ECG). Postoperative heart catheterization is recommended for evaluation of the patient who has had surgery for pulmonary valve stenosis or aortic stenosis and is necessary after tetralogy of Fallot or transposition of the great arteries repair to identify the important postoperative residua and sequelae.

The term "curative" surgery probably should be reserved for operation for division of ductus arteriosus unassociated with pulmonary hypertension and performed in childhood.

After closure of ASD, patients should continue to be observed for late development of arrhyth-

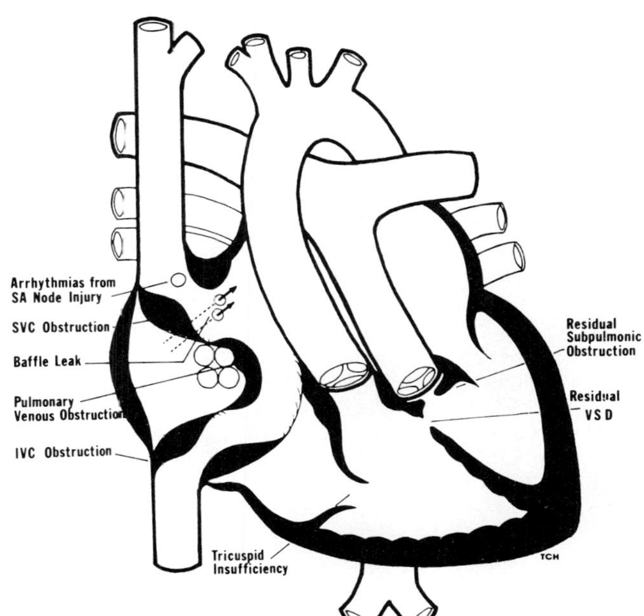

Fig. 15. Sites of possible postoperative residua and sequelae after Mustard procedure.

mias and persistent cardiac enlargement, although the incidence of these problems is low.

After VSD closure the patient is still followed at intervals for possible ill effects of the ventriculotomy scar, manifest as arrhythmias, ventricular aneurysm or myocardial insufficiency.

The patient with coarctation repair must be observed for a possible late complication from one of the several clinically silent cardiovascular or cerebrovascular anomalies as well as for the chance of restenosis or unrelieved hypertension.

Patients who have had an effective relief of the pressure gradient from pulmonary valve stenosis have a good outlook but should be observed for signs of myocardial insufficiency or the possible effects of increased load on the right heart resulting from pulmonary insufficiency.

The high incidence of some degree of aortic insufficiency after valvotomy for aortic valve stenosis as well as the slight chance of restenosis necessitates follow-up examinations for these patients.

After tetralogy of Fallot repair partially unrelieved infundibular stenosis or pulmonary annular stenosis and/or persistent VSD may require some limitation of physical activities even though the patient feels much improved because of disappearance of the cyanosis. Whether there are residual defects or not, patients should continue to be re-examined annually for an indefinite period of time because of possible myocardial insufficiency or arrhythmias.

The problems after transposition repair include arrhythmias, right ventricular myocardial insufficiency, tricuspid insufficiency, persistent communications around the atrial baffle, and vena caval and/or pulmonary vein stenosis. Despite the frequent residua and sequelae of surgery, most patients with transposition obtain remarkable relief of symptoms.

The use of exercise stress testing should increase the reliability of clinic assessment of the operative result. In those patients at risk for arrhythmias after surgery, electrophysiological studies at the time of postop cath may contribute to the management of the patient. The addition of ultrasound in the pre and postoperative evaluation of patients will aid the identification of certain clinically silent associated defects and some of the postoperative sequelae.

The risk of subacute bacterial endocarditis remains in most patients after intracardiac repair of defects and, with few exceptions, patients who have had definitive surgery require long-term follow-up despite relief of symptoms and the disappearance of clinical manifestations of cardiovascular dysfunction.

It is reasonable to expect that with improvement in diagnostic and surgical technique, many of the currently acceptable residua and sequelae of surgery for congenital heart disease will, in the future, be designated as avoidable complications in these patients. With the current healthy interest in long-term postoperative results there is a good chance that more precise information will become available to guide in the selection for surgery of the patient with congenital heart disease.

REFERENCES

1. Young D: Later results of closure of secundum atrial septal defect in children. Am J Cardiol 31:14, 1973

2. McDonald A, Harris A, Jefferson K, et al: Association of prolapse of posterior cusp of mitral valve and atrial septal defect. Br Heart J 33:373, 1971

3. Allen H, Harris A, Leatham A: Significance and prognosis of an isolated late systolic murmur: a 9- to 22-year follow-up. Br Heart J 36:525, 1974

4. Hynes KM, Frye RL, Brandenburg RO, et al: Atrial septal defect (secundum) associated with mitral regurgitation. Am J Cardiol 34:333, 1974

5. Kaplan BM, Langendorf R, Lev M, et al: Tachycardia-bradycardia syndrome (so called "Sick Sinus Syndrome"). Am J Cardiol 31:497, 1973

6. Allen HD, Anderson RC, Noren GR, et al: Postoperative follow-up of patients with ventricular septal defect. Circulation 50:465, 1974

7. Shah P, Singh WSA, Rose V, et al: Incidence of bacterial endocarditis in ventricular septal defects. Circulation 34:127, 1966

8. Edwards JE: Coarctation of aorta, in Pathology of the Heart (ed 2). Springfield, Ill., Thomas, 1965, p 677

9. Simon AB, Zloto AE: Coarctation of the aorta: Longitudinal assessment of operated patients. Circulation 50:456, 1974

10. Freed MD, et al: Coarctation of the aorta with congenital mitral regurgitation. Circulation 49:1175, 1974

11. Karnell J: Coarctation of the aorta. Circulation 38 (Suppl 5):35, 1968

12. Gutgesell HP: Personal communication of unpublished data

13. Ruzyllo W, Nihill MR, Mullins CE, et al: Hemodynamic evaluation of 221 patients after intracardiac repair of tetralogy of Fallot. Am J Cardiol 34:565, 1974

14. Donahoo JS, Brawley RK, Gott VL, et al: Reoperation after total correction of tetralogy of Fallot. J Thorac Cardiovasc Surg 68:466, 1974

15. Malm JR, et al: Factors that modify hemodynamic results in total correction of tetralogy of Fallot. J Thorac Cardiovasc Surg 52:502, 1966

16. Kirklin J, Karp R: The Tetralogy of Fallot. Philadelphia, Saunders, 1970

17. Reitman MJ, Galioto FM, El-Said GM, et al: Ascending aorta to right pulmonary artery anastomosis. Circulation 49:952, 1974

18. Moss AJ, Klyman G, Emmanouilides GC: Late onset complete heart block. Am J Cardiol 30:884, 1972

19. Tandon R, Nadas AS, Gross RE: Results of open-heart surgery in patients with pulmonic stenosis and intact ventricular septum. Circulation 31:190, 1965

20. Stone FM, Bessinger FB, Jr, Lucas RV, Jr, et al: Pre- and postoperative rest and exercise hemodynamics in children with pulmonary stenosis. Circulation 49:1102, 1974

21. McIntosh HD, Cohen AI: Pulmonary stenosis: The importance of the myocardial factor in determining the clinical course and surgical results. Am Heart J 65:715, 1963

22. Stark J, Tynan MJ, Ashcraft KW, et al: Obstruction of pulmonary veins and superior vena cava after Mustard operation for transposition of the great arteries. (Abstr) Circulation 44 (Suppl II): 11–91, 1971

23. Stark J, de Leval MR, Waterston DJ, et al: Corrective surgery of transposition of the great arteries in the first year of life. J Thorac Cardiovasc Surg 67:673, 1974

24. Tynan M, Aberdeen E, Stark J: Tricuspid incompetence after the Mustard operation for transposition of the great arteries. Circulation 45 (Suppl I):1–111, 1972

Radiographic Changes in the Postoperative Patient

Kurt Amplatz, Augustin Formanek, Laura Knight, S. Murphy Tadavarthy, Gernot Gypser, and Gerhard Bardach

IN RECENT YEARS many papers have appeared dealing with the clinical and hemodynamic changes associated with surgical correction of congenital heart disease. However, very little information is available concerning the radiographic and angiographic changes following corrective or palliative cardiac surgery. It is the purpose of this communication to fill in this gap and emphasize the importance of cardiovascular radiology in the postoperative management of these patients. Only the most important cardiac defects will be discussed.

The postero-anterior (PA) and lateral film of the chest with the barium-filled esophagus is one of the simplest, most important noninvasive technique to follow these patients. Hemodynamic changes, chamber enlargement, and complications of surgery may be visualized leading to a more definitive diagnosis by angiocardiography. Radiographic observations which can be readily made on follow-up chest examinations are concerned with: (1) changes of the thoracic cage, (2) the change in cardiac configuration due to alteration of chamber size, (3) changing left atrial size, (4) decrease or increase of central or peripheral pulmonary arteries, and (5) changing appearance of the mediastinum.

Follow-up roentgenograms are useful for comparison only if all technical factors are kept constant.[1–6] Attention should be paid to the position of the diaphragm which may significantly alter the radiographic size of the cardiac silhouette and the appearance of the vasculature. This factor alone is more important than the measurement of the cardiac–thoracic ratio which is conveniently used in follow-up examinations to determine heart size.[7,8] Overexposure and underexposure should be strictly avoided.

From the Department of Radiology, University of Minnesota Hospitals, Minneapolis, Minn.

Reprint requests should be addressed to Kurt Amplatz, M.D., Department of Radiology, University of Minnesota Hospitals, Minneapolis, Minn. 55455.

LEFT-TO-RIGHT SHUNTS

General Remarks

The radiologic features of surgically corrected left-to-right shunts are concerned with the changes of the thoracic cage, changes of cardiac silhouette, great vessels, and particularly of the pulmonary vascular bed.

Thorax. Radiographic evidence of corrective surgery are wire sutures in the sternum, symmetrical rib changes in cases of transverse thoracotomies, or unilateral rib regeneration. Regeneration of the left upper ribs should immediately suggest surgical correction of patent ductus arteriosus. Radiographic evidence for a midline sternotomy should suggest surgical correction of ventricular or atrial septal defect very rarely rib regeneration on the right may be due to closure of an atrial septal defect.

There may be an amazing decrease of the antero-posterior (AP) diameter of the thoracic cage with disappearance of the anterior chest bulge following successful cardiac surgery (Figs. 1 and 2). Scoliosis of the thoracic spine either developing following surgery (Fig. 2) or progressing (Fig. 3) may make follow-up examination of heart size very difficult. Persistent cardiomegaly or even progressive left ventricular enlargement may be erroneously diagnosed on the basis of progressing spine deformity, due to the associated rotation of the heart.

Changes in the mediastinum. The appearance of the mediastinum may be altered by the decrease of the size of the main pulmonary artery. Also, there may be postoperative mediastinal widening suggesting complications of cardiac surgery such as mediastinal hematomas or abscesses. In the severely diseased baby with left-to-right shunts, stress from surgery may cause disappearance of the thymus. Following surgery there may be "rebound" growth of thymus, which is most marked in surgical correction of transposition of the great vessels (Fig. 4).

Changes in the peripheral pulmonary vasculature. The fastest and most striking improvement noted radiographically may be the decrease of the

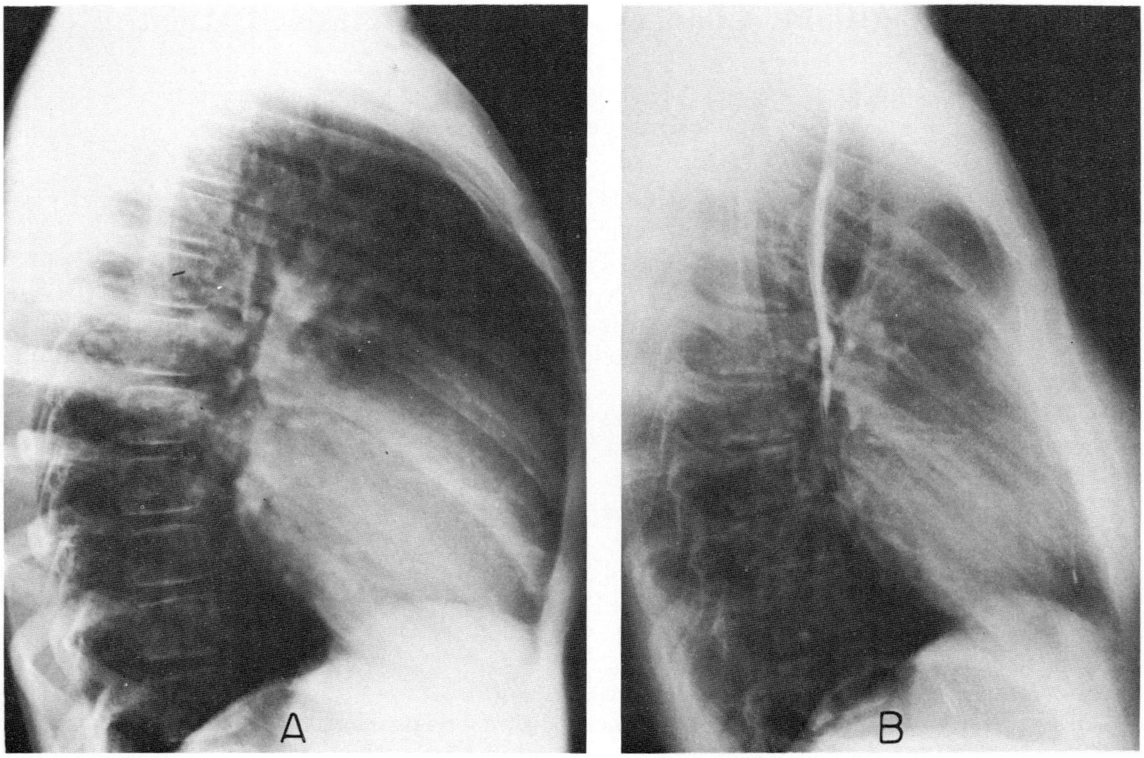

Fig. 1. (A) Preoperative lateral view in patient with ostium primum defect showing prominent bulge of the anterior chest wall. (B) Postoperatively marked decrease in heart size and disappearance of bulge.

peripheral pulmonary vasculature. This obviously does not only involve a decrease of the peripheral pulmonary arteries but also peripheral pulmonary veins. These signs of improvement are most dramatically demonstrated in high-flow, low-resistant shunts. In the older patients, decreasing pulmonary vasculature can be radiographically detected by comparing arteries "on end." The bronchus and accompanying artery of the anterior segment of the right upper lobe may be well seen in left-to-right shunts (Fig. 5A). Following surgery (Fig. 5B), the diminution in size of the same artery may be striking.

Changes of the central pulmonary vasculature. It has to be emphasized that sometimes the pulmonary vasculature may be radiographically normal pre- and postoperatively in spite of the presence of a large left-to-right shunt through an atrial septal defect.[9] Therefore, a "normal" chest roentgenogram cannot rule out an atrial septal defect. In the vast majority of the cases, however, the radiographic diagnosis can be readily made on plain films.

Postoperatively, the decrease of the size of the main pulmonary artery segment depends on the hemodynamics, particularly the association of pulmonary hypertension. High-pressure and high-resistant shunts may show little or no change of the size of the main pulmonary artery. On the other hand, low-resistant, high-flow shunts tend to show a rather rapid decrease in size of the main right and left central pulmonary arteries (Fig. 6).

Change in heart size. Successful, uncomplicated correction of left-to-right shunts is followed by radiographic decrease in heart size. This change in heart size, however, depends largely on the hemodynamic status, particularly the presence or absence of pulmonary hypertension. In high-flow, low-resistant shunts, the decrease of heart size and particularly left atrial enlargement may be rapid. Although the decrease of ventricular chamber size may involve primarily the right or left ventricles,

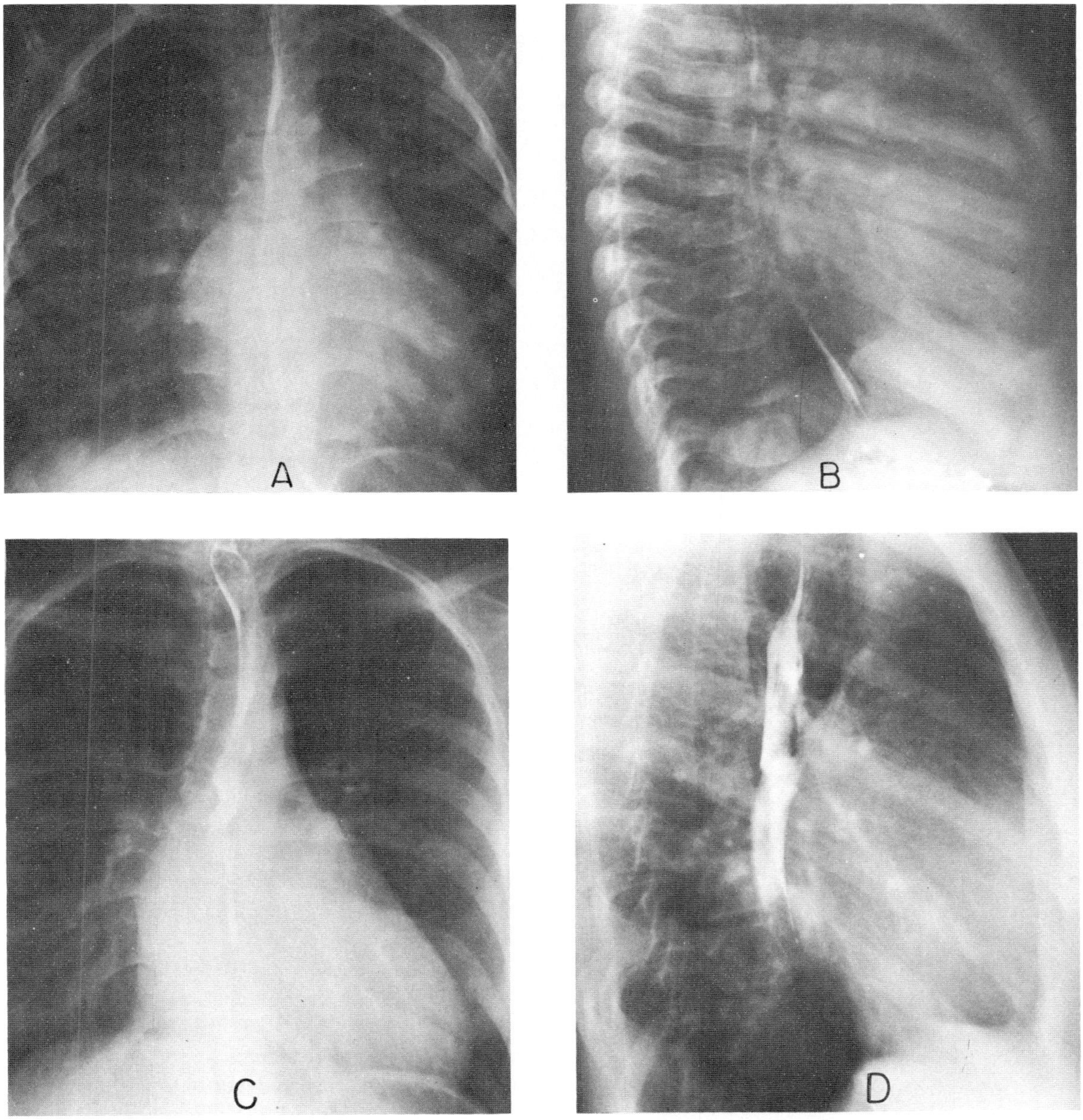

Fig. 2. (A and B) AP and lateral views of the chest show the typical findings of complete AV canal. (C and D) Following complete repair, marked decrease in size on the lateral view with decrease of AP diameter of the chest. PA film, however, suggests erroneously persistent cardiomegaly due to mild scoliosis.

as for example in atrial septal defect or patent ductus, the overall shape of the heart does not change significantly. Rarely the overall heart size does not decrease in spite of uncomplicated, successful surgical closure of left-to-right shunts. Under those circumstances the heart size remains unchanged but becomes relatively smaller due to normal growth of the thoracic cage.

Atrial Septal Defects

Atrial communications of the secundum and sinus venosus type account for the vast majority of

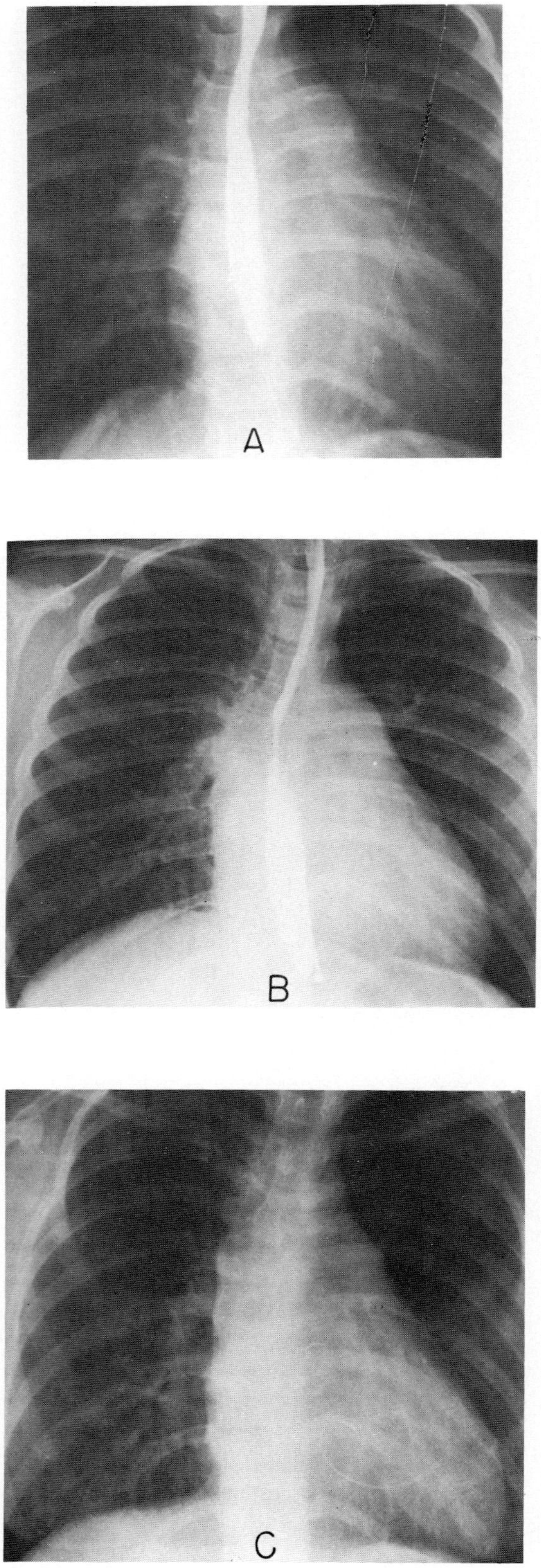

persistent atrial communications. The uncomplicated atrial septal defect in childhood with large flow and increased pulmonary vasculature shows a most rapid and striking postoperative decrease of the peripheral pulmonary vessels. This can almost invariably be noticed during the first week following surgery.[1,3,10] The most dramatic improvement of the radiographic findings can be expected if not only the atrial septal defect but also an associated mitral disease are surgically corrected as in Lutembacher syndrome.

Although there is usually a marked decrease of the overall pulmonary artery size, the central pulmonary arteries may remain prominent (Fig. 7). Some enlargement of the main pulmonary artery may be seen after years in spite of postoperative normal hemodynamic findings.[3,11] In spite of a persistent prominence of the central pulmonary arteries, their hilar pulsations as seen on fluoroscopy become normal immediately postoperatively.[12]

Decrease in heart size occurs slower, primarily involving the right ventricle. Consequently, the change in heart size may be best appreciated on the lateral chest x-ray and may actually result in decrease of AP diameter of the thoracic cage. Rarely cardiomegaly may persist postoperatively, which may be the case if the atrial septal defect was complicated by high pulmonary vascular resistance.[11] The possibility of concomitant myocardial disease caused by long standing volume and pressure overload of the right ventricle was suggested by Young.[11]

Complicated atrial septal defect with increased pulmonary resistance as sometimes found in the adult patients may not show the above mentioned favorable radiographic findings. Rarely vascular disease may progress and actually result in progressively increasing heart size and more prominence of the central pulmonary arteries (Fig. 8).

Complications. Persistent increase of peripheral pulmonary vasculature following surgery or the appearance of increased flow on follow-up examinations should suggest the dehiscence of the suture line. Fortunately, this occurrence is rare nowadays.

Fig. 3. (A) Preoperative chest of patient with ostium primum defect, mild scoliosis. (B) Progression of the scoliosis mimicking left ventricular enlargement. (C) Postoperative chest (complete correction, no shunt). The marked scoliosis simulates persistent cardiomegaly, pacemaker wires.

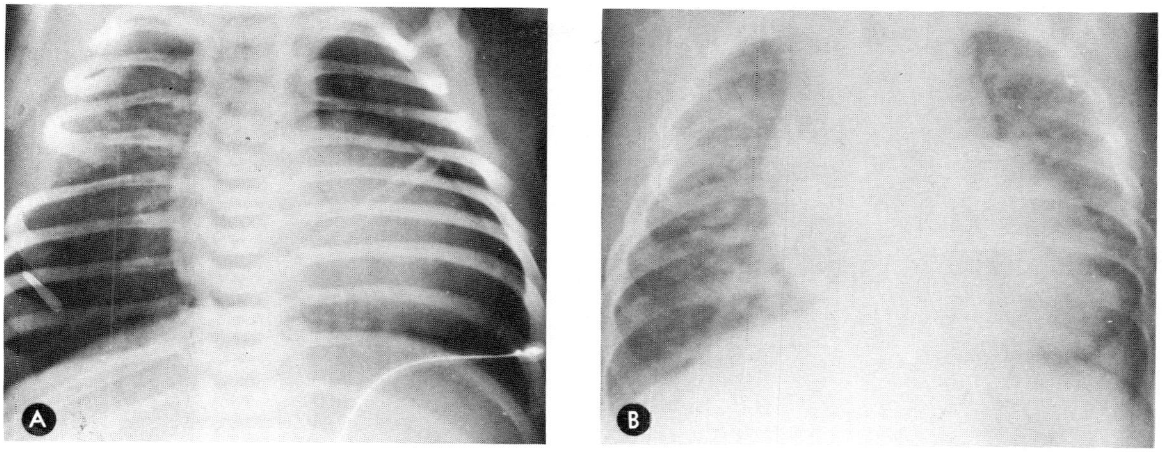

Fig. 4. (A) Complete transposition with narrow mediastinum immediately at the Blalock–Hanlon procedure. (B) One yr later, rebound growth of thymus.

Persistent cardiomegaly and appearance of left atrial enlargement should strongly suggest an additional hemodynamic left-sided lesion. The importance of radiographic follow-up examinations is demonstrated in one patient who had an uncomplicated atrial septal defect repaired. Three yr following surgery, an RAO (right anterior oblique) view with barium showed clearly left atrial enlargement (Fig. 9). Because of this finding, a pulmonary arteriogram was performed which demonstrated a filling defect in the left atrium (Fig. 10), thought to be a thrombus or less likely left-atrial myxoma. A myxoma was successfully removed at time of surgery!

Lack of surgical correction of an anomalous pulmonary vein does usually not account for persistent increased pulmonary vasculature.[11,13–18] Anomalous venous connection to the superior vena

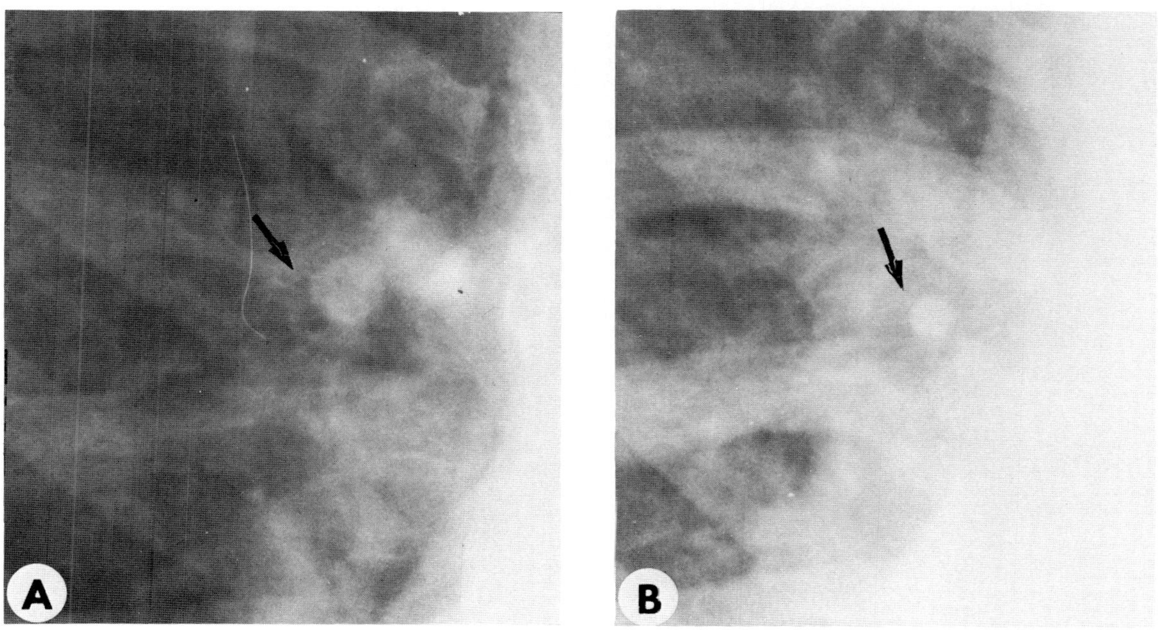

Fig. 5. (A) Close-up view of the right mid-lung field showing markedly enlarged pulmonary artery on end. Artery to anterior segment of right upper lobe (arrow). Note much smaller adjacent bronchus. (B) Postoperatively marked reduction in size of the same pulmonary artery (arrow).

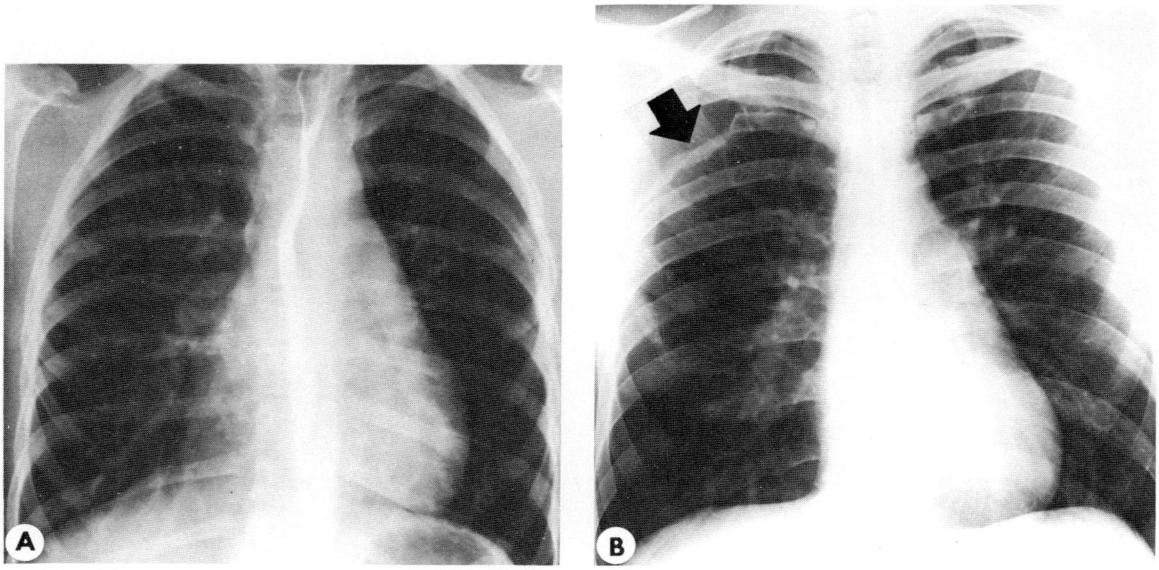

Fig. 6. (A) Preoperative chest x-ray shows slight cardiomegaly, increased pulmonary vasculature in patient with ASD. (B) One yr following surgery the findings were normal. The arrow points to a regenerated rib (a right-sided surgical approach was made).

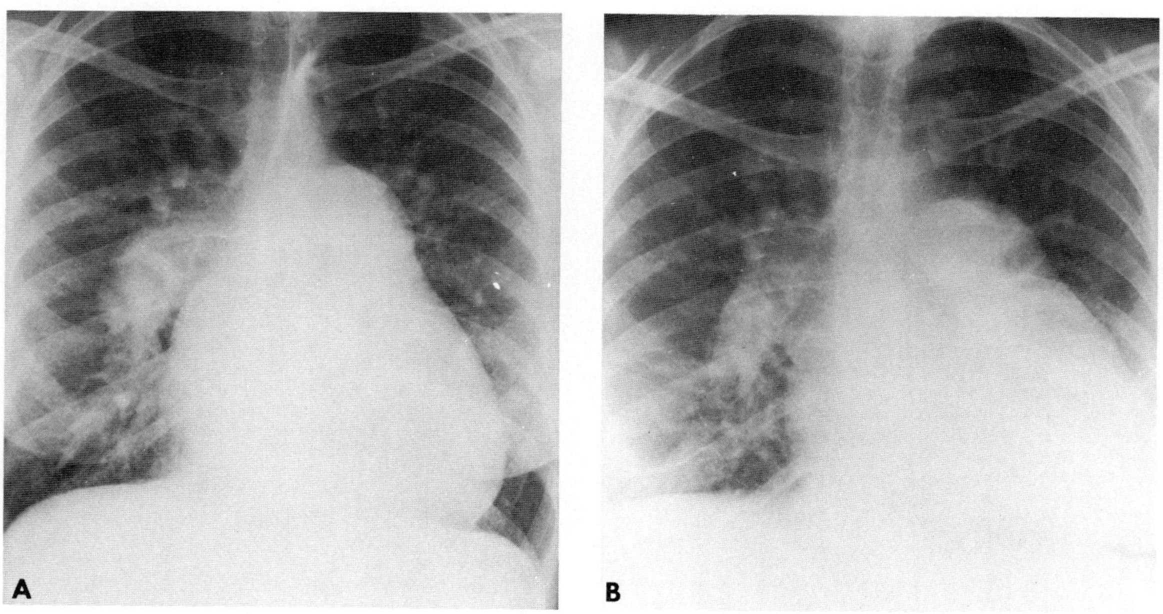

Fig. 7. (A) ASD with markedly increased central pulmonary artery. (Comparatively normal peripheral pulmonary arteries suggest associated pulmonary hypertension). (B) Three wk after surgery the size of the right pulmonary artery has decreased but still remains prominent.

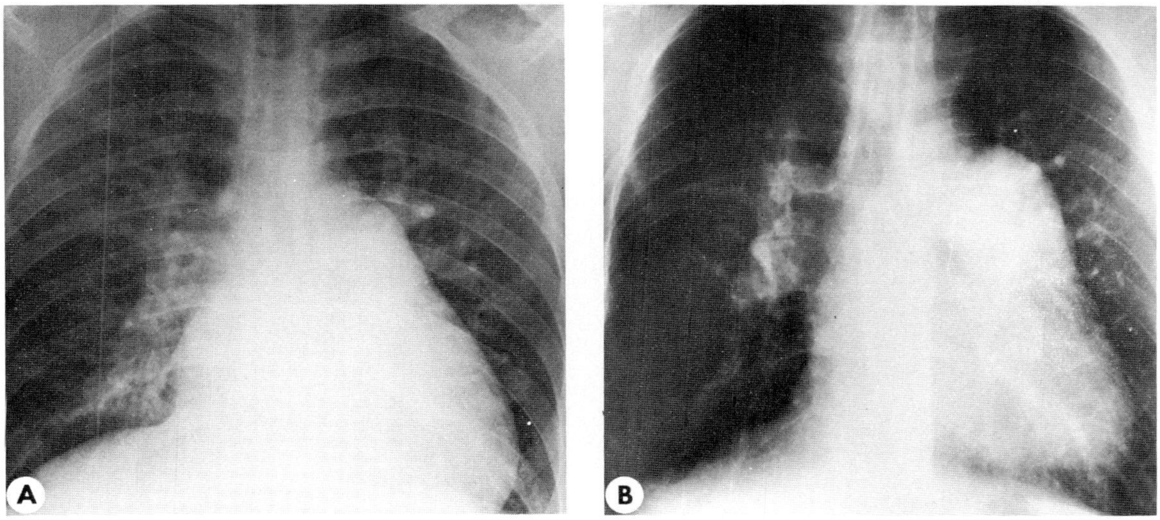

Fig. 8. (A) Preoperative PA chest roentgenogram shows marked cardiomegaly and increased pulmonary vasculature as in ASD with pulmonary hypertension. (Pulmonary hypertension was found at the time of catheterization.) (B) Fifteen yr following surgical correction. There is decrease in heart size but persistent enlargement of the pulmonary arteries due to pulmonary hypertension.

cava may be very high and, therefore, intentionally ligated. Sometimes this may result in right upper lobe infarction and cavitation (Fig. 11).

The appearance of desaturation or frank cyanosis following atrial septal defect repair is almost pathognomonic of incorporation of the inferior vena cava into the left atrium. At the time of surgery, the Eustachian valve is mistaken for the lower border of the atrial septal defect; and the patch is sewn to the valve. At time of catheteriza-

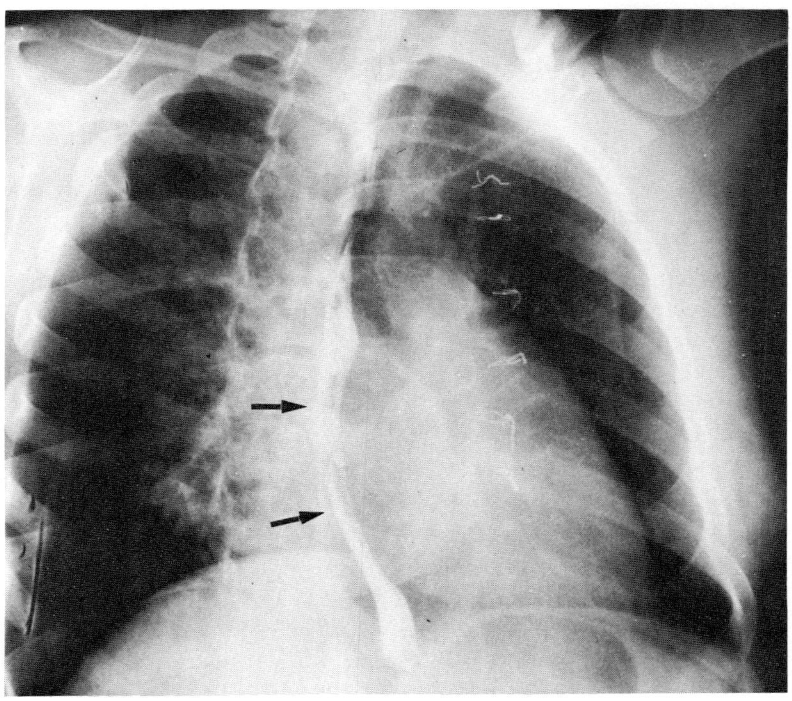

Fig. 9. RAO view of the patient 3 yr following ASD repair. Note appearance of left atrium (arrow).

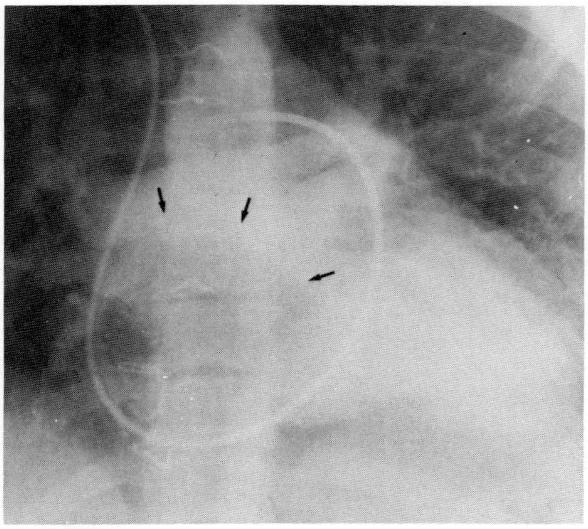

Fig. 10. Levogram following pulmonary artery injection shows large filling defect (arrows) in the left atrium.

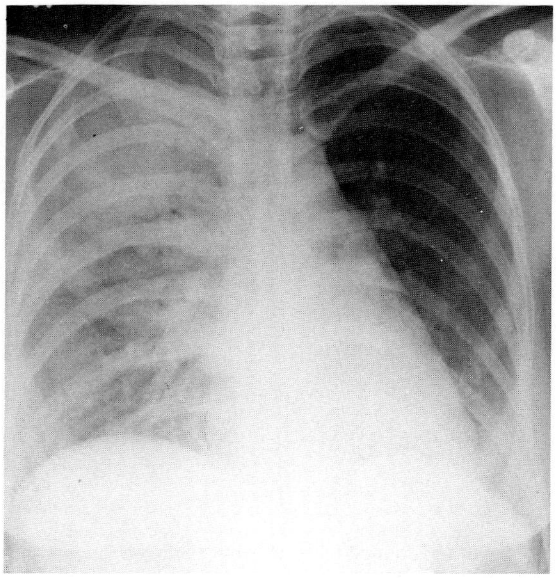

Fig. 11. PA chest following ASD repair and ligation of right-upper-lobe pulmonary vein. Note consolidation of the right-upper-lobe due to infarction.

tion, the catheter can be passed from the inferior vena cava to the left atrium; and the lesion is unequivocally demonstrated by angiography (Fig. 12).

Ventricular Septal Defects

The surgical treatment for ventricular septal defects is either palliative (banding) or corrective (closure).

Pulmonary banding. None of the materials used (umbilical tape, teflon, nylon, silk, dacron, etc.) are radiopaque; and, therefore, pulmonary bands are not visible on plain chest roentgenograms. One of the complications of banding, namely slippage,[19–23] cannot be diagnosed without angiography. The introduction of radiopaque banding materials as suggested by Patterson[24] has not found widespread acceptance.

The postoperative changes of the pulmonary vasculature following banding depend primarily on its hemodynamic effectiveness and the preoperative hemodynamic status of the ventricular septal defect. In large-flow shunts and tight bands, diminution of peripheral pulmonary arteries may be seen during the first postoperative weeks or months. Decrease of pulmonary flow may also be strikingly evidenced by diminution of left atrial size. (This rapid response to banding is rare.) Signs of congestive heart failure and repeated pulmonary complications may clear dramatically.[25] Cardiomegaly may diminish but tends to persist to some degree.[19,22,26–29]

Very commonly, however, the pulmonary band is not tight enough to cause immediate postoperative radiographic signs of improvement. Months and years may elapse until obvious signs of decreased pulmonary flow are visible, and sometimes the radiographic picture may be unchanged until corrective surgery is carried out. In patients with effective bands there is a general slow trend in decrease in heart size over the years. Since the band cannot grow and cardiac output increases with the patient's growth, pulmonary banding becomes hemodynamically more and more obvious. Finally, bidirectional or a frank right-to-left shunt may occur which may be evidenced by the appearance of cyanosis. Left-atrial enlargement is absent, the heart decreases markedly in size, and the pulmonary vasculature appears decreased.[19,27]

Complications. Gradual sudden enlargement of the mediastinum may suggest erosion of the pulmonary artery with the formation of a false aneurysm due to pressure necrosis or complicating infective endocarditis.

Improper surgical placement of a band may result in infundibular pulmonary stenosis[22,23,30,31] or pulmonary insufficiency.[22] If the band is placed in close proximity to the pulmonary valve leaflets, thickening of the valve leaflet may be observed

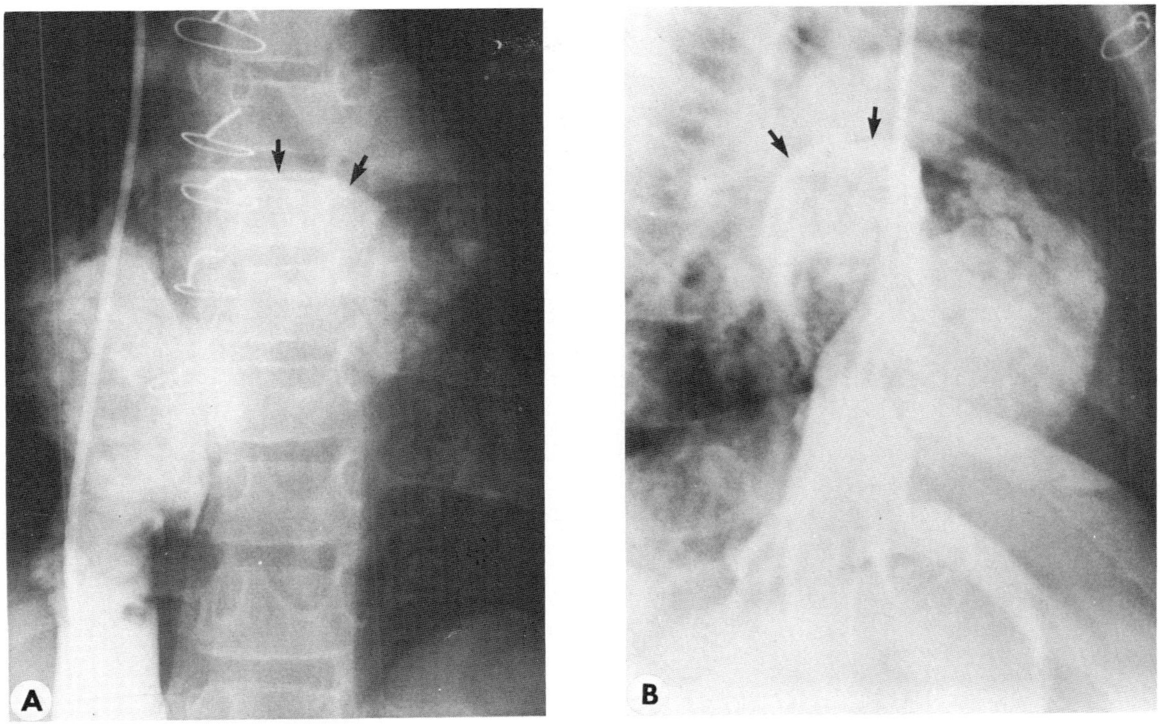

Fig. 12. (A and B) AP and lateral views of inferior vena cavogram showing opacification of the left atrium (arrows) due to incorporation of the inferior vena cava at the time of surgery.

angiographically (Fig. 13). This is very likely due to impingement of the valve against the banding site.

A much more common and more serious complication is application of the pulmonary band too far distal on the main pulmonary bifurcation or possibly slippage of the band towards the bifurcation. This may result in severe stenosis or complete obstruction of the right pulmonary artery. Sometimes this complication can be suspected on plain films by decreasing pulmonary vasculature in the right lung (Fig. 14). Such stenoses involving the

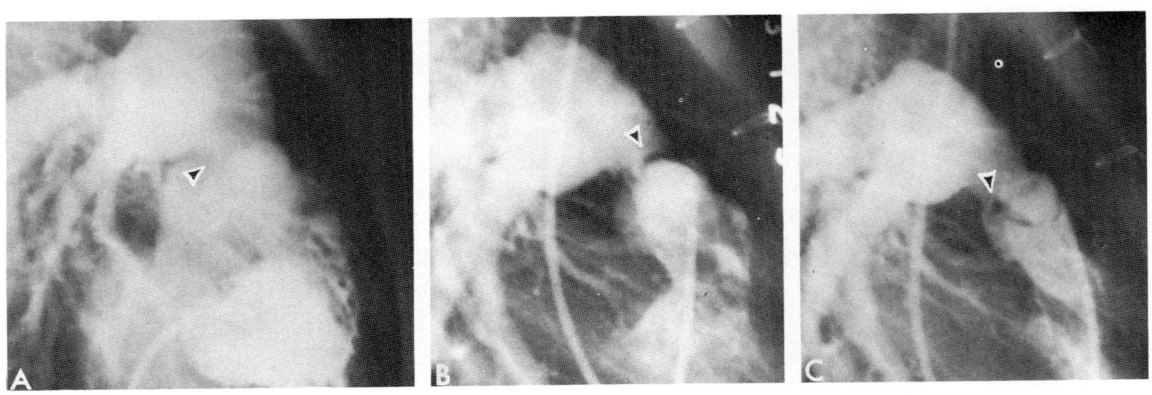

Fig. 13. (A) Tight pulmonary band (arrow) resulting in right-to-left shunt at the ventricular level and opacification of the aorta. (B) Following closure of VSD and removal of band, marked thickening of the pulmonary valve is well seen (arrow) in systole. (C) Markedly thickened valve tissue with nodules at the free edges well seen in diastole (arrow).

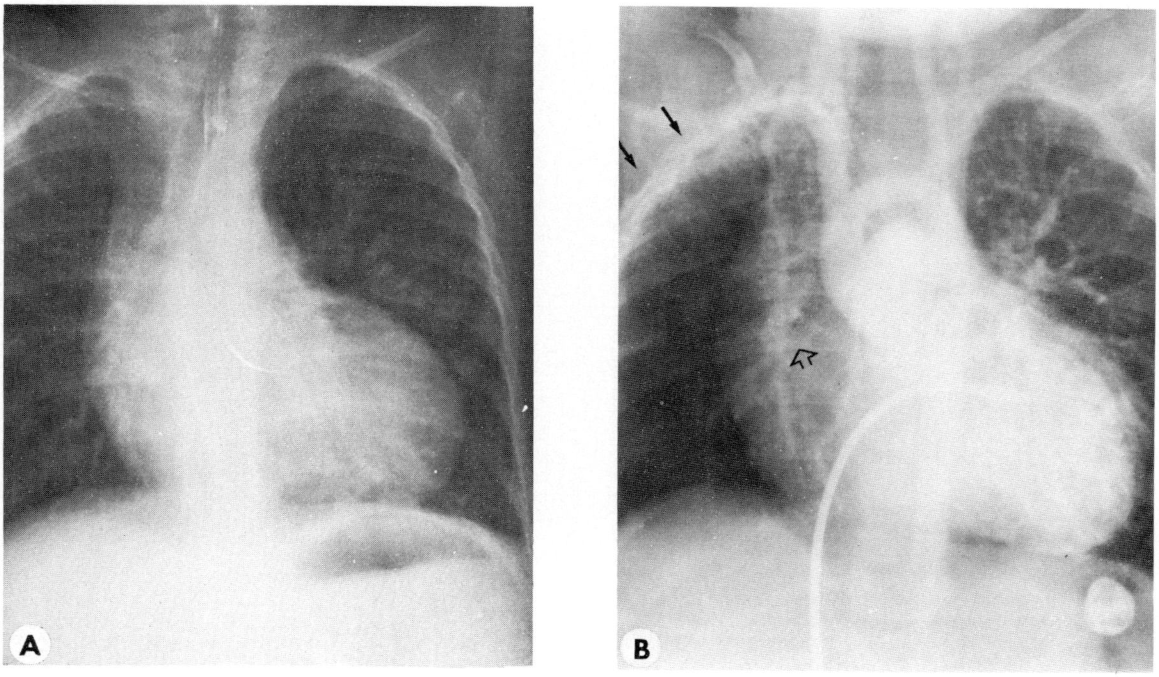

Fig. 14. (A) Mild cardiomegaly with increased pulmonary vasculature on the left and markedly decreased pulmonary vasculature in the right lung. Pleural thickening in the right upper chest. (B) Levophase of right ventriculogram showing opacification only of the left pulmonary artery and occlusion of the right pulmonary artery by banding. Right pulmonary artery opacifies late (arrow) by extensive transpleural collaterals (arrows).

right pulmonary artery may persist following removal of the band requiring a patch graft. Persistent stenosis of the main pulmonary artery following removal of bands has also been observed.[1,20–22,32–34]

An interesting but rare radiographic observation is gradual right heart enlargement following pulmonary banding which is due to spontaneous closure of a ventricular septal defect.[35–38]

Closure of ventricular septal defect. Depending on the type of ventricular septal defect, the hemodynamic and radiographic postoperative changes may differ. Small defects with no significant increase in pulmonary resistance and shunts in less than 50% may have a normal heart size and normal pulmonary vasculature preoperatively. Ventricular septal defects with large flows and low pulmonary resistance show the most dramatic immediate postoperative change in decrease of left atrial enlargement, decrease in peripheral pulmonary vasculature, and gradual decrease of the main pulmonary segment and heart size. A slow decrease of cardiomegaly may continue for several years.[3,39,40]

The least dramatic postoperative response may be expected in ventricular septal defect with markedly elevated pulmonary arteriolar resistance. The size of the main pulmonary arteries is usually out of proportion in relation to pulmonary flow preoperatively. The large size of the central pulmonary arteries tends to persist or may even progress after surgery.[13,39,41–44]

Rarely the interventricular patch may calcify and become visible on roentgenograms. This calcification, however, is of no clinical significance.

Complications. Incomplete closure of ventricular septal defect was more common in the early days of cardiac surgery especially seen in patients with severe pulmonary hypertension and simple suture closure of the defect.[13,32,33,39,40]

A fortunately rare finding is the dehiscence of the patch as may be evidenced radiographically and particularly clinically by the reappearance of a murmur. Since recurrent or residual shunts tend to be rather small, they are commonly missed on plain films.

If surgical closure of the ventricular septal defect is complicated by postoperative heart block, the heart may remain significantly enlarged in spite of complete correction of the ventricular communication (Fig. 15).

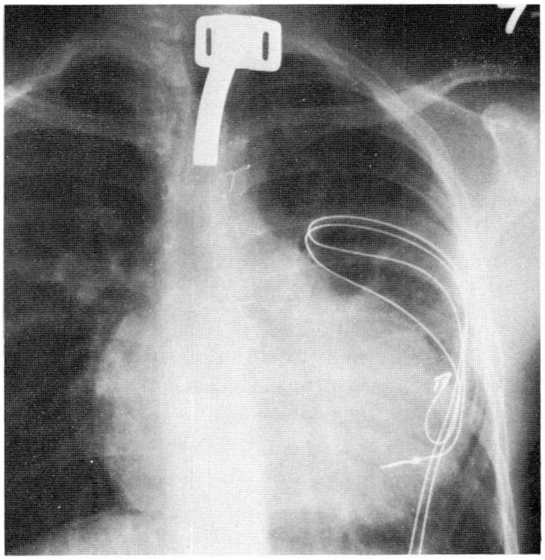

Fig. 15. Six yr following successful closure of VSD and ASD. Slightly accentuated vasculature and marked cardiomegaly persists due to complete heart block. (Note epicardial pacemaker wires.) Tracheal tube in place following postintubation-subglottic stenosis.

Atrioventricular Canal

Atrioventricular canal is a complex, anatomic and hemodynamic lesion. Basically a left-to-right shunt at the atrial and ventricular levels is complicated by mitral insufficiency or pulmonary hypertension of varying degrees. Therefore, no generalized statements can be made as to the postoperative appearance of the chest with this complicated congenital cardiac defect. Clues as to the predominant hemodynamic lesion, however, can be obtained from plain roentgenograms.

The patients with ostium primum defect without significant mitral regurgitation display the same postoperative heart changes as the patients with ostium secundum defect, namely fast decrease of pulmonary vasculature and somewhat slower decrease in heart size. The heart size of patients with significant mitral regurgitation and cardiomegaly diminishes much slower after complete repair (Fig. 16A and B) but eventually will resume a normal size. Persistent cardiomegaly or postoperatively increasing cardiomegaly indicates either persisting mitral insufficiency or a surgically created mitral reflux (Fig. 17A and B).

One of the complications of corrective surgery is complete atrioventricular block which can be suspected radiographically by the presence of pacemaker wires.

Postoperative angiocardiography may demonstrate complete correction of the defects, but the basic angiocardiographic deformity of the left ventricular outflow tract remains (Fig. 16C).[45]

Postoperative angiography may be necessary to locate the site of a residual shunt or quantitate the mitral regurgitation (Fig. 17C and D). In patients with ostium primum defect and mitral regurgitation, no reliable technique is available to quantitate the degree of the regurgitation.[46–48] After closure of the septal defect, however, angiocardiography becomes a sensitive method to detect and to estimate the degree of mitral incompetence since the regurgitant contrast medium is no longer shunted into the right atrium.

Extracardiac Left-to-Right Shunts

All extracardiac left-to-right shunts as patent ductus arteriosus, AP window, ruptured sinus of Valsalva aneurysm, ventricular septal defect with associated aortic insufficiency have in common increased pulsations of the aorta. In large shunts, this can be readily detected by fluoroscopy, cine fluoroscopy, or kymography. Following complete surgical correction, this increased pulsation disappears postoperatively. Otherwise, the changes of heart size, left atrial enlargement, and pulmonary vasculature depend largely on hemodynamics and are very similar as described in closure of ventricular septal defects.

Complications. The operative procedure of obliteration of a ductus arteriosus has a very low complication rate. Several authors[49–52] reported no lethal case in their series irrespective of the technique used.

Documented complications in literature include: (1) recanalization of a ligated ductus, (2) rupture, and (3) aneurysm. Other complications are pneumonia, pulmonary infarction, lobular atelectasis, and chylothorax.[49] Since these pulmonary complications are nonspecific, they are not discussed any further.

Recanalization happens only in cases where the ligature method is applied. Even then this complication indicates poor technique.[53] The roentgen signs are the reappearance of the shunt vasculature and cardiac enlargement. Clinically the typical murmur at the left sternal border persists or reappears.

Rupture of a ductus arteriosus can occur either at the time of the operation or postoperatively. The clinical signs of patients with rupture of the

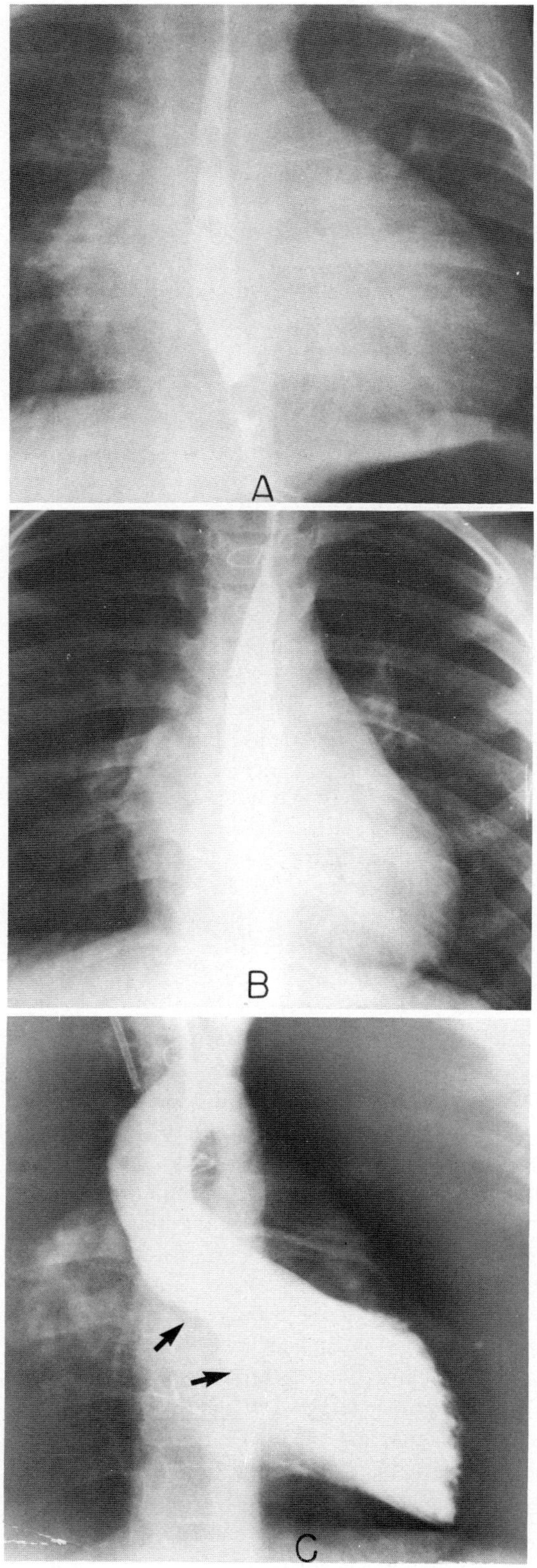

Fig. 16. (A) Marked cardiomegaly, increased vasculature and left atrial enlargement as in complete AV canal. (B) Chest findings completely normal only 4 yr following complete repair. (C) Left ventriculogram demonstrating no shunt or mitral reflux but persistent deformity of the left ventricular outflow tract (arrows).

previously closed pulmonary ductus arteriosus include hemoptysis and hoarseness due to recurrent nerve palsy. X-ray examination reveals a widened mediastinum above the left hilum due to hemorrhage.[53]

The postoperative appearance of an aneurysmal dilatation at the ductal area can be caused either by a residual leak leading to the formation of a pulsatile hematoma or more often by a local staphylococcus aureus infection. These patients present postoperatively with intermittent pyrexia and a loud continuous murmur. Radiographically a mediastinal shadow, inseparable from the great vessels, can be seen at the site of the ligated pulmonary ductus arteriosus. The opacity has a convex outer border which may be irregular in outline due to pleural reaction. This opacity may enlarge rapidly. Contrast studies performed from the left ventricle or aorta may show passage of contrast medium into the aneurysmal cavity with opacification of the pulmonary artery.[54]

Total Anomalous Pulmonary Venous Return

Although hemodynamically a cyanotic condition, this abnormality is discussed here because of its radiographic similarity to left-to-right shunts. The experience with postoperative radiologic findings in patients with total anomalous pulmonary venous return is limited because this congenital defect is rather rare. (The overall frequency is 1% of all congenital heart diseases).

The postoperative x-ray findings can be divided into: (1) the changes of the chest, and (2) cardiovascular changes.

Chest changes. With successful surgical correction of this lesion, the anterior bulge of the chest wall may regress during the first postoperative year with resulting decrease of the AP chest diameter (Fig. 18).

Cardiovascular changes. Normalization of heart size occurs within months or at the latest in a year (Fig. 19A). The persistence of cardiomegaly indicates a significant residual left-to-right shunt or postsurgical hemodynamic problem (Fig. 20). The

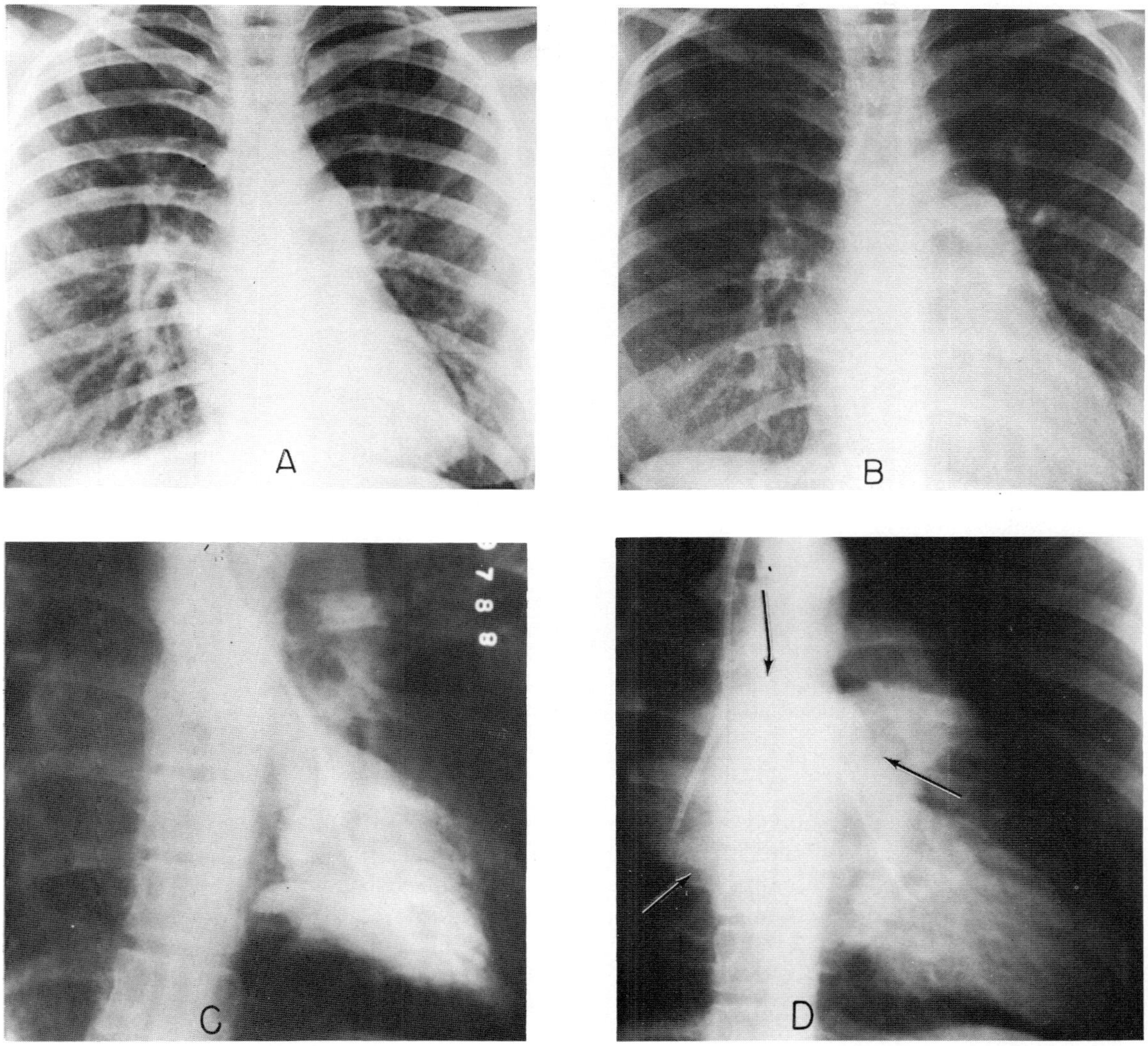

Fig. 17. (A) Marked cardiomegaly and increased vasculature in patient with ostium primum defect and no mitral reflux. (B) Following correction of atrial shunt, vasculature decreased but cardiomegaly persists due to mitral reflux created at time of surgery. (C) Preoperative angiogram demonstrating a typical left ventricular outflow tract deformity but no mitral reflux. (D) Postoperative left ventriculogram shows considerable mitral reflux outlining densely the left atrium (arrows).

postsurgical regression of the pulmonary vasculature seems to be dependent on the age of the patient and presence of pulmonary hypertension. If the operation was performed prior to adolescence, the pulmonary vascular tree can assume the normal pattern within a short period of time. On the other hand, increased pulmonary vasculature can persist in patients operated upon in adulthood, particularly if pulmonary hypertension was present (Fig. 21).

Postoperatively the appearance of the mediastinum may change dramatically. The density of the left vertical vein disappears completely, and the size of the right superior vena cava can diminish considerably (Fig. 20B). Persistent prominence of the left vertical vein may suggest persistence of some partial anomalous connection to this vein.

In some patients the anastomosis of the common pulmonary vein with the left atrium may be stenotic. In these patients signs of venous congestion with pulmonary hypertension can be found (Fig. 19B and C). An uncommon complication of

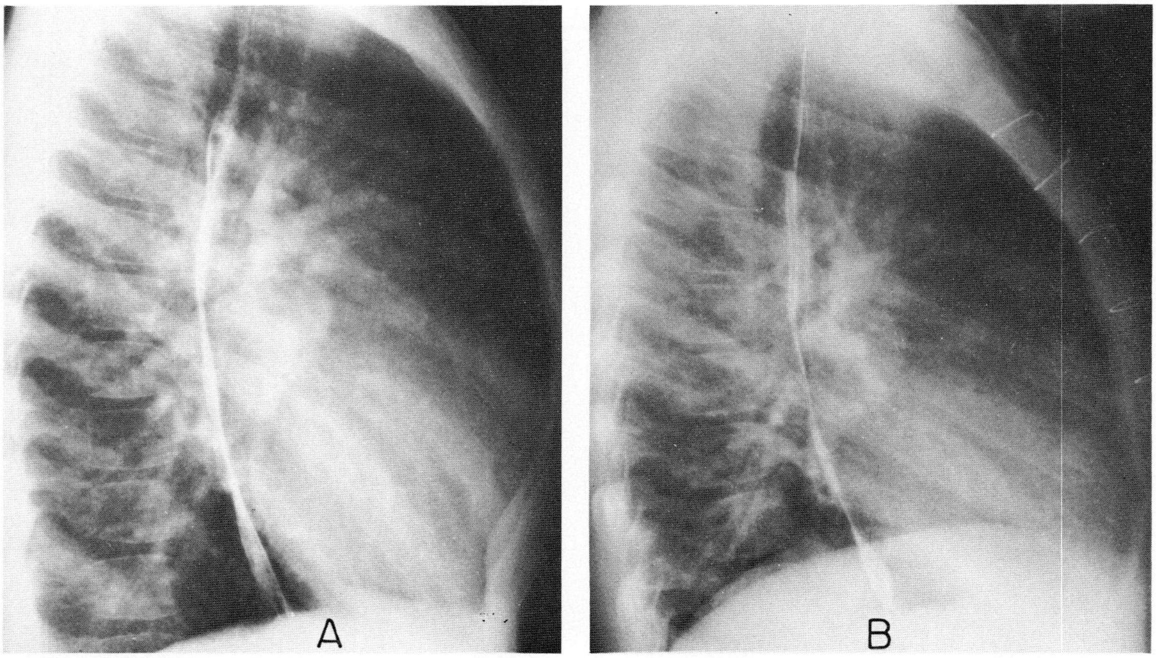

Fig. 18. (A) Lateral view of patient with total anomalous venous return. Note markedly increased vasculature and lacking left atrial enlargement. Prominent precordial bulge of the thoracic cage. (B) Precordial bulge disappears following corrective surgery within 1 yr.

surgery is incorporation of the inferior vena cava in the left atrium during the closure of the atrial septal defect. This complication results in cyanosis and is identical to a complication occurring in closure of atrial septal defects.

TETRALOGY OF FALLOT

Most patients with tetralogy of Fallot can be anatomically corrected by cardiac surgery with low-operative mortality[55-59] and improvement of the cardiac status.[58,60-66] Although most patients are clinically markedly improved, many have residual hemodynamic abnormalities which are reflected both by the chest roentgenograms and postoperative angiocardiograms.

Plain Chest Roentgenograms

In the immediate postoperative period, some mediastinal widening is usually present. Progressive and excessive mediastinal widening or accumulation of pleural fluid should suggest excessive hemorrhage which may require reoperation. Other complications during this period may be cardiac tamponade, pulmonary edema, pneumothorax, and atelectasis.

In the immediate postoperative period the most consistent change in the chest roentgenogram is an increase in cardiac size.[67-70] This increase in heart size is probably due to increased blood flow through the left side of the heart following corrective surgery. This usually occurs within the first 6 mo without further progression in the presence of a good hemodynamic result. Most patients have a postoperative cardiothoracic ratio (CTR) of 0.51-0.60. A progressive increase in cardiac size points to a significant hemodynamic problem such as a residual ventricular septal defect, residual outflow tract obstruction, outflow tract aneurysm, severe pulmonary or tricuspid insufficiency, atrioventricular dissociation, complete heart block, or a combination of these.

Some authors indicate that the CTR tends to be greater in patients with patches across the pulmonary annulus than in those without.[55-58] It is suggested that this may be due to pulmonary insufficiency created by extension of the patch across the annulus.[71] Among our group of 108 patients

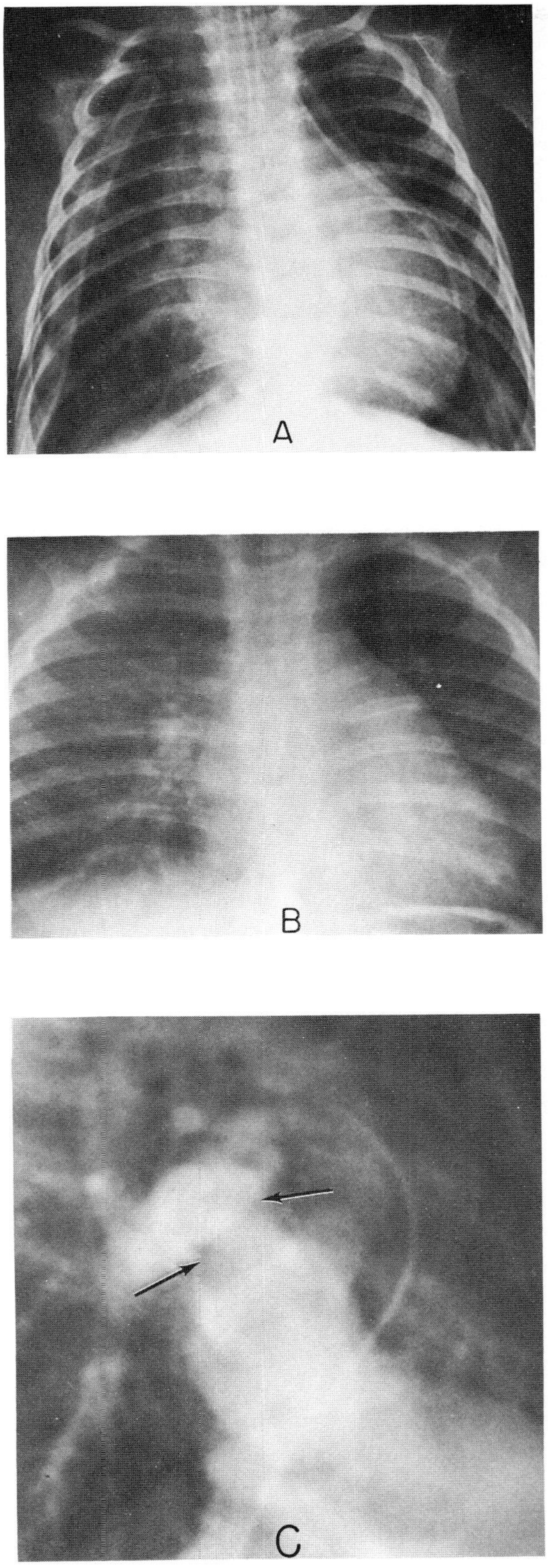

whose postoperative plain films were studied, no such correlation was found.

Postoperatively there is an increased prominence of the outflow tract area (Fig. 22).[67,70,71] In our group, this degree of prominence was not greater in patients with outflow tract reconstruction than in those with only ventriculotomy and infundibulectomy. The type of ventriculotomy did not appear to affect the degree of this prominence. It is, to be sure, difficult to distinguish from a single postoperative thoracic roentgenogram, or even a series of them, whether a prominent "outflow tract" represents the infundibulum or pulmonary artery which is dilated or whether there is actually a postoperative aneurysm. Angiocardiography is needed for definitive diagnosis.

In our group of patients, we found no significant one-to-one correlation between the degree of postoperative cardiomegaly or degree of prominence of the outflow tract and such parameters as peak right ventricular systolic pressure, size of residual shunt or residual gradient across the right ventricular outflow tract. It may be, that in any one case, an abnormal degree of cardiomegaly is caused by a combination of factors rather than by one particular factor alone.

Postoperatively, the pulmonary vasculature usually appears increased as compared with the preoperative film. When increased above the normal, the possibility of a residual left-to-right shunt or dehiscence of the ventricular septal defect patch should be considered.

Calcifications in Ivalon and pericardial outflow patches are not rare and have been previously reported by various authors (Fig. 23).[71–74] These calcifications are of no hemodynamic consequence.

Angiocardiography

Residual ventricular septal defect is one of the common residual hemodynamic abnormalities

Fig. 19. (A) Total anomalous venous return 1 day postop showing decrease in vasculature and heart size as compared with the preoperative film. (B) Three yr postoperatively. Some cardiomegaly persists and increased wedge pressure was noted at time of recatheterization. (C) Lateral projection of angiogram shows narrowing at the anastomotic site between the common pulmonary vein and left atrium (arrows). Angiographically the degree of narrowing appears to be mild.

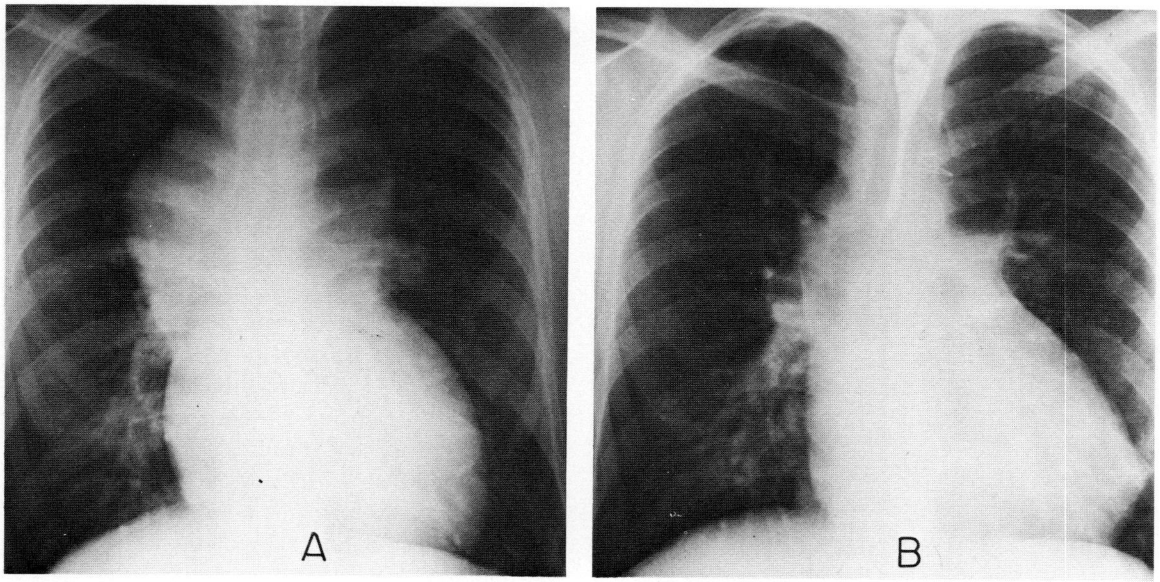

Fig. 20. (A) Total anomalous venous return showing typical "snow man" (Figure of 8) configuration. (B) Three yr following complete correction. The left superior vena cava density has completely disappeared. Moderate cardiomegaly persists due to postoperatively appearing severe arrhythmias and cardiac failure.

which occurs postoperatively. Its incidence varies widely among the reported series and appears to depend on the operating surgeon and the type of diagnostic tool used in evaluating the patients. In Malm's series of 100 patients, 65 were catheterized; and of these, nine (10.9%) and left-to-right shunts by oximetry.[59] Burnell found three residual ventricular septal defects among thirteen cases (23%),[63] and Kirklin and co-workers found residual ventricular septal defects in eight out of 92 patients (8%).[59] Lillehei and his group found fifteen residual shunts in thirty patients (50%), but these were done early in their experience of total correction and some of the septal closures had been done by direct suture.[64] Complete closure of ventricular septal defects without the creation of heart block remains a technical challenge for the surgeon.

In our group of 108 patients who had undergone postoperative catheterization, 76 had postoperative

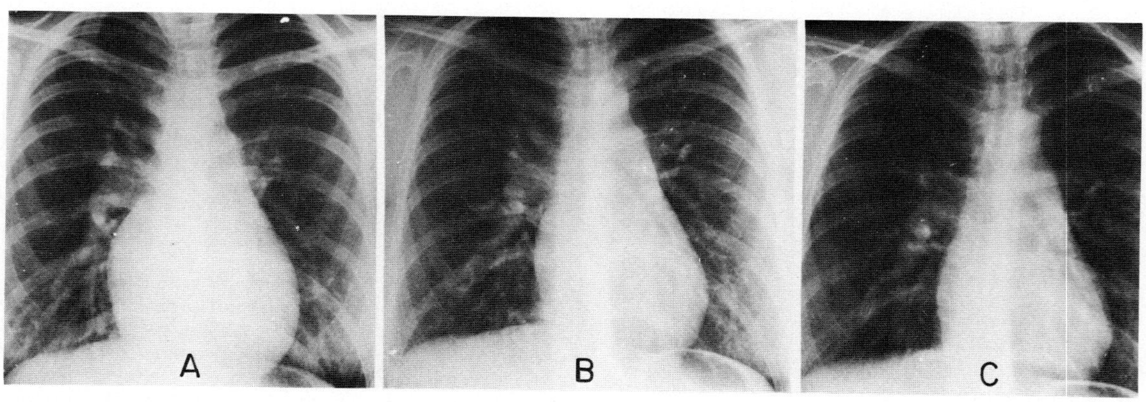

Fig. 21. (A) AP view in patient with total anomalous return directly to the right atrium showing cardiomegaly and markedly increased vasculature. (B) One yr postoperatively the heart size is almost normal but some prominence of vasculature remains. (C) Six yr later, normal heart size and still mild prominence of the central pulmonary vasculature.

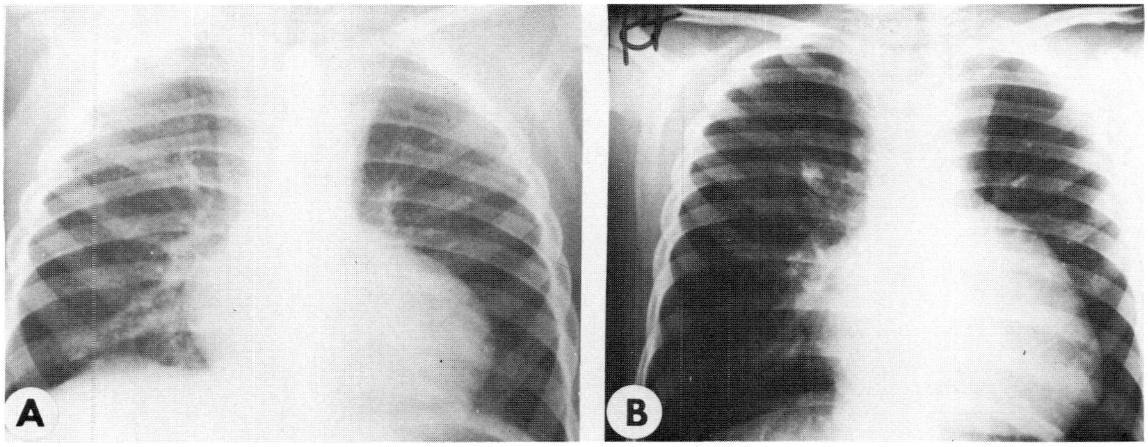

Fig. 22. Preoperative (A) and postoperative (B) roentgenograms show increased prominence of the outflow tract region.

angiocardiography also. Of the total of 108, 40 (37%) had residual shunts. Many of these shunts were not detectable by oximetry but were either detected only by the Freon method[75] or seen transiently at angiography. Angiographically, the most common site of the residual or recurrent ventricular septal defect in this group was at the superoposterior aspect of the patch. This is in contrast to Malm's series in which most postoperative ventricular shunts were in the inferoposterior aspect of the ventricular septal defect patch. A variation in surgical technique may account for this difference.

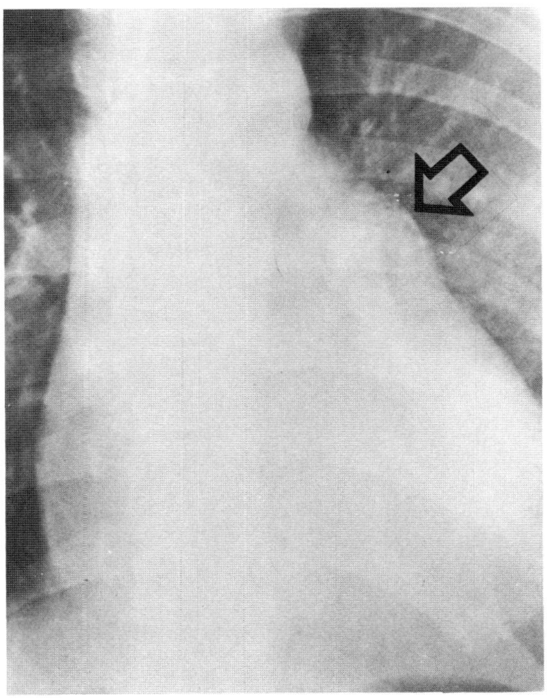

Fig. 23. Postoperative roentgenograms show curvilinear calcification in a pericardial patch (arrow).

Another common postoperative angiographic finding is the change in the outflow tract and main pulmonary artery. After ventriculotomy and infundibulectomy, the infundibular region appears irregular; and its anterior wall may show areas of akinesia or hypokinesia. This region may well be adherent to the posterior aspect of the sternum, thus being rendered immobile and fixed during angiography (Fig. 24). True and false aneurysm formation may occur (Figs. 25 and 26). A total of nine right ventricular aneurysms were observed among our 76 patients with postoperative angiocardiograms (13.8%). Six of these aneurysms were in patients without outflow tract reconstruction. Of these six aneurysms, three were false and three were true aneurysms.

After reconstruction of the outflow tract, the patch may dilate and show various degrees of bulges to frank true aneurysms (Fig. 27). In our series, three of the nine aneurysms observed were in patients with outflow tract reconstruction. The incidence of aneurysm of the outflow tract in these patients varies widely in the reported series depending primarily on the material used for the patch graft. In Hawe's series,[56] the incidence of aneurysm formation in the outflow tract in cases with Ivalon patches was 33%, 9% in cases with

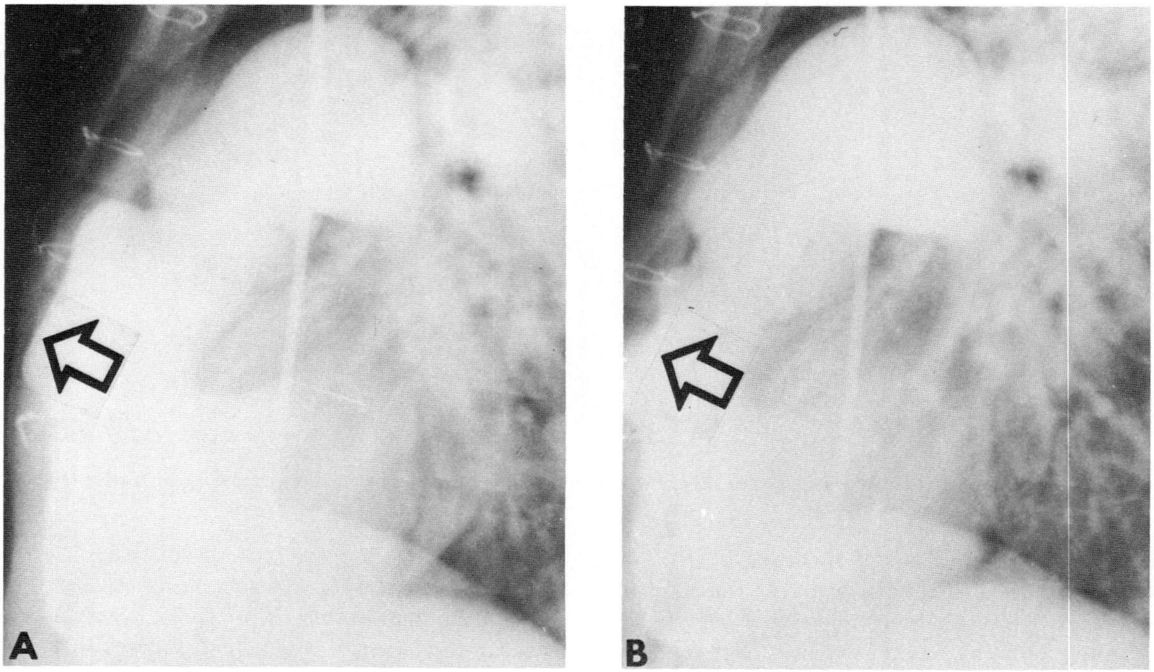

Fig. 24. Lateral views of right ventriculogram [diastole (A) and systole (B)]. Partial adhesion of anterior aspect outflow tract to the sternum (arrow) after infundibulectomy.

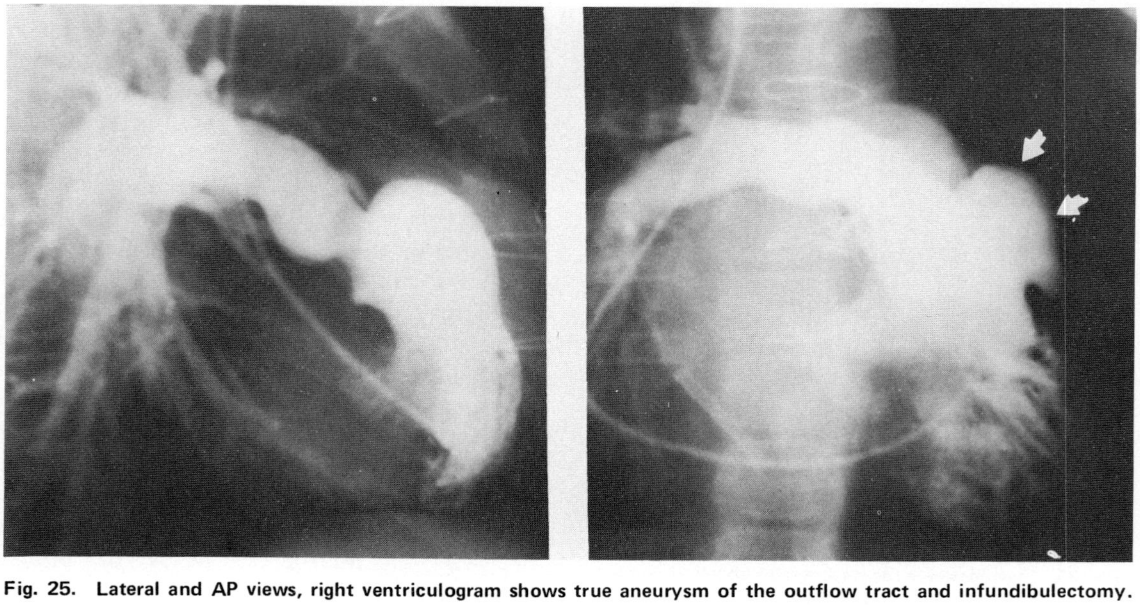

Fig. 25. Lateral and AP views, right ventriculogram shows true aneurysm of the outflow tract and infundibulectomy.

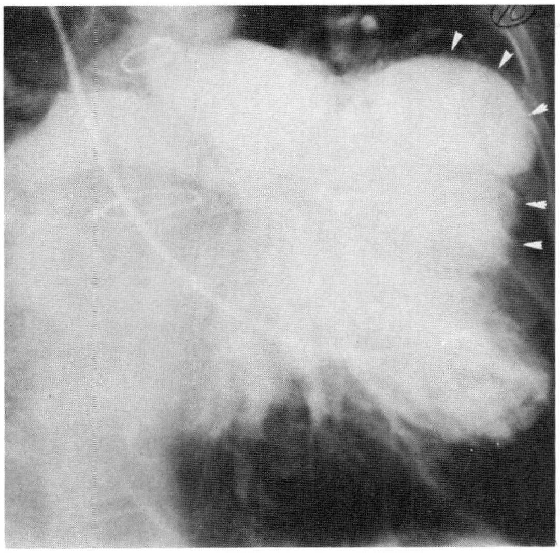

Fig. 26. AP view of right ventriculogram shows false aneurysm of the outflow tract (arrows).

teflon patches, and 8% in those with autogenous pericardial tissue patches. Rosenthal[76] reported a 7% incidence of outflow tract aneurysm in patients with pericardial outflow tract patches.

In contrast to most series, we observed a higher incidence of aneurysm formation in patients who had undergone ventriculotomy and infundibulectomy rather than in those with outflow tract reconstruction. This may be due again to a difference in surgical technique with possibly our group having a more "thorough" resection of infundibular muscle.

Pulmonary insufficiency is commonly seen in the postoperative tetralogy patient, particularly after outflow tract reconstruction with extension of the patch across the annulus. In these cases, depending on the degree of insufficiency, the main pulmonary artery and the right ventricle dilate and show active pulsation during fluoroscopy. There is usually no correlation between symptoms and the degree of insufficiency observed angiographically. Pulmonary regurgitation is well tolerated by most patients.[11]

The most common site for residual outflow tract obstruction is at the valve and valve ring area. However, the severity of the residual stenosis, whether infundibular, valvular, or supravalvular, cannot be determined postoperatively by the angiographic appearance alone. Complete catheterization data are needed to determine the significance of such residual stenotic areas.

SYSTEMIC-PULMONARY-ARTERIAL SHUNTS

Systemic-pulmonary-arterial shunts are widely used as a palliative measure for incorrectable, complex cardiac lesions as well as correctable lesions such as tetralogy of Fallot. Ebert and Sabiston[77] have concluded that patients with previous shunt procedures have a lower mortality and that a shunt may exert a favorable influence on subsequent

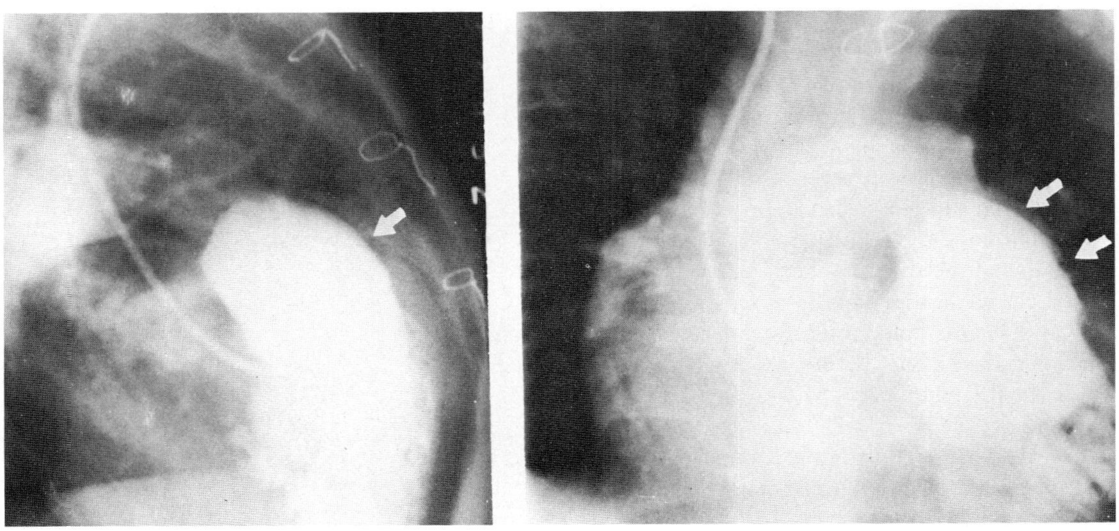

Fig. 27. Typical smooth appearance of the outflow tract following adequate reconstruction by pericardial patch (arrows).

total corrective procedures. Although recently Pacifico[78] reported only a 4.5% mortality rate for correction of tetralogy in infants and small children less than 4 yr of age, it is still presumed that systemic-pulmonary shunts will be continued, particularly for complex cyanotic heart lesions such as common ventricle, pulmonary atresia, complete atrioventricular canal with pulmonary stenosis, tricuspid atresia, or as a preparatory phase prior to correction.

Superior Vena Cava to Right Pulmonary Artery Anastomosis—Glenn Procedure

Anastomosis of the superior vena cava to the right pulmonary artery was first described by Carlson,[79] subsequently developed by Glenn,[80] Bakulev, and Kolesnikov.[81] As suggested by Glenn, the cardiac anomalies that could benefit from circulatory bypass of the right side of the heart include tricuspid atresia, pulmonary atresia, Ebstein's anomaly, single ventricle with pulmonary stenosis, and transposition with pulmonary stenosis. Classically the Glenn procedure is a pulmonary artery-superior vena cava end-to-side anastomosis with ligation of the superior vena cava at its entrance into the right atrium. An end-to-end anastomosis has been proposed by Bakulev and Kolesnikov (Fig. 28).[81,82] There are various advantages that could be attributed to the Glenn procedure: (1) 30%–40% of total systemic venous return flows through the shunt, thereby decreasing the work load of the right heart.[80] (2) Pulmonary blood flow is increased with low saturation venous blood.[83] (3) The amount of blood shunted right-to-left at the atrial level is decreased.

Glenn's procedure is only carried out as a palliative procedure because it is technically difficult to take down the superior vena cava-right pulmonary artery anastomosis. The higher mortality rate of 45% of Glenn procedures has been reduced to 8.6% by the delayed ligation of the azygous vein proposed by Edwards[82] and intensive, improved postoperative management. Before a Glenn procedure is attempted, pulmonary arterial hypertension should be excluded as well as a persistent left superior vena cava. This venous anomaly provides an escape of blood from the shunt unless ligated as shown in Fig. 29.

The late complications of the Glenn procedure include:

Superior vena cava obstruction. Late superior

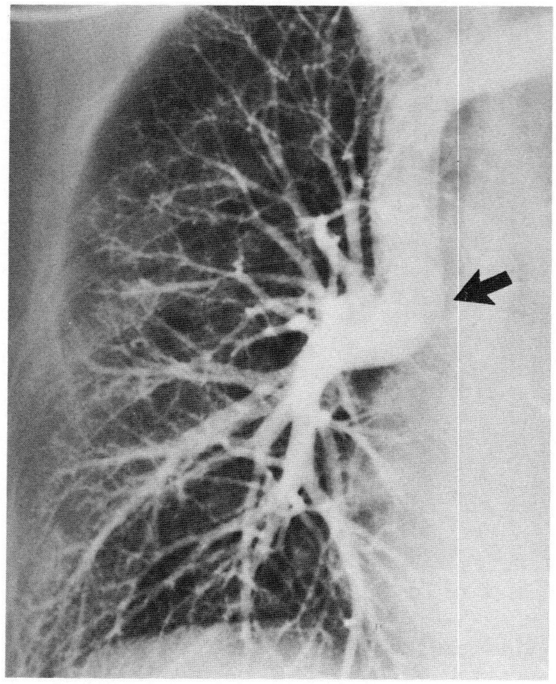

Fig. 28. Superior vena cavogram nicely reveals normally patent end-to-end Glenn anastomosis.

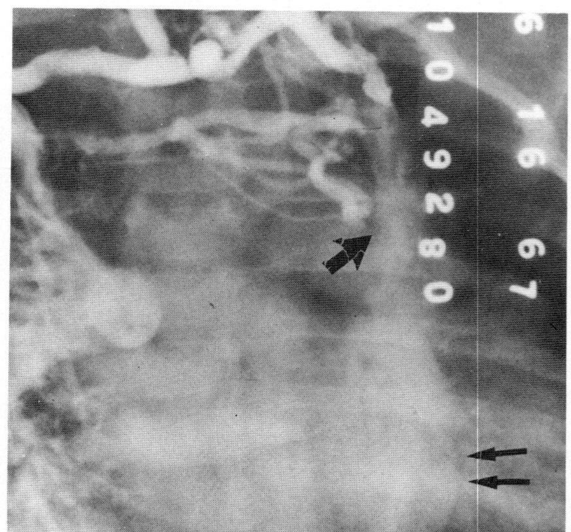

Fig. 29. Late phase of superior vena cavogram shows good filling of right pulmonary artery via Glenn anastomosis. Collateral flow across the mediastinum to persistent left superior vena cava (arrow) which empty into the left atrium (arrows).

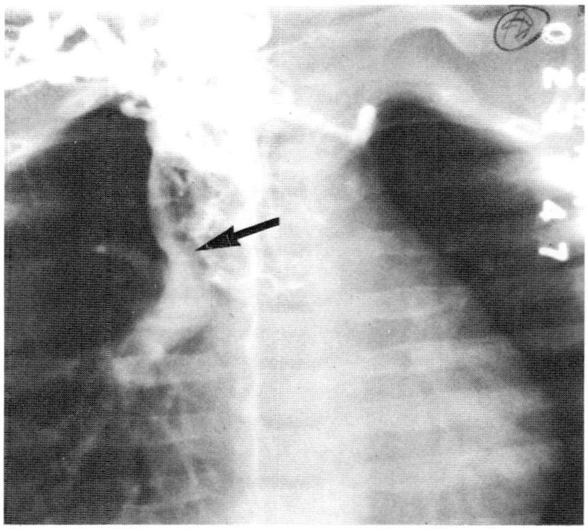

Fig. 30. Stenosis of the superior vena cava (↗) at the anastomotic site to the pulmonary artery.

vena cava syndrome includes facial edema,[84] headaches, abnormal enlargement of the head with increased cyanosis, and a rise in the hematocrit. This may be due to stenosis at the anastomotic site (Fig. 30) or thrombus formation. Extensive collaterals may develop from the superior vena cava to the inferior vena cava, right atrium, azygous or hemiazygous, and internal mammary system due to stenosis at the anastomotic site (Fig. 31). When

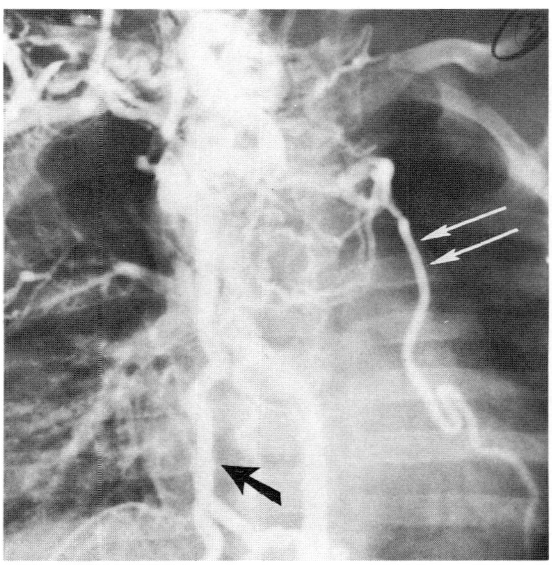

Fig. 31. Extensive collaterals to the internal mammary (single black arrow) and hemiazygous system (two white arrows) due to stenosis at Glenn's anastomosis.

such collaterals are formed, blood flow through the shunt into the right pulmonary artery decreases.[85]

Early superior vena cava syndrome can be secondary to elevated pulmonary resistance.

Progression of pulmonary stenosis. Sometimes infundibular pulmonary stenosis may progress to pulmonary atresia. This development is also seen in association with other systemic-pulmonary shunts such as Potts and Blalock–Taussig anastomoses.

Reversal of pulmonary blood flow into the superior vena cava. A modified Glenn procedure was performed on an infant with transposition, single ventricle, and pulmonary stenosis. Instead of ligation, the superior vena cava was banded below the anastomosis.

The patient returned with increasing exertional dyspnea. A superior vena cavogram (Fig. 32) revealed banding of the superior vena cava with drainage of contrast medium into the right atrium. In the delayed phase a negative filling defect in the

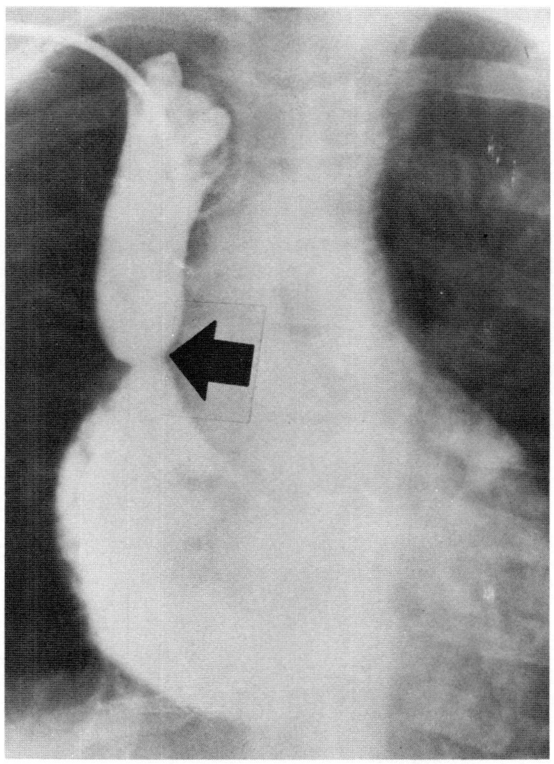

Fig. 32. Superior vena cavogram in a patient with modified Glenn operation and distal banding of superior vena cava. No antegrade flow into the pulmonary artery seen.

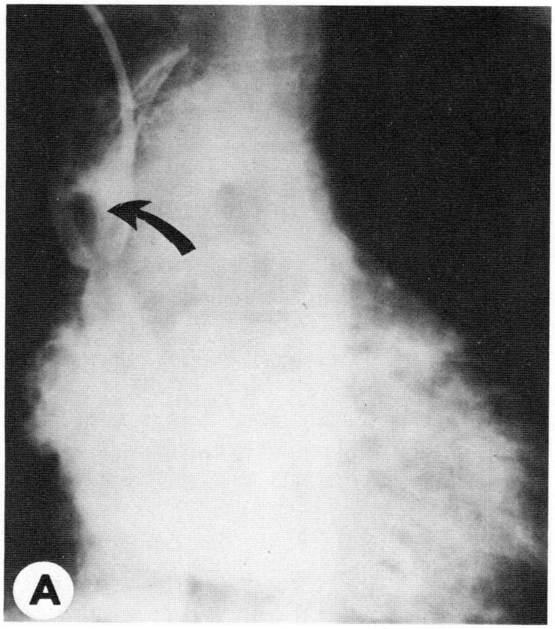

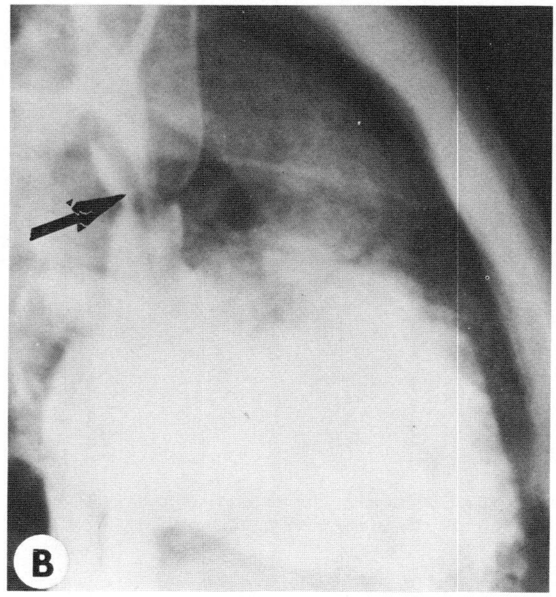

Fig. 33. (A and B) Same patient as in Fig. 5. AP and lateral superior vena cavogram showing washout in the superior vena cava due to reversal of blood flow in the right pulmonary artery.

superior vena cava was demonstrated (Fig. 33A and B). This was the result of reversed blood flow in the right pulmonary artery due to intercostal artery anastomoses. An aortogram revealed hypertrophied intercostal collaterals and filling of the right pulmonary artery (Fig. 34).

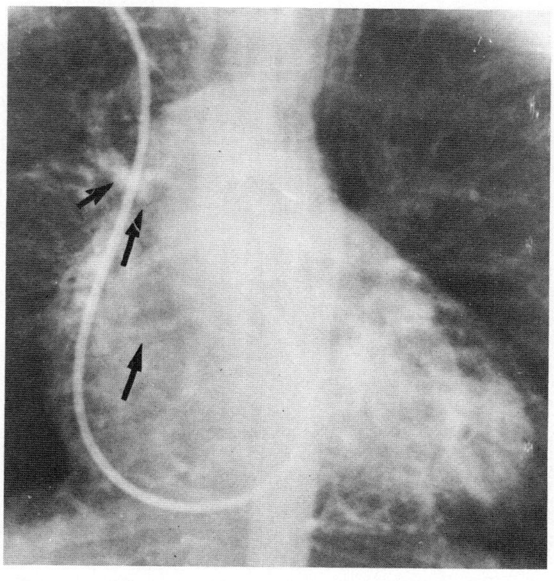

Fig. 34. Aortogram reveals hypertrophied intercostal collaterals (single arrow) with retrograde filling of the pulmonary artery (two arrows) via transpleural collaterals.

At time of surgery, occlusion of the superior vena cava by a balloon catheter improved the arterial oxygen saturation from 71% to 84%. The superior vena cava pressure increased from 9 to 18 mm of mercury, and the patient's color improved. A total permanent occlusion of the superior vena cava was accomplished by ligation.

To our best knowledge, this case represents the

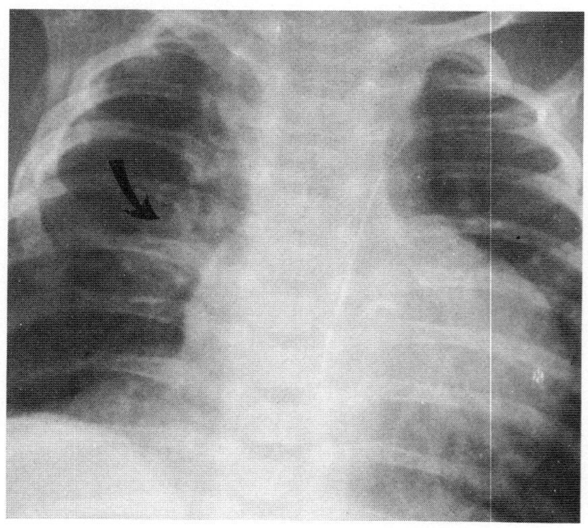

Fig. 35. Chest of a patient with Waterston anastomosis. Vasculature in the right lung is (↗) more prominent than the left.

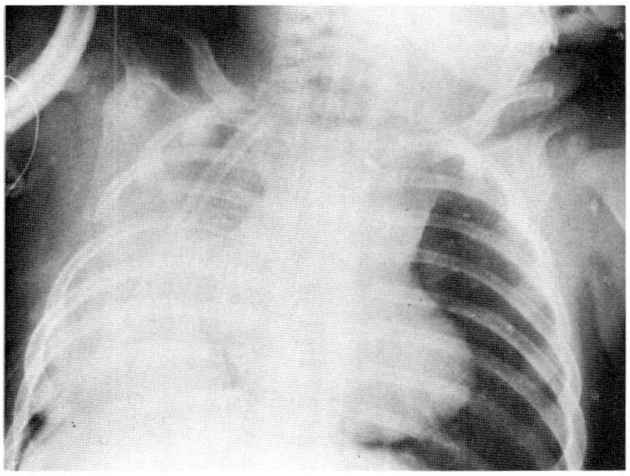

Fig. 36. Chest of a patient with pulmonary atresia and a recent Waterston anastomosis. Postoperatively pulmonary edema developed in the right lung.

first description of reversal of blood flow from intercostal arteries into the right pulmonary following a Glenn procedure.

Waterston–Cooley Anastomosis

Waterston described a technique in 1962 consisting of a side-to-side anastomosis of the right pulmonary artery to the ascending aorta by an extrapericardial approach.[86] Subsequently, the same procedure was carried out intrapericardially by Cooley and Hallman.[87]

Some of the advantages of the Waterston-Cooley procedure are: (1) It can be performed in infants under 6 mo of age when the Blalock–Taussig anastomosis is technically difficult because of the small size of the arteries and a high incidence of thrombosis.[83] (2) The Waterston shunt can be carried out in patients with atresia or stenosis of the subclavian arteries.[87] (3) The shunt is easily closed at the time of corrective surgery.[87]

According to Sommerville,[88] the size of anastomosis should be tailored to the size of the patient. They suggest a 5-mm shunt in patients be-

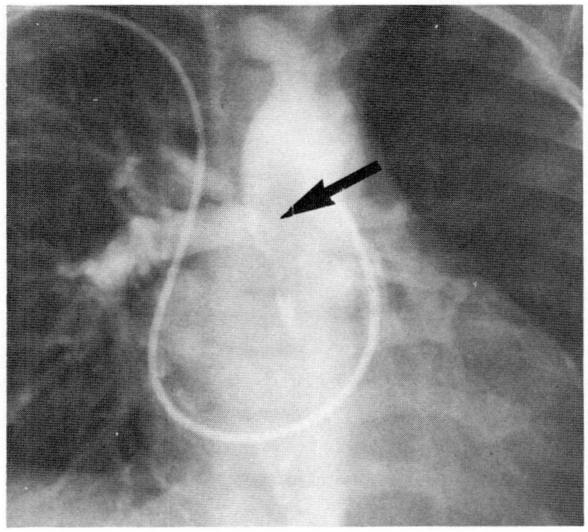

Fig. 38. Aortogram reveals narrowing (arrow) of the proximal portion of the right pulmonary artery following Waterston–Cooley anastomosis.

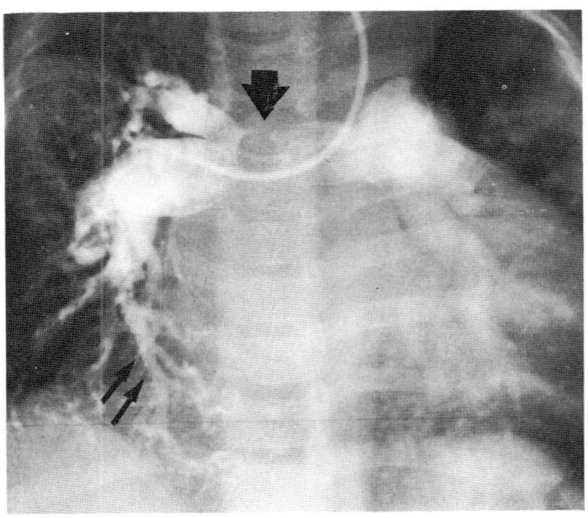

Fig. 37. Pulmonary arteriogram with Waterston shunt demonstrated as negative filling defect (arrow) (8 mm size). Tortuosity of peripheral pulmonary arteries (arrows) suggesting pulmonary hypertension.

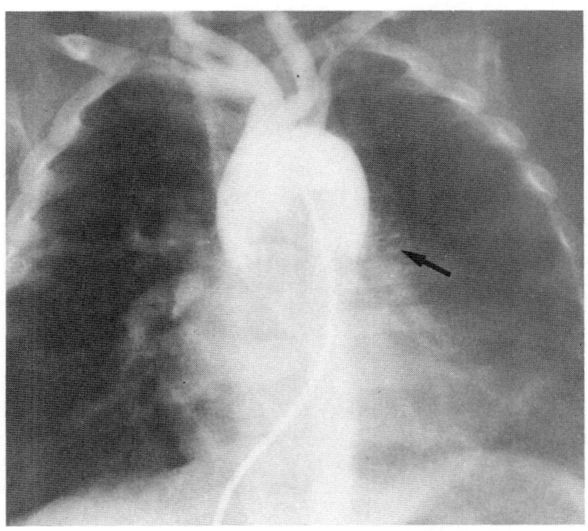

Fig. 39. Aortogram reveals filling of right pulmonary artery following Waterston–Cooley anastomosis and no filling of the left pulmonary artery which is occluded. Small collateral vessels are seen in the region of the left hilum (arrow).

tween the ages of 9–14 yr, 3–4 mm in patients of 2–9 yr and 2–3 mm in infants. The same group reports bilaterally equal increase of pulmonary flow in 50% of these; the rest showing a predominant increase in right pulmonary vasculature (Fig. 35). The studies on experimental animals reported by Oldham et al.[89] show preferential blood flow through the anastomosis to the right lung in the range of 65%–82%. On the other hand, blood flow through the right ventricle was directed primarily to the left lung.

Some of the roentgen findings of Waterston–Cooley anastomosis include:

Localized edema or pulmonary hemorrhage. In the immediate postoperative period (Fig. 36), there is a tendency for opacification of the right lung due to pulmonary edema or hemorrhage. The explanation of localized edema may be the direct transmission of systemic arterial pressure to the pulmonary vasculature with associated venous congestion secondary to a large shunt.[88,90] In the case shown in Fig. 36, the autopsy specimen showed hemorrhagic infarction of the lung secondary to rupture of smaller arterioles and capillaries probably due to the sudden increase in pressure.

Pleural effusion and pulmonary edema. A higher incidence of right sided pleural effusion and pulmonary edema has been reported, especially in patients with large anastomoses and those with contralateral pulmonary artery occlusion or hypoplasia.[90] The mechanism of unilateral pleural effusion is probably similar to localized pulmonary edema.

Other pulmonary findings. Comparatively few of the cases with postoperative systemic-pulmonary shunts show complications such as atelectasis, pneumothorax, pneumonia, chylorthorax, or empyema.

Development of pulmonary arterial hypertension. A direct transmission of systemic arterial pressure with excessive pulmonary arterial blood flow due to large shunts (Fig. 37) may cause pulmonary arterial hypertension. In the case demonstrated in Fig. 37, the pulmonary artery pressure was equal to systemic.

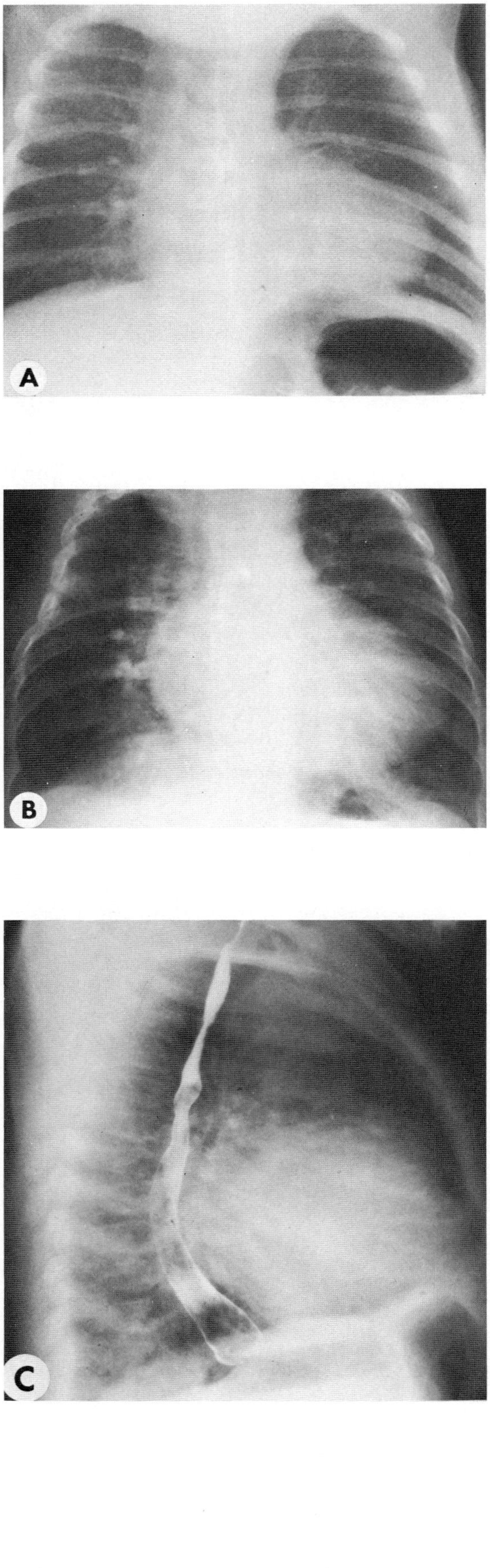

Fig. 40. (A) Preoperative roentgenogram in a patient with double outlet right ventricle and pulmonary stenosis. (B) Pulmonary vasculature and heart size increased following widely patent Waterston anastomosis. (C) Left atrial enlargement due to increased pulmonary flow.

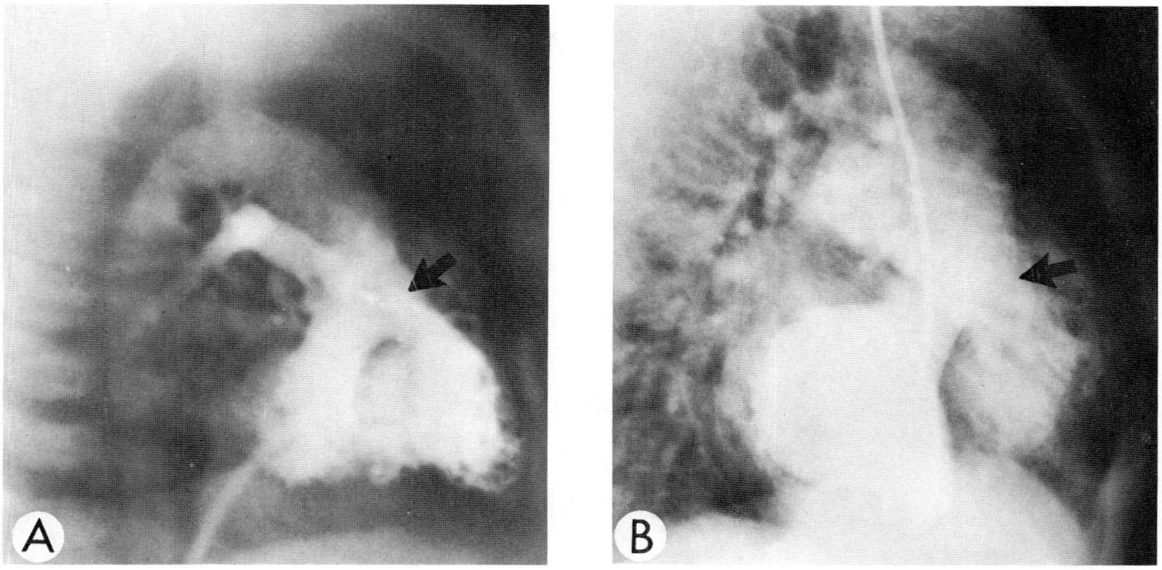

Fig. 41. (A) Narrowing of infundibulum (arrow) and pulmonary valvular stenosis in a case of double outlet right ventricle preoperatively. (B) Following Waterston-Cooley anastomosis, there is increase in size of the infundibulum and pulmonary artery. This finding is uncommon.

Angiographic visualization of the size of the shunt is best accomplished by selective injection of the main pulmonary artery. In the case of pulmonary atresia this can only be done by passing the catheter through the Waterston anastomosis. The negative filling defect due to washout of blood from the aorta can be exactly measured (8 mm in this case) (Fig. 37).

Narrowing of the proximal portion of the right pulmonary artery. The side-to-side anastomosis of the ascending aorta and right pulmonary artery should be made as far posteriorly as possible behind the aorta to prevent forward kinking and subsequent stenosis (Fig. 38).[88] The kinking of the anastomotic site can be responsible for prefer-

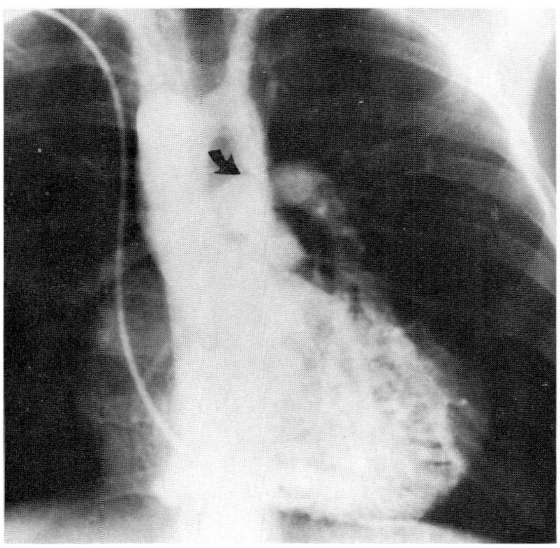

Fig. 42. Note the end-to-side anastomosis of the left subclavian artery with predominant flow into the pulmonary artery and normal appearing Blalock–Taussig anastomosis.

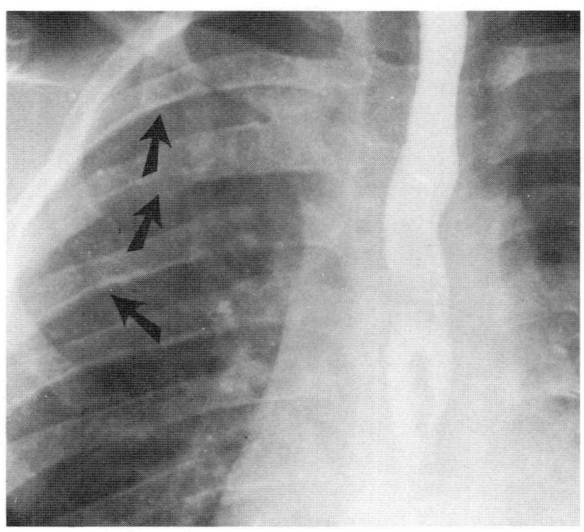

Fig. 43. Note the typical rib notching (arrow) on the right ribs following Blalock–Taussig anastomosis.

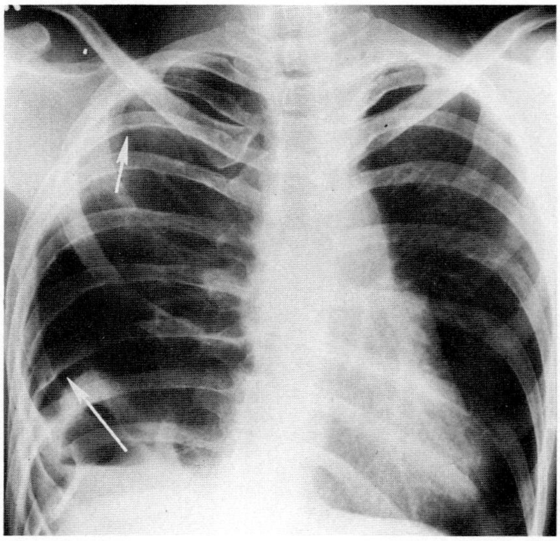

Fig. 44. In addition to the right upper ribs (↗) notching due to Blalock–Taussig anastomosis, note the lower rib notching (↗) at the 7th and 8th ribs due to intercostal hypertrophy as a result of pulmonary artery thrombosis.

ential flow of blood from the aorta into the right pulmonary artery. There is commonly less flow into the left pulmonary artery which may become completely occluded (Fig. 39).

Increase in heart size. There may be increase in the size of the heart, especially involving the left atrium and left ventricle due to increased pulmonary venous return (Fig. 40A, B, and C).

Development of progressive pulmonary stenosis. Eight out of ten cases of tetralogy that underwent Waterston-Cooley shunt developed progressive pulmonary stenosis due to lack in growth of the infundibulum and pulmonary annulus.[91] This progressive infundibular pulmonary narrowing, however, may be seen with any systemic pulmonary shunt. Sometimes, however, the infundibulum may show a normal growth as demonstrated in Fig. 41A and B.

Blalock–Taussig Anastomosis

In 1945, Blalock and Taussig developed an operation wherein the subclavian artery is anastomosed to the side of the pulmonary artery. This is a palliative procedure performed in patients with cyanosis and decreased pulmonary flow such as pulmonary atresia and tetralogy of Fallot.[92] The anastomosis is usually performed opposite to the aortic arch to avoid kinking of the base of the subclavian artery (Fig. 42). Sometimes an anastomosis

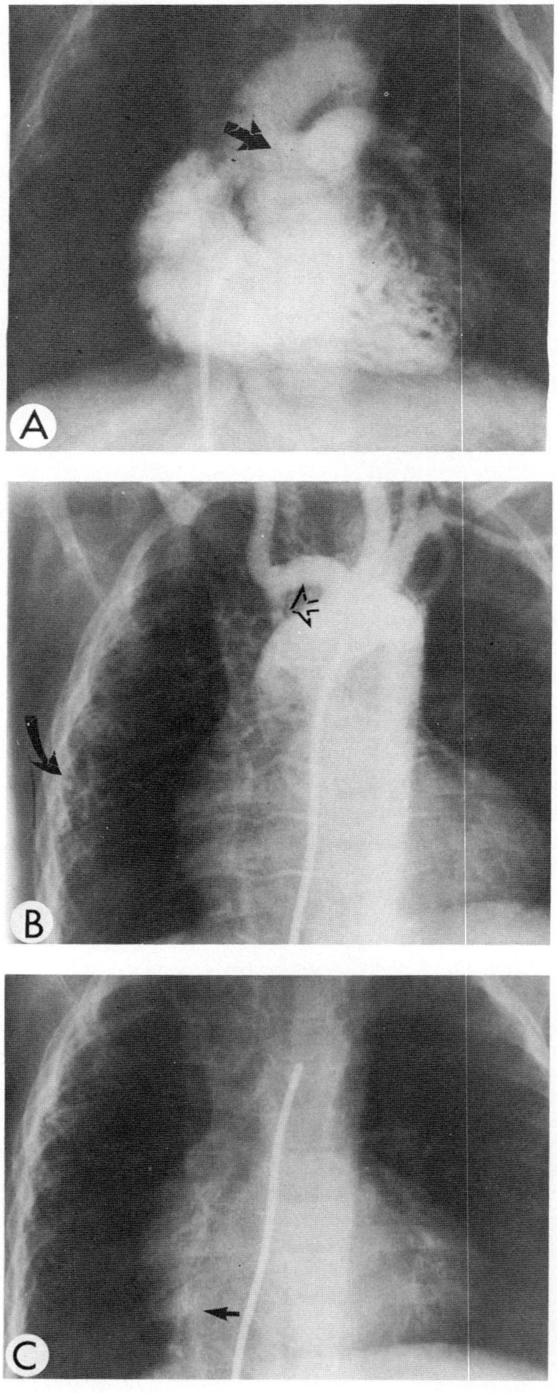

Fig. 45. (A) Right ventriculogram in a patient with tetralogy of Fallot following Blalock–Taussig shunt showing thrombosis of the right pulmonary artery. (B) Aortogram reveals occluded right Blalock–Taussig anastomosis (open arrow), prominent hypertrophied intercostal arteries along with transpleural collaterals (curved arrow). (C) Later phase shows opacification of the distal right pulmonary artery (arrow) via intercostal anastomosis.

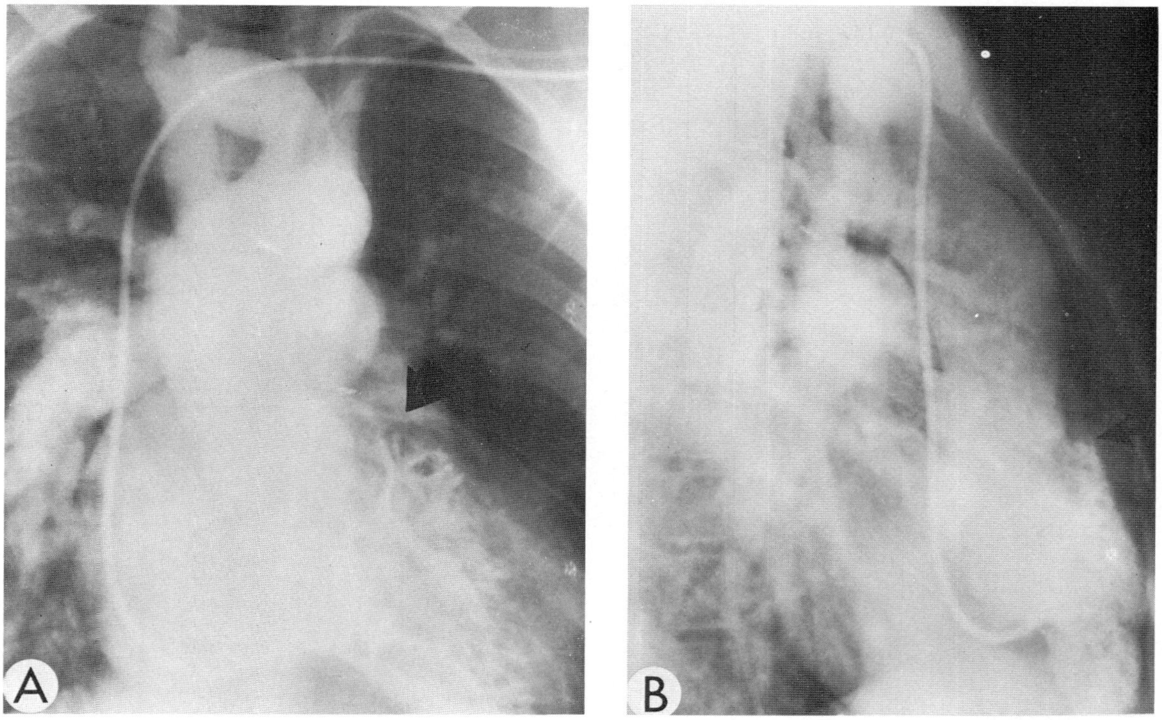

Fig. 46. (A and B) AP and lateral right ventriculogram reveal widely patent Blalock anastomosis with predominant filling of the right pulmonary artery. Severe narrowing of infundibulum (arrow) with no antegrade flow from the right ventricle.

is performed on the same side of the aortic arch or bilaterally to increase pulmonary blood flow.

Blalock–Taussig anastomosis may not be technically feasible in the following circumstances: (1) Infants under 6 wk of age with small subclavian arteries and a higher incidence of thrombosis, (2) Aberrant subclavian arteries wherein the anastomosis to the pulmonary artery could result as a sling formation around the trachea and esophagus.

Some of the postoperative roentgen findings include:

Rib notching. Interruption of the subclavian artery causes the development of intercostal collaterals as evidenced radiographically by rib notching generally in the upper 2nd to 6th ribs (Fig. 43). In some cases of Blalock–Taussig shunts, thrombosis of the shunt may also involve the right pulmonary artery. This serious complication can be suspected from plain roentgenograms by rib notching involving the upper as well as *lower ribs.* This is due to extensive intercostal collaterals bridging the pleura and supplying the thrombosed pulmonary artery in retrograde fashion. Pleural thickening is usually also present as shown in Fig. 44.

Thrombosis of the anastomosis and failure of growth. Blalock–Taussig anastomosis may thrombose, especially if done under the age of 1 yr. Some cases of shunt thrombosis extend into the proximal right pulmonary artery (Fig. 45) leading to occlusion. Usually the right pulmonary artery downstream to the occluded shunt may remain patent via transpleural and bronchial collaterals. According to Taussig et al.[93] less than 5% of patients require a second operation at the end of the 5 yr, and another 20% require a second operation following the next 5 yr.

Pulmonary arterial hypertension. Only two cases of Blalock–Taussig anastomosis wherein large subclavian arteries were anastomosed to pulmonary arteries were associated with pulmonary hypertension with marked enlargement of the pulmonary arteries.[94] As the pulmonary arterial resistance rises, the pulmonary artery becomes more dilated, the pressure in both great vessels equalizes, and the flow murmur disappears.

Acquired pulmonary atresia. Following any

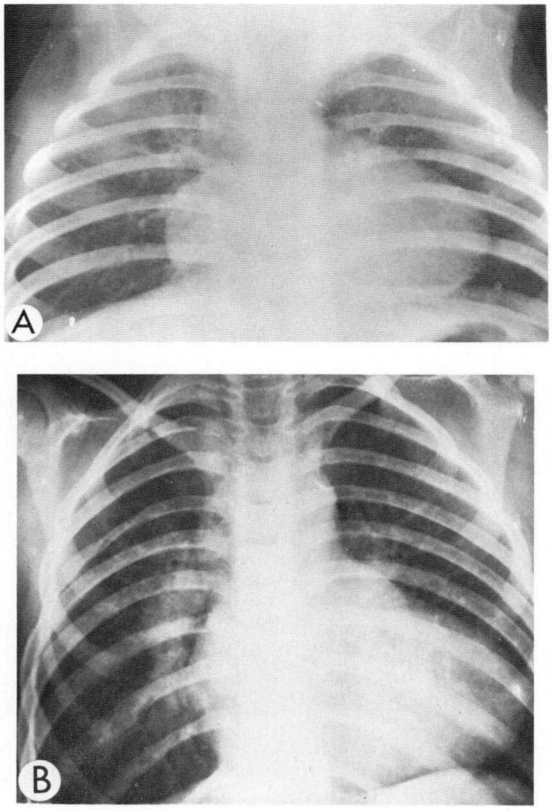

Fig. 47. (A) Preoperative chest x-ray in a patient with pulmonary atresia and ventricular septal defect revealing small heart and decrease in pulmonary vasculature. (B) Following Blalock–Taussig anastomosis there is increase in size of heart and large right pulmonary artery (arrow) indicating functioning anastomosis.

systemic-pulmonary anastomosis, there is a decrease in blood flow across the pulmonary valve resulting in progressive infundibular narrowing. At the time of operation, however, these patients have patent but very narrow infundibula and are potentially curable (Fig. 46A and B).

Heart size. Typically the heart size will be larger following Blalock–Taussig anastomosis or any other systemic-pulmonary shunt because of increase in flow through the left side of the heart (Fig. 47A and B). Helen B. Taussig et al.[97] believed that cyanosis, small size of the heart, and decrease in the pulmonary vasculature indicate surgical failure.

Potts Anastomosis

Following the principles set forth by the Blalock–Taussig procedure, in 1946 W. P. Potts et al.[95]

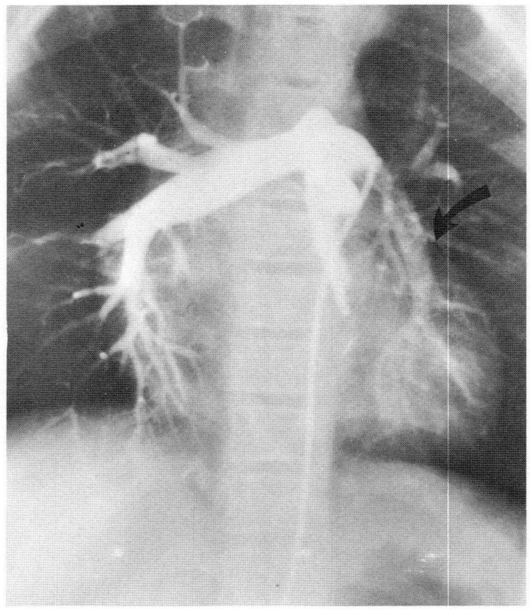

Fig. 48. AP pulmonary arteriogram via Potts anastomosis in a patient with pulmonary atresia. Note dilution of contrast in left pulmonary artery (curved arrow) by the shunt.

proposed a side-to-side anastomosis of aorta to left pulmonary artery. In recent years Potts anastomosis has not been widely practiced because of difficulties in taking down the anastomosis[96] when corrective surgery is contemplated as well as a higher incidence of pulmonary hypertension.[97] Kirklin reported a mortality rate of 20% in 35 patients with a previous Potts anastomosis and corrective surgery.[98]

Roentgen findings associated with Potts anastomosis include:

Pulmonary vasculature. There is increase in pulmonary vasculature, more so in the left lung. In cases of pulmonary atresia the pulmonary artery can be demonstrated by passing the catheter through the Potts anastomosis (Fig. 48). Rarely Potts anastomosis are associated with aneurysmal dilatation of the pulmonary artery.[96] Pulmonary vascular obstructive disease is present in 50% (13/26) of patients with tetralogy of Fallot and Potts anastomosis.[99]

Occluded right sided Potts anastomosis. Potts anastomoses associated with right aortic arch are associated with a higher incidence of thrombosis because of technical difficulties.[96] In one of our

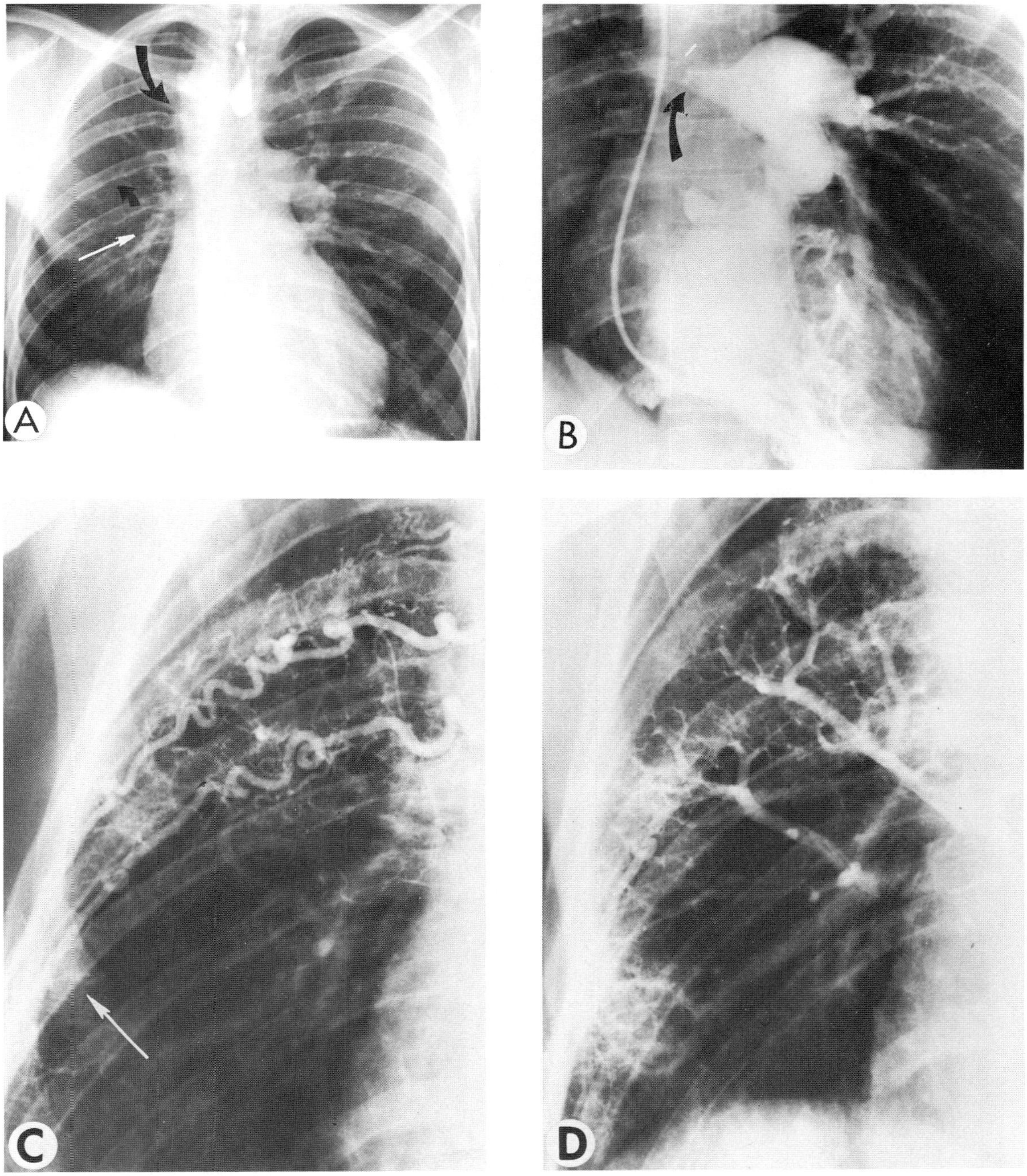

Fig. 49. (A) Note the right aortic arch (curved black arrow), diminution in size of the right pulmonary artery (white arrow), notching of several ribs on right hemithorax (small black arrow) in a patient with Potts anastomosis. (B) Right ventriculogram reveals thrombosis of right pulmonary artery (arrow) at the anastomotic site to the ascending aorta (right-sided Potts procedure). (C and D) Same patient, simultaneous selective injection of two right intercostal arteries showing dense filling of pulmonary artery via transpleural collaterals (↗).

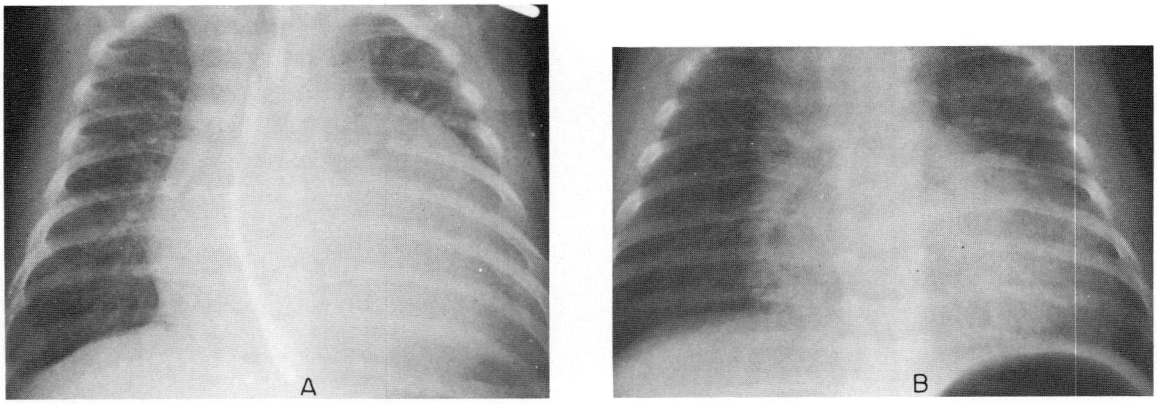

Fig. 50. (A) Severe cardiomegaly with displacement of the esophagus by a large left atrium and venous congestion in a patient with coarctation. (B) Six days following correction, considerable decrease in heart size and disappearance of congestive changes.

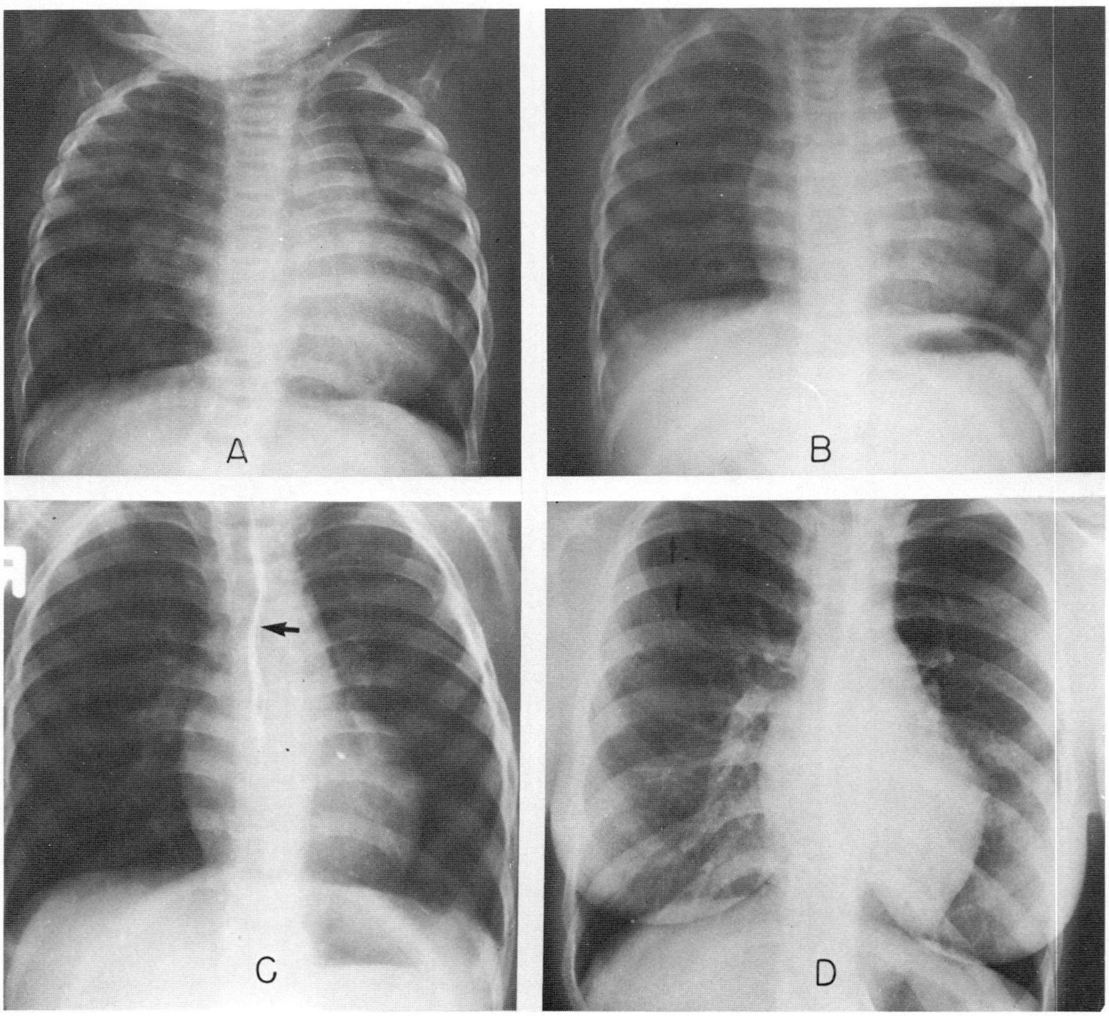

Fig. 51. (A) PA chest in patient with coarctation showing mild cardiomegaly. (B) Seven mo following corrective surgery there is considerable decrease in heart size but a peculiar roundness of the left ventricle persists. (C) Three yr later, normal heart size but displacement of the esophagus by persistent poststenotic dilatation (arrow). (D) Fourteen yr later, rib notching appeared about the right upper ribs (arrows) indicating recoarctation.

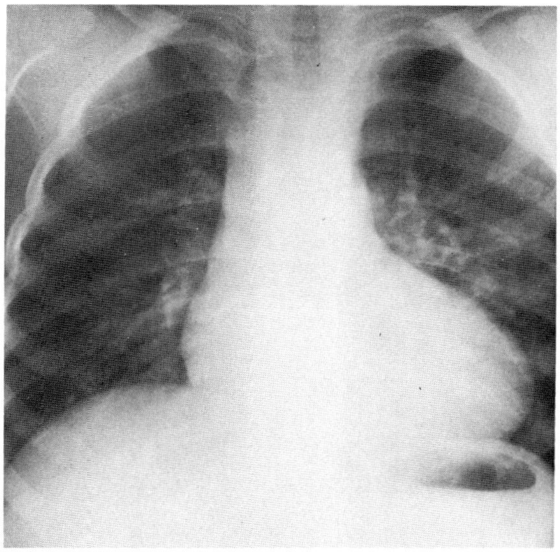

Fig. 52. PA chest $3\frac{1}{2}$ yr after coarctation repair showing persistent roundness of the left ventricle and mild cardiomegaly. No gradient across the coarctation was found at time of catheterization.

cases a selective right ventriculogram showed thrombosis of the right pulmonary artery at its proximal portion. The selective simultaneous injection of right intercostal arteries proved patency of the right pulmonary artery via retrograde flow of contrast medium through transpleural collaterals (Fig. 49A and B).

COARCTATION OF THE AORTA

The postoperative radiographic changes following the surgical correction of coarctation of the aorta can be subtle or dramatic. Immediate postoperative improvement is due to improved heart function as a result of relief of the hemodynamic burden. Marked decrease in heart size and diminution of the left atrial enlargement can be noted during the first 10 postoperative days (Fig. 50), particularly in early childhood. In some patients the heart size may not return to normal before 6 mo or even 3 yr (Fig. 51). It is important to realize that mild cardiomegaly with a peculiar rounded apex may remain even after surgery without residual stenosis (Fig. 52).

A radiographically striking change may be the disappearance of the thymic shadow as a result of the surgical stress. Regrowth of the thymus is usually complete within 3 mo after surgery (Fig. 53).

Persistence of cardiomegaly suggests an additional lesion (aortic stenosis and ventricular septal defect being the most common) or persistence or recurrence of coarctation (Fig. 54). Poststenotic dilatation of the descending aorta persists in spite of surgery but does not correlate with persistent hemodynamic coarctation. This anatomical deformity without gradient could be observed even 13 yr following surgery (Fig. 55). Therefore, no hemodynamic conclusions can be drawn from

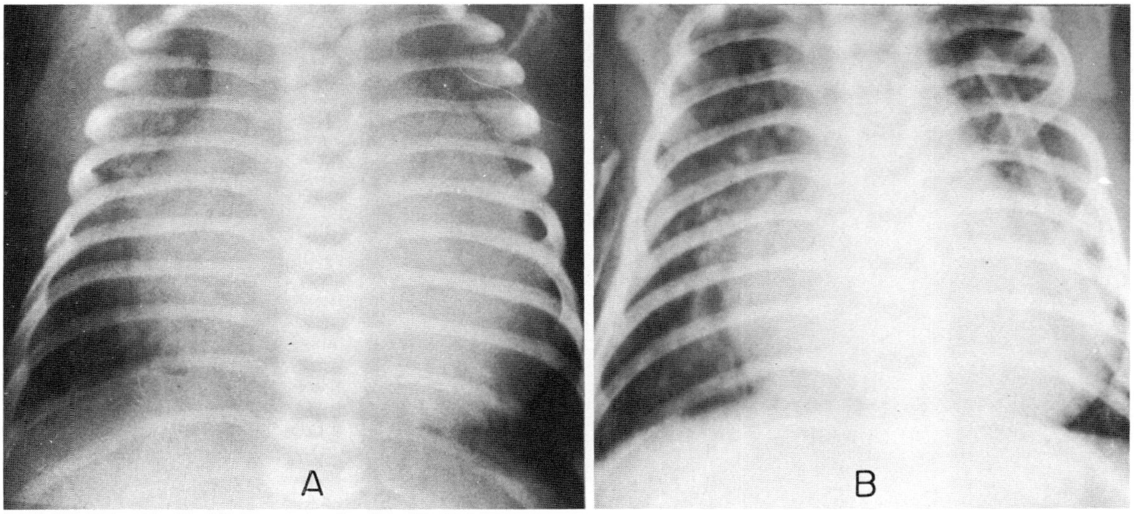

Fig. 53. (A) Preoperative chest in patient with coarctation showing cardiomegaly and large thymus. (B) Two days postop, thymus has disappeared apparently due to surgical stress.

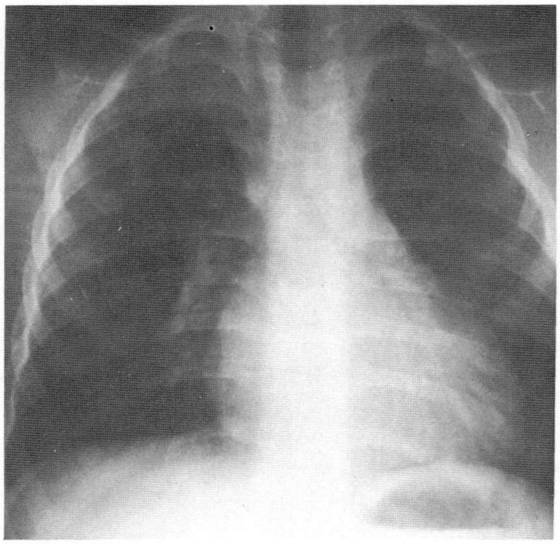

Fig. 54. PA chest 3 yr following coarctation repair showing persistent cardiomegaly, strongly suggesting persisting obstruction. (Gradient 65 mm at time of catheterization).

demonstration of poststenotic dilatation. The failure to pass a catheter across the stenotic segment does not necessarily indicate an obstruction of a significant degree (Fig. 56).

Postoperative widening of the mediastinum is an indication for aortography since such changes may represent a postsurgical complication, as the for-

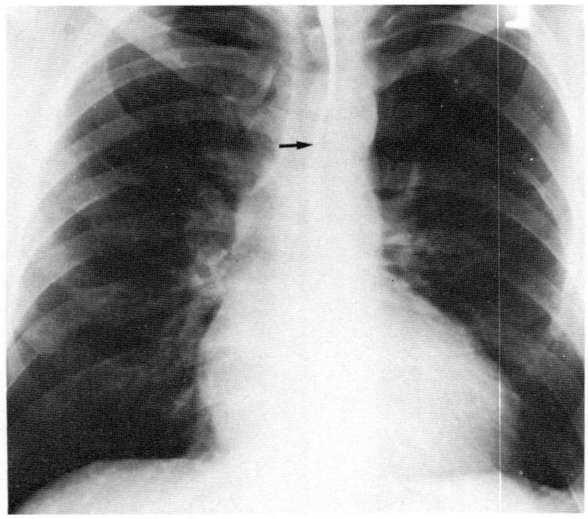

Fig. 55. Thirteen yr postop coarctation repair. Poststenotic displacement of the esophagus persists (arrow).

mation of true and false aneurysms. In our series of 1400 patients with surgical correction of coarctation of the aorta, we could find only one adult patient with an aneurysm at the site of the coarctation (Fig. 57).

In the adolescent or adult, rib notching, if present, tends to persist; but the bony changes may regress to some extent (Fig. 57). If corrective

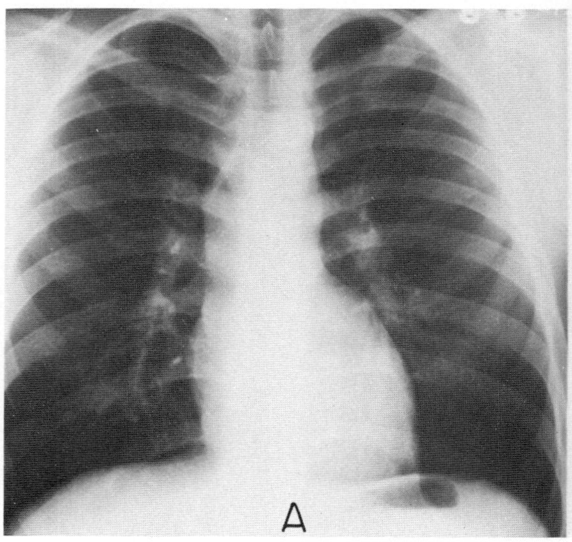

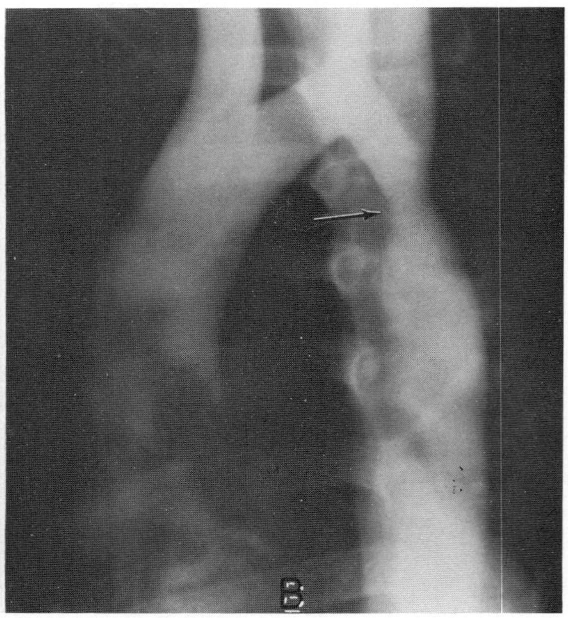

Fig. 56. Thirteen yr following surgery, aortogram shows persistent tubular hypoplasia and poststenotic dilatation (arrow) but no significant gradient at time of catheterization. The catheter could not be advanced through the area of narrowing.

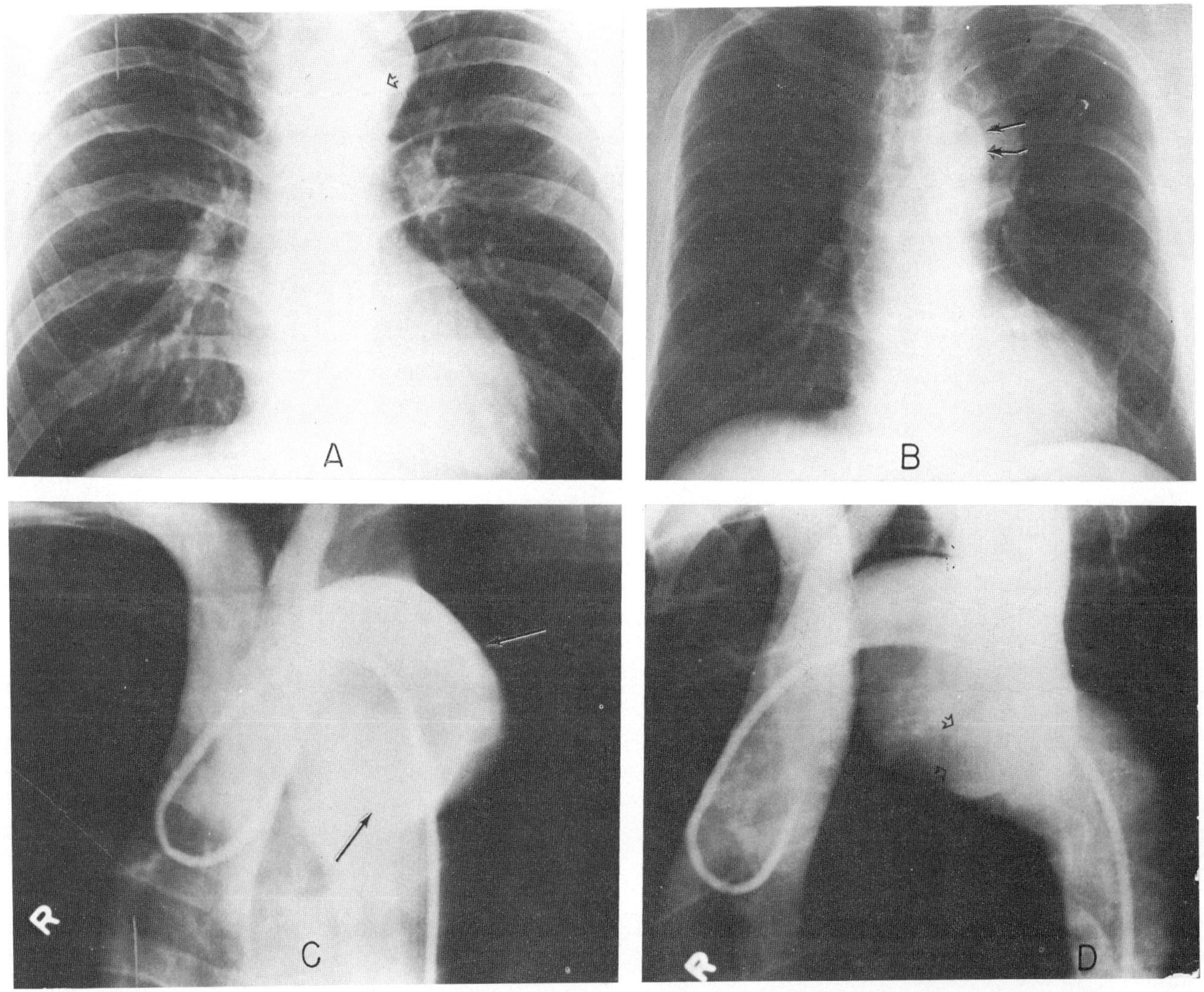

Fig. 57. (A) Preop chest in patient with coarctation showing rib notching and an aneurysm of the arch and left subclavian artery. The poststenotic segment can be seen through the aneurysm (arrow). (B) Nine yr postoperatively, poststenotic segment unchanged (double arrows) and regrowth of the aneurysm. (C and D) Oblique and lateral projections of aortogram show large aneurysm of the distal arch and origin of the left subclavian artery (aneurysm successfully removed).

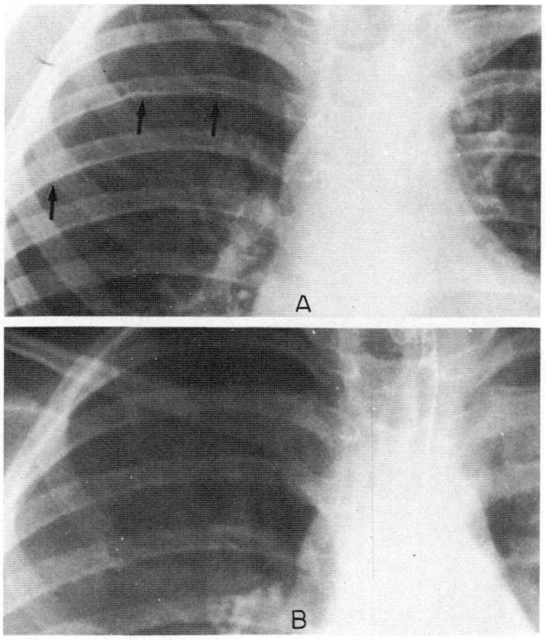

Fig. 58. (A) Patient with coarctation showing rib notching of the right upper ribs. (B) One yr postoperative, almost complete disappearance of rib notching.

surgery is carried out in childhood, however, rib changes are usually minor and may disappear completely (Fig. 58). The reappearance of rib notching, even without concommitant cardiomegaly, should suggest recoarctation (Fig. 51). It is important to emphasize that rib notching involves only the upper ribs. If prominent rib notching is seen about the lower ribs, abdominal coarctation should be considered.

REFERENCES

1. Strickland B: The postoperative heart. Br J Radiol 39:403–413, 1966

2. Sigmann JM, Stern AM, Sloan HE: Early surgical correction of large ventricular septal defects. Pediatrics 39: 4–13, 1967

3. Silbiger ML, Stewart S, Morrow AG, et al: Correlation of chest roentgenograms and hemodynamic findings following surgical closure of secundum atrial septal defects. Radiology 91:42–45, 1968

4. Winchell P, Bashour F: Some physiologic features of atrial septal defect. Observations in 38 adult patients. Am J Cardiol 2:687–693, 1958

5. Park CD, Nicodemus H, Downes JJ, et al: Changes in pulmonary vascular resistance following closure of ventricular septal defects. Circulation 39 and 40 (Suppl 1): 193–200, 1969

6. Beck W, Swan HJC, Burchell HB, et al: Pulmonary vascular resistance after repair of atrial septal defects in patients with pulmonary hypertension. Circulation 22: 938–946, 1960

7. Caffey J: Pediatric X-Ray Diagnosis (ed 4). Chicago, Year Book, 1961, p. 437

8. Schad N, Juenzler R, Onat T: Differentialdiagnose Kongenitalen Hertzfehler. Georg Thieme (ed). Stuttgart, 1963

9. Baltaxe HA, Amplatz K: The normal chest roentgenogram in the presence of large atrial septal defects. Am J Roentgenol Radium Ther Nucl Med 107:322–327, 1969

10. Peterson PO: Atrial septal defect of secundum type. A clinical study before and after operation with special reference to hemodynamic function. Acta Paediatrica Scand (Suppl) 174:1–96, 1967

11. Young D: Later results of closure of secundum atrial septal defect in children. Am J Cardiol 31:14–22, 1973

12. Blount SG, Swan H, Gensini G, et al: Atrial septal defect. Clinical and physiologic response to complete closure in five patients. Circulation 9:801–812, 1954

13. Kirklin JW, Dushane JW: Indications for repair of right ventricular septal defects. Am J Cardiol 12:75–79, 1963

14. Kay EB, Zimmerman HA: Surgical treatment of atrial septal defects. Open versus closed technics. Am J Cardiol 2:732–734, 1958

15. Pieroni DR, Strife JL, Donahoo JS, et al: Postoperative assessment of residual defects following cardiac surgery in infants and children. III. Atrial septal defects. Johns Hopkins Med J 133:287–294, 1973

16. Lawrence K, Grimshaw VA, Hoyle G, et al: Surgical treatment of atrial septal defect and partial anomalous pulmonary venous drainage. J Thorac Cardiovasc Surg 43:622–633, 1962

17. Friedli B, Guerin R, Davignon A, et al: Surgical treatment of partial anomalous pulmonary venous drainage. A long-term follow-up study. Circulation 45:159–170, 1972

18. Dave KS, Brojesh CP, Geoffrey HW, et al: Atrial septal defects in adults. Clinical and hemodynamic results of surgery. Am J Cardiol 31:7–13, 1973

19. Gyepes MT, Abrams HL, Shumway NE: Radiologic aspects of operable heart disease. Radiology 88:466–472, 1967

20. Hunt CE, Formanek G, Levin MA, et al: Banding of the pulmonary artery. Results in 111 children. Circulation 43:395–406, 1971

21. Hunt CE, Formanek G, Castaneda A, et al: Closure of ventricular septal defect and removal of pulmonary arterial band. Am J Cardiol 26:345–350, 1970

22. Ebert PA, Canent RV, Spach M, et al: Late cardiodynamics following correction of ventricular septal defects with previous pulmonary artery banding. J Thorac Cardiovasc Surg 60:516–522, 1970

23. Rohmer J, Brom AG, Nauta J: Bands inside the pulmonary artery. A complication of the Dammann–Muller procedure. Ann Thorac Surg 3:449–454, 1967

24. Patterson MWH: A radiopaque pulmonary artery band. J Thorac Cardiovasc Surg 61:975–976, 1971

25. Craig TW, Sirak HD: Pulmonary artery banding. J Thorac Cardiovasc Surg 45:599–604, 1963

26. Goldblatt A, Bernhard WF, Nadas AS, et al: Pulmonary artery banding. Circulation 32:172–184, 1965

27. Grainger RG, Nagle RE, Pawidapha C, et al: Pulmonary artery banding for ventricular septal defect. Br Heart J 29:289–298, 1967

28. Takahashi M, Lurie PR, Petry EL, et al: Clinical and hemodynamic effects of pulmonary artery banding. Am J Cardiol 21:174–184, 1968

29. Therkelsen F, Boessen I: Ventricular septal defects in infancy. Late results of artificial stenosis of the pulmonary artery and indications for radical operation. Acta Chir Scand 124:188–193, 1962

30. Parameswaran R, Maranhao V, Ablaza SGG, et al: Calcification of the pulmonary artery: A complication of the banding procedure. Chest 57:577–579, 1970

31. Osborn JR, Hall RJ, Winn DF, et al: An unusual late complication of pulmonary artery banding. Circulation 34:61–64, 1966

32. Hallman GL, Cooley DA, Bloodwell RD: Two-stage surgical treatment of ventricular septal defect: Results of pulmonary artery banding in infants and subsequent open-heart repair. J Thorac Cardiovasc Surg 52:476–485, 1966

33. Hallman GL, Cooley DA, Wolfe RR, et al: Surgical treatment of ventricular septal defect associated with pulmonary hypertension. J Thorac Cardiovasc Surg 48:588–600, 1964

34. Dobell ARC, Murphy DA, Poirier NL, et al: The pulmonary artery after debanding. J Thorac Cardiovasc Surg 65:32–36, 1973

35. Stark J, Tynan M, Aberdeen E: Spontaneous closure of ventricular septal defect following pulmonary artery constriction (banding). Am Heart J 79:548–551, 1970

36. Edgett JW, Nelson WP, Hall RJ, et al: Spontaneous closure of a ventricular septal defect after banding of the pulmonary artery. Am J Cardiol 22:729–732, 1968

37. Mesko ZG, Jones JE, Nadas AS: Diminution and closure of large ventricular septal defects after pulmonary artery banding. Circulation 48:847–855, 1973

38. Wada J, Iwa T: Two-stage treatment of ventricular septal defect with pulmonary hypertension. Ann Thorac Surg 8:415–424, 1969

39. Cartmill TB, Dushane JW, McGoon DC, et al: Results of repair of ventricular septal defect. J Thorac Cardiovasc Surg 12:1–10, 1971

40. Coleman EN, Reid JM, Inall JA, et al: Ventricular septal defect repair in childhood. Br Heart J 30:845–849, 1968

41. Hallidie-Smith KA, Hollman A, Abbott JA, et al: Long-term results of closure of ventricular septal defects in patients with pulmonary vascular disease. Br Heart J 29:939, 1967

42. Ho CS, Krovetz LJ, Strife JL, et al: Postoperative assessment of residual defects following cardiac surgery in infants and children: II. Ventricular septal defects. Johns Hopkins Med J 133:278–286, 1973

43. Ching E, Dushane JW, McGoon DC, et al: Total correction of ventricular septal defect in infancy using extracorporeal circulation. Ann Thorac Surg 12:1–10, 1971

44. Gotsman MS, Beck W, Barnard CN, et al: Haemodynamic studies after repair of ventricular septal defect. Br Heart J 31:63–71, 1969

45. Randall PA, Goodman DJ, Schweder JS: Left ventricular angiographic anatomy of ostium primum defect in the adult. Am J Roentgenol Radium Ther Nucl Med 121:597–605, 1974

46. Braunwald SN, Morrow AG: Incomplete persistent atrioventricular canal. J Thorac Cardiovasc Surg 51:71–80, 1966

47. McMullan MH, McGoon DC, Wallace RB, et al: Surgical treatment of partial atrioventricular canal. Arch Surg 107:705–710, 1973

48. McMullan MH, Wallace RB, Weidman WH, et al: Surgical treatment of complete atrioventricular canal. Surgery 72:905–912, 1972

49. Thomson NB: Patent ductus arteriosus in infancy. J Cardiovasc Surg 11:7–14, 1970

50. Glenn WWL, Bloomer WE, Spear HC: Operative closure of the patent ductus arteriosus. A report of 110 operations without mortality. Ann Surg 143:471–480, 1956

51. Porstmann W, Wierny L, Warnke H, et al: Catheter closure of patent ductus arteriosus. Radiol Clin North Am 9:203–218, 1971

52. McGoon DC: Closure of patent ductus during open heart surgery. J Thorac Cardiovasc Surg 48:456–464, 1964

53. Sheldon WA, Windsor HM: The complicated patent ductus arteriosus. Med J Aust Dec:1161–1165, 1969

54. Payne RF, Jordan SC: Postoperative aneurysms following ligation of the patent ductus arteriosus. Br J Radiol 41:858–861, 1968

55. Gersony W, Batthany S, Bowman F Jr, et al: Late follow-up of patients evaluated hemodynamically after total correction of tetralogy of Fallot. J Thorac Cardiovasc Surg 66:209–213, 1973

56. Hawe A, Rastelli G, Ritter D, et al: Management of the right ventricular outflow tract in severe tetralogy of Fallot. J Thorac Cardiovasc Surg 60:131–143, 1970

57. Kirklin JW: The tetralogy of Fallot. Am J Roentgenol Radium Ther Nucl Med 102:253–266, 1967

58. Kirklin JW, Wallace RB, McGoon DC, et al: Early and late results after intracardiac repair of tetralogy of Fallot. Ann Surg 162:578–587, 1965

59. Malm JR, Blumenthal S, Bowman FO, et al: Factors that modify hemodynamic results in total correction of tetralogy of Fallot. J Thorac Cardiovasc Surg 152:502–513, 1966

60. Beach M, Jr, Bowman F, Kaiser G, et al: Total correction of tetralogy of Fallot in adolescents and adults. Circulation 43:I-37–43, 1971

61. Bristow JD, Adroundy Z, Porter G, et al: Hemodynamic studies after total correction in tetralogy of Fallot. Am J Cardiol 9:924–932, 1962

62. Bristow JD, Kloster F, Lees M, et al: Serial cardiac catheterizations and exercise hemodynamics after correction of tetralogy of Fallot. Circulation 41:1057–1066, 1970

63. Burnell R, Woodson RD, Lees M, et al: Results of correction of tetralogy of Fallot in children under four years of age. J Thorac Cardiovasc Surg 57:153–159, 1969

64. Lillehei CW, Levy MJ, Adams P, et al: Corrective surgery for tetralogy of Fallot. J Thorac Cardiovasc Surg 48:556–576, 1964

65. Sunderland CO, Matarazzo RG, Lees MH, et al: Total correction of tetralogy of Fallot in infancy. Circulation 48:398–405, 1973

66. Zenher R, Klinner W: Total correction of tetralogy of Fallot. Dis Chest 5:311–314, 1967

67. Bristow JD, Menashe V, Griswold H, et al: Total correction of tetralogy. Am J Cardiol 8:358–368, 1961

68. Hallidie-Smith K, Dulake M, Wong M, et al: Ventricular structure and function after radical correction of the tetralogy of Fallot. Br Heart J 29:533–547, 1969

69. Knight L, Joransen J, Marin-Garcia J, et al: Roentgenographic and angiocardiographic changes after total correction of the tetralogy of Fallot. Am J Roentgenol Radium Ther Nucl Med (in press)

70. Walzen DE, Singleton EB: Tetralogy of Fallot: Radiologic evaluation before and after surgical treatment. Am J Roentgenol Radium Ther Nucl Med 81:760–768, 1963

71. Ellis K: Postoperative roentgen evaluation of total correction of tetralogy of Fallot. Circulation 47:1335–1348, 1973

72. Hipona F, Bloom D: Postoperative aneurysm of the right ventricle. Am J Roentgenol Radium Ther Nucl Med 95:642–654, 1965

73. Jones E, Conti C, Neill C, et al: Long-term evaluation of tetralogy patients with pulmonary valvular insufficiency resulting from outflow-patch correction across the pulmonic annulus. Circulation 47:III-11–18, 1973

74. Payne WS, Kirklin JW: Late complications after plastic reconstruction of outflow tract in tetralogy of Fallot. Ann Surg 154:53–57, 1961

75. Amplatz K, Jeffery RF, Gobel FL, et al: The freon test. A new sensitive technic for the detection of small cardiac shunts. Circulation 39:551–556, 1969

76. Rosenthal A, Gross RE, Pasternac A: Aneurysms of right ventricular outflow patches. J Thorac Cardiovasc Surg 63:735–740, 1972

77. Ebert PA, Sabiston DC: Surgical management of the tetralogy of Fallot: Influence of a previous systemic-pulmonary anastomosis on the results of open correction. Ann Surg 165:806–813, 1967

78. Pacifico AD, Bargeron LM, Kirklin JW: Primary total correction of tetralogy of Fallot in children less than four years of age. Circulation 48:1085–1091, 1973

79. Carlson CA, Mondini PG, De Marchie R: Surgical treatment of some cardiovascular diseases (a new vascular anastomosis). J Int College Surg (Bull) 16:1–10, 1951

80. Glenn WWL: Circulatory bypass of the right side of the heart. IV. Shunt between superior vena cava and distal right pulmonary artery—report of clinical application. New Engl J Med 259:117–120, 1958

81. Bakulev AN, Kolesnikov SA: Anastomosis of superior vena cava and pulmonary artery in the surgical treatment of certain congenital defects of the heart. J Thorac Surg 37:693–702, 1959

82. Edwards WS, Bargeron LM: The superiority of the Glenn operation for tricuspid atresia in infancy and childhood. J Thorac Cardiovasc Surg 55:60–69, 1968

83. Litwin SB, Fellows K: Systemic to pulmonary arterial shunts for patients with cyanotic congenital heart disease: Current status. Pediatr Radiol 1:41–46, 1973

84. Buruchow IB, Bartley TD, Elliott LP, et al: Late superior vena cava syndrome after superior vena cava—right pulmonary artery anastomosis. Report of four cases. New Engl J Med 281:646–650, 1969

85. Bargeron LM, Karp RB, Barcia A, et al: Late deterioration of patients after superior vena cava to right pulmonary artery anastomosis. Am J Cardiol 30:211–216, 1972

86. Waterston DJ: Treatment of Fallot's tetralogy in children under 1 year of age. Rozhl Chir 41:181–183, 1962

87. Cooley DA, Hallman GL: Intrapericardial aortic-right pulmonary arterial anastomosis. Surg Gynecol Obstet 122:1084–1086, 1966

88. Somerville J, Yacoub M, Ross DN, et al: Aorta to right pulmonary artery anastomosis (Waterston's operation) for cyanotic heart disease. Circulation 39:593–602, 1969

89. Oldham HN, Simpson L, Jones RH, et al: Differential distribution of pulmonary blood flow following aorto-pulmonary anastomosis. Surg Forum 21:201–202, 1970

90. Albers WH, Nadas AS: Unilateral chronic pulmonary edema and pleural effusion after systemic-pulmonary artery shunts for cyanotic congenital heart disease. Am J Cardiol 19:861–866, 1967

91. Tay DJ, Engle MA, Ehlers KH, et al: Early results and late developments of the Waterston anastomosis. Circulation 50:220–229, 1974

92. Blalock A, Taussig HB: The surgical treatment of malformations of the heart. JAMA 128:189–202, 1945

93. Taussig HB, Crawford H, Pelargonio S, et al: Ten to thirteen year follow-up on patients after a Blalock-Taussig operation. Circulation 25:630–634, 1962

94. Hancock EW, Hultgren HN, March HW: Pulmonary hypertension after Blalock–Taussig anastomosis. Am Heart J 67:817–823, 1964

95. Potts WJ, Smith S, Gibson S: Anastomosis of the aorta to a pulmonary artery. Certain types in congenital heart disease. JAMA 132:627–631, 1946

96. Paul MH, Miller RA, Potts WJ: Long-term results of aortic-pulmonary anastomosis for tetralogy of Fallot. An analysis of the first 100 cases eleven to thirteen years after operation. Circulation 23:525–533, 1961

97. Wagenvoort CA, DuShane JW, Edwards JE: Cardiac clinics. 151. Hypertensive pulmonary arterial lesions as a late result of anastomosis of systemic and pulmonary circulations. Staff Meetings of the Mayo Clinic 35:186–191, 1960

98. Kirklin JW, Wallace RB, McGoon DC, et al: Early and late results after intracardiac repair of tetralogy of Fallot. Ann Surg 162:578–589, 1965

99. VonBermuth G, Ritter DG, Frye RL, et al: Evaluation of patients with tetralogy of Fallot and Potts anastomosis. Am J Cardiol 27:259–263, 1971

Electrocardiographic Changes Following Surgical Treatment of Congenital Cardiac Malformations

Daniel S. Clark, Henry D. Hirsch, Dolores M. Tamer, and Henry Gelband

IMPROVEMENTS in surgical techniques in the past 20 yr have brought a significant decrease in operative mortality and the survival of many more patients with congenital cardiac malformations into adulthood.[1] Various electrocardiographic (ECG) patterns evolve postoperatively in these patients. Cardiac surgery per se or the natural postoperative history of the defect may be responsible for these ECG changes. Regardless of the cause of these changes, the evaluation of the postoperative ECG is important in the clinical assessment of these patients. Many of these ECG changes are easily understood, but in some, controversies exist as to their etiology and their relationship to prognosis.

Because of these controversies we will review the late and persistent postoperative ECG findings in congenital cardiac lesions, with particular reference to: (1) resolution of abnormal preoperative findings, (2) the development of new abnormal postoperative patterns, and (3) chronic rhythm disturbances. The following *isolated* congenital cardiac malformations will be considered: valvar aortic stenosis, valvar pulmonic stenosis, simple coarctation of the aorta, complete transposition of the great arteries, atrial septal defects (primum and secundum), patent ductus arteriosus, ventricular septal defects, and tetralogy of Fallot.

VALVAR AORTIC STENOSIS

The presence of aortic stenosis (AS) results in left ventricular systolic hypertension and subsequent left ventricular hypertrophy (LVH). The degree of abnormalcy of the preoperative ECG in patients with AS is largely dependent upon the degree of this hypertrophy. There is general agreement that the ECG is valuable in estimating the severity of the hemodynamic abnormality.[2] It has been shown that the ECG in the majority of patients with a gradient across the aortic valve of less than 40 mm Hg does not demonstrate LVH, while if an aortic valve gradient exceeding 40 mm Hg is present, ECG evidence of LVH occurs in 75% of the patients.[3] A superimposed strain pattern over the left precordial leads may occur with severe gradients. It should be noted that exceptions do occur. LVH can occur with a small gradient, and more importantly some patients with severe gradients may have a normal ECG.[3] These exceptions appear to be more frequent in the adult than in the pediatric patient.[4] Thus, the scalar preoperative ECG although valuable in estimating the severity of AS, does have its limitations. The vectorcardiogram may be a better tool to assess the preoperative hemodynamic abnormality.[5]

Postoperatively the ECG may well be an unreliable tool in assessing the postoperative change in hemodynamics. Despite adequate relief of the obstruction many patients continue to demonstrate LVH and ischemic changes on the ECG.[6–9] This is demonstrated in a series of patients followed at the Boston Childrens Hospital from 1959 to 1972. In this series, a persistant postoperative strain pattern existed in 50% of the patients despite a residual aortic valve gradient of 30 mm Hg or less.[9] In fact, a few cases have been reported demonstrating no resolution of abnormal ECG changes in spite of a complete lack of postoperative gradients.[7] A likely explanation for this lack of ECG resolution despite adequate hemodynamic relief is the development of irreversible myocardial and endocardial damage. A recent animal study[10] has demonstrated that in response to aortic outflow obstruction and resultant left ventricular hypertrophy, the concentration of cardiac connective tissue increases and that this concentration is slow to regress upon release of the obstruction and apparently is related to the duration of the pressure overload.

On the other hand, regression of LVH and the disappearance of a strain pattern are nearly always indicative of an adequate surgical repair. These changes may occur over a variable period of time. When strain changes are associated with LVH,

From the Division of Pediatric Cardiology, Department of Pediatrics, and the Division of Cardiology, Department of Medicine, University of Miami School of Medicine, Miami, Fla.

Reprint requests should be addressed to Henry Gelband, M.D., Division of Pediatric Cardiology, University of Miami Hospital and Clinics, 1475 N.W. 12 Avenue, P.O. Box 236217, Station B, Miami, Fla. 33123.

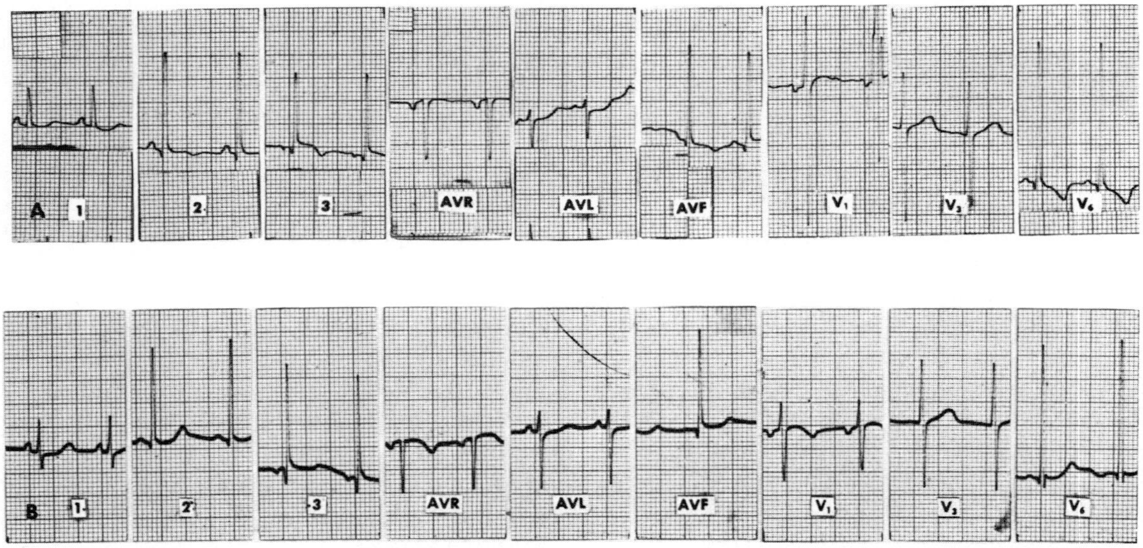

Fig. 1. Preoperative (A) and 4-yr postoperative (B) electrocardiograms in an 8-yr-old boy with severe valvar aortic stenosis. The preoperative ECG demonstrates LVH by voltage criteria and strain (ST-T changes). Note that although LVH by voltage is still present, the strain pattern has resolved. Postoperative hemodynamic studies revealed only a 10-mm Hg gradient across the aortic valve.

these usually resolve before there is any decrease in the left ventricular potentials (Fig. 1). LVH with an associated strain pattern may revert to normal as early as 6-mo postoperatively,[11] however, it has been noted that these changes may take much longer to normalize.[6,7,12–14]

In summary, while regression of LVH and strain is nearly always indicative of an adequate repair, the persistence of these abnormal findings may represent: (1) an adequate hemodynamic repair with associated irreversible changes of the endocardium and/or myocardium, (2) an inadequate surgical relief, or (3) the presence of moderate or severe postoperative aortic regurgitation.[15] Evaluation in such cases by postoperative cardiac catheterization is recommended.

VALVAR PULMONIC STENOSIS

The principle hemodynamic derangement of valvar pulmonic stenosis (PS) is obstruction to ejection of blood from the right ventricle. This leads to the development of right ventricular systolic hypertension which is proportional to the degree of obstruction. The preoperative ECG abnormalities in PS are very closely related to the systolic pressure measured in the right ventricle.[2,16–19] This relationship appears to be better in children than in adults.

A rsR′, RS, or rR′ configuration of the QRS complex in the right precordial leads is indicative of mild to moderate right ventricular hypertrophy (RVH). These correlate well with mild to moderate increases in the right ventricular systolic pressure. In children under 10 yr of age the presence of an upright T wave in V_1 in an otherwise normal ECG may be the only evidence of RVH.[20] Preoperatively both right axis deviation and delayed right ventricular depolarization are observed.[21] As the obstruction increases in severity a pure R wave or qR pattern may be observed in the right precordial leads. The presence of RVH, associated with ST-T wave changes and right atrial enlargement, as evidenced by increased P wave voltage, is found in the ECG of patients with severe PS. The more severe the PS, the more striking are these ECG changes, except in neonates with a diminutive right ventricle.[22]

Operative release of right ventricular obstruction leads to resolution of right ventricular hypertrophy with its ECG counterparts. The ECG abnormalities may show improvement within 3 mo and may continue to improve up to 3 yr postoperatively.[23] There is resolution of abnormal ST-T changes, and a decrease in right ventricular activation time. A postoperative decrease in the right ventricular potentials[21–28] is to be expected after a satisfac-

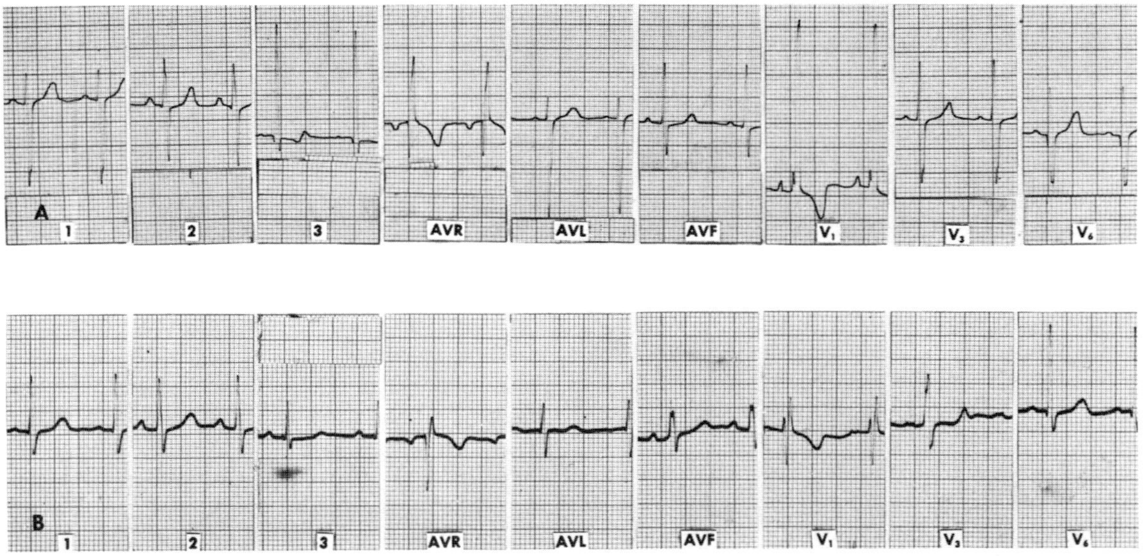

Fig. 2. Preoperative (A) and 5-yr postoperative (B) electrocardiograms in a boy with valvar pulmonic stenosis. Preoperatively significant right ventricular hypertrophy (RVH) is evident (rR′) in V_1. Following surgery there is an obvious leftward shift of the frontal plane QRS axis from +150° to +60° and a decrease in the right precordial anterior potentials. The ECG pattern regressed to a rSR′ in lead V_1 suggestive of mild RVH. Additionally the R wave in lead I increased in amplitude while the S wave in V_6 decreased. This correlated with mild residual pulmonary stenosis and insufficiency documented during postoperative cardiac catheterization.

tory surgical result (Fig. 2). There apparently is a close correlation between the decrease in amplitude of the R wave in the right precordial leads and the diminished right ventricular systolic pressure.[24] The postoperative frontal plane QRS axis demonstrates a more leftward trend;[21,25,29] this axis shift, however, fails to show any linear relationship to changes in right ventricular systolic pressure.[25] A decrease in the amplitude of the P wave is also noted after satisfactory surgical correction.[21,24,25]

Though supraventricular arrhythmias are not uncommon in the immediate postoperative period, they rarely persist or recur years after surgery.[30] Significant residual PS must be considered whenever there is a lack of improvement of the ECG within 3 yr postoperatively; hemodynamic reevaluation is mandatory in such cases.

COARCTATION OF THE AORTA

The basic hemodynamic alteration in simple, uncomplicated coarctation of the aorta (CoA) is similar to that seen in AS. There is obstruction to outflow which results in pressure overloading of the left ventricle. This obstruction is distal to the coronary ostia so that the LVH that develops is usually associated with a more adequate coronary blood flow. No correlation has been found between the severity of the CoA and the presence or degree of LVH. There may be a wide variation in the preoperative electrocardiographic features. The tracing may range from normal to LVH with a QRS axis abnormally deviated to the left for the patient's age.[31] Frequently the presence of LVH with a strain pattern in an infant or young child with the physical signs of coarctation suggests the presence of associated severe aortic stenosis. RVH and right axis deviation are rare in the absence of associated lesions except within the first few months of life.[2,31]

Adequate resection of the coarctation usually leads to improvement in the ECG pattern if it initially demonstrated LVH. Landtman has noted changes to start as early as 3-mo postoperatively.[31] These changes included: (1) resolution of abnormal preoperative ST-T changes, (2) a decrease in QT intervals from abnormally prolonged preoperative values, (3) a rightward shift in the frontal plane QRS axis, although this was usually still within the normal range, and (4) a significant decrease in the R wave amplitude in V_5. In an analysis of postoperative ECGs, Shuster[32] noted that 67% of the tracings reverted to normal, 7% "improved" showing regression of left ventricular potentials, 17%

remained abnormal, and 7% showed progression of left ventricular hypertrophy.

In summary, the reversion of the ECG toward a normal axis associated with the regression of the ECG evidence of left ventricular hypertrophy with or without strain would lead one to expect a favorable surgical and hemodynamic result. Persistent gradients across the coarctation or associated congenital cardiac lesions such as AS and aortic or mitral regurgitation may explain the persistent abnormal postoperative ECG findings. Obviously long-term hemodynamic and ECG correlation is necessary.

TRANSPOSITION OF THE GREAT ARTERIES

There is no specific ECG pattern for transposition of the great arteries (TGA). The ECG may be considered normal in the immediate neonatal period. Depending upon the specific anatomical lesions and subsequent hemodynamics, two ECG patterns may evolve.[33,34] The first occurs in infants with intact ventricular septum, in which case the ECG usually demonstrates a normal or rightward frontal-plane QRS axis, right atrial and right ventricular hypertrophy. When TGA is associated with a ventricular septal defect of significant size, biatrial and biventricular hypertrophy usually occur. Rhythm or conduction disturbances are rare preoperatively in either instance.[34]

The Mustard procedure for correction of TGA produces few major changes in the ECG. Khoury et al.[35] noted an increase in P wave duration, P wave notching, and a decrease in P wave amplitude postoperatively. These changes were seen in 90% of cases. He felt that these were suggestive of left atrial enlargement. However, the P wave notching and increased duration may be due to interruption of internodal conduction pathways. It should be noted that in some patients, the PR interval was slightly prolonged postoperatively, although still remaining within normal limits. No significant changes occur in the QRS frontal plane axis or in the degree of RVH since the right ventricle remains the systemic ventricle postoperatively.

The most common ECG abnormality noted after the Mustard repair is the occurrence of arrhythmias.[35–46] The majority are supraventricular in origin and include premature atrial extrasystoles, sick sinus syndrome, paroxysmal atrial tachycardia, junctional tachycardia, and atrial flutter-fibrillation. There are additional reports of varying degrees of transient or persistent heart block.[43] The incidence of these arrhythmias is approximately 10% immediately postoperatively; but some suggest that as many as 36% of patients following surgical repair will have arrhythmias as late as 3 yr following surgery.[47]

Much has been written about the etiology of the rhythm disturbances. Pathological studies have shown interruption of the internodal conduction pathways,[45] acute sinoatrial nodal hemorrhage and inflammation, chronic sinoatrial node fatty degeneration and fibrosis, and arteriosclerosis of the sinus node artery.[44,46] Additionally, histologic studies of the atrioventricular node have shown evidence of acute and chronic inflammatory changes.[48] All of these have been implicated in the genesis of the above arrhythmias.

Gillette,[39] utilizing His bundle electrograms has demonstrated that these postoperative patients have normal intraatrial, atrioventricular, and intraventricular conduction times. The only abnormality noted was a prolonged sinoatrial node recovery time suggesting sinoatrial node disease. Supportive evidence that the major electrophysiologic abnormality occurs in the sinoatrial node was also suggested by Rodriquez-Fernandez,[38] who found only one patient with atrioventricular node disease, while his remaining patients demonstrated sinoatrial node dysfunction.

In an attempt to decrease this high incidence of postoperative arrhythmias, the Mustard procedure has been modified. Areas near specialized conduction tissue, specifically the coronary sinus and atrioventricular node are avoided.[40,49] This has resulted in a significant decrease in postoperative rhythm disturbances,[40] although a longer period of evaluation is necessary to determine whether this observation is valid.

SECUNDUM ATRIAL SEPTAL DEFECT

The major hemodynamic alteration in secundum atrial septal defects (SASD) consists of an increase in the volume of blood delivered to the right atrium and right ventricle resulting in right atrial and right ventricular overloading. The usual ECG manifestations in association with this defect include: (1) right axis deviation, with the majority of patients having a mean QRS axis greater than +90°, (2) right ventricular hypertrophy as evidenced by an rsR′ pattern or variant in the right precordial leads, and (3) right and left atrial enlargement in up to 36% of cases.[50]

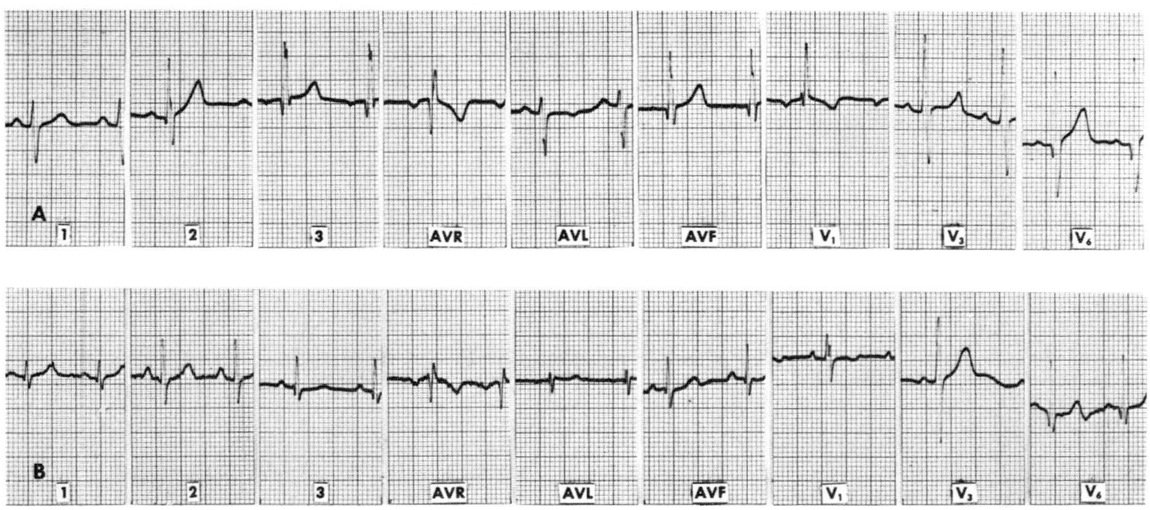

Fig. 3. Preoperative (A) and 3-yr postoperative (B) electrocardiograms in a girl with secundum atrial septal defect (SASD). The preoperative ECG demonstrates the typical pattern of SASD including an rsR′ configuration in lead V_1. Postoperatively a leftward shift of the frontal plane QRS axis from +120° to +60° and a significant decrease in the right precordial anterior potentials is observed. The ECG pattern in lead V_1 regressed to a rr′S pattern. Additionally there is a decrease in the amplitude and the duration of the S wave in lead I and V_6.

The PR interval in patients with SASD, although usually within normal limits, is significantly longer than in other children with congenital heart disease without atrial septal abnormalites. By utilizing intracardiac electrograms, the components of the PR interval have been measured, and have shown that patients with SASD have normal atrioventricular and His–Purkinje conduction times. However, the intraatrial conduction time in these patients is prolonged to twice the control values.[51] The cause of this prolongation may simply be right atrial enlargement. However, because of the anatomical location of the defect, alteration of atrial conduction pathways by disruption or displacement may also be responsible for the delay. These electrophysiologic observations may also explain the occurrence of the prolonged PR interval observed in 10% of children with SASD and suggests that these patients do not have "first degree heart block" in the classical sense since the delay may be within the atria and not the atrioventricular node.

Arrhythmias are not common in patients with SASD preoperatively. However, in the adult, atrial fibrillation is not uncommon, being reported in the range of 20%–50%.[52–58] It has been suggested that the occurrence of this arrhythmia may be related to the duration of established pulmonary hypertension.[59]

Surgical closure of the defect with normalization of the hemodynamics results in the changes observed in the postoperative ECG. Adequate repair results in a leftward shift of the frontal plane QRS axis from its preoperative rightward displacement, as well as a minor decrease in P wave amplitude and duration. An insignificant decrease in the QRS duration has been noted in the pediatric patient.[59] The amplitude of the R′ in the right precordial leads usually decreases within the first 6 mo after surgery (Fig. 3). This is associated with a decrease in the amplitude and duration of the S wave in leads I, aVL, V_5, and V_6. We have noted such changes in 84% of our postoperative population. Failure of the R′ in the right precordial leads to decrease significantly postoperatively should suggest a persistent defect or pulmonary artery hypertension.[60] However, the ECG need not return entirely to normal in order to reflect a good surgical result.[61,62]

Chronic arrhythmias following the repair of SASD are not common, occurring in about 5% of patients.[63] The spectrum of arrhythmias include sick sinus syndrome, junctional tachycardia, supraventricular tachycardia, and atrial flutter-fibrillation.[64–70] These arrhythmias have been observed more frequently after correction of SASD of the sinus venosus variety. Additionally complete heart block (CHB) though rarely encountered, has been reported.[64] The vast majority of these arrhythmias

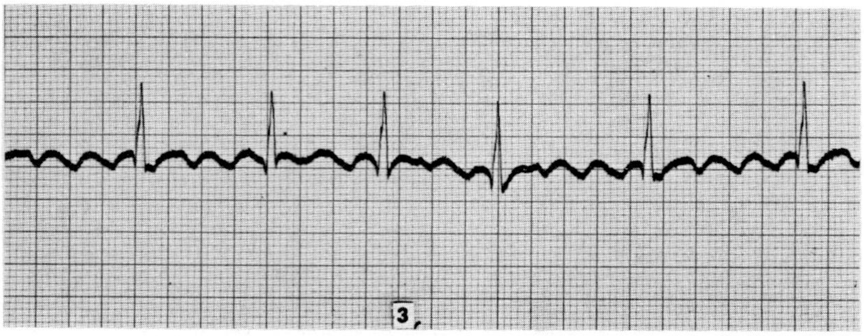

Fig. 4. Rhythm strip (lead III) in a 5-yr-old girl who developed atrial flutter 4 mo after repair of an atrial septal defect. She has remained in this rhythm for 6 yr despite attempts at medical conversion. No residual cardiac defect is present.

start within the immediate postoperative period, although some have been noted to begin several weeks to months following surgery (Fig. 4).[64–66] Young has recently described some patients with chronic arrhythmias (junctional bradycardia with or without multifocal ventricular ectopic beats) whose ECGs spontaneously reverted to normal sinus rhythm as late as 9 yr postoperatively.[71] The mechanism for this late reversion remains unclear.

As a general rule the adult patient demonstrates similar ECG changes as the pediatric patient. The only differences are minor and they include a decrease of about 10% in the QRS duration,[72] and a much higher incidence of atrial fibrillation postoperatively.

PRIMUM ATRIAL SEPTAL DEFECTS

Characteristic ECG findings are present in the majority of patients with primum atrial septal defects (PASD). These include: (1) a left axis deviation (LAD) where the mean QRS frontal axis ranges from −30° to −170°, (absent on rare occasions),[73,74] (2) a counterclockwise frontal plane QRS loop, (3) rsR′ pattern or variant in the right precordial leads, indicative of delayed right ventricular depolarization secondary to overloading of the right ventricle, (4) evidence of biventricular hypertrophy in the presence of associated mitral regurgitation,[75–79] (5) a prolonged PR interval occurring in 40%–50% of the patients, and (6) an increase in P wave amplitude and occasionally duration suggesting right and/or left atrial enlargement.

Controversy over the etiology of the LAD still exists. Electrophysiologic studies in these patients have concluded that the posterobasal portion of the left ventricle is the first to be activated.[80,81] This early activation results in displacement of the maximal QRS vector superiorly and to the left. Anatomic studes have reported variations in the location of the fascicles of the left bundle branch which additionally support this concept. These anatomic variations may either be a displaced, abnormally long anterior fascicle,[82,83] or a short abnormal left posterior fascicle.[80,84] Thus, the LAD may be due to anatomic variations in location of the left bundle branch and not due to intrinsic disease as observed in other conditions (myocardial infarction). Borkon et al.[84] believe that this anatomic variation of the left posterior fascicle may only partially explain the abnormal LAD. The presence of abnormal hemodynamics (i.e., elevated right ventricular pressure and a large left-to-right shunt), as well as LVH, and right bundle branch block may exaggerate the axis superiorly. Further study will be necessary to resolve this question.

In the right precordial leads, the common ECG patterns are rsR′, rsr′ or rR′. However rS and qR patterns have also been noted. The amplitude of the right precordial anterior forces has been observed to correlate well with right ventricular systolic pressure but poorly with the magnitude of the left-to-right shunt at the atrial level. It has been noted that patients with complete endocardial cushion defects generally demonstrate a more severe degree of RVH on the ECG than patients with partial defects.[85] Arrhythmias in patients with PASD, as in patients with SASD, are uncommon except in the adult.[74]

The etiology of the prolonged PR interval in patients with PASD is controversial. Waldo and coworkers recently demonstrated an intraatrial conduction delay in patients with PASD.[86] The atrio-

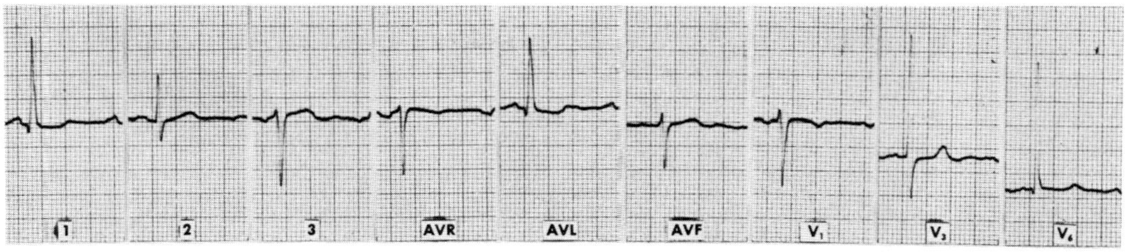

Fig. 5. The postoperative electrocardiogram of a 10-yr-old girl who underwent cardiac surgery for a primum atrial septal defect. This ECG was recorded 5 yr postoperatively. It still demonstrates an abnormal left axis deviation of −15° with evidence of persistent left ventricular hypertrophy. Clinically, she demonstrated severe residual mitral insufficiency.

ventricular and His–Purkinje conduction times were normal. They felt that interruption or displacement of the internodal tracts by the anatomical location of the septal defect may be responsible for this prolongation of the PR interval. However, we are following a family in which three members have PASD. Two members have associated congenital complete heart block. It is obvious that these patients must have a conduction block at or distal to the atrioventricular node. The precise etiology of this abnormality remains undetermined, and further evaluation is required.

Postoperatively there is little change in the frontal plane QRS axis. A rightward shift of the left superior QRS axis is to be expected, but usually it remains greater than −30°.[73,84] No significant changes occur in the PR interval or the right precordial QRS pattern. Persistence of LVH on the ECG may be related to the presence of residual mitral regurgitation (Fig. 5). Supraventricular tachyarrhythmias, such as junctional tachycardia and atrial fibrillation, have been described but are not common problems.[64,73,87]

The most serious postoperative ECG manifestation is the development of complete heart block. This block may be transient; present only in the immediate postoperative period and reverting to sinus rhythm usually within days or as late as 25 mo.[74,86–88] Permanent CHB occurred more frequently in the early years of open heart surgery,[89] and is less common today. Hopefully by the utilization of intraoperative electrogram monitoring and identification of the atrioventricular conduction system, this complication will be avoided in the future.[90]

PATENT DUCTUS ARTERIOSUS

The major hemodynamic stress imposed by a simple patent ductus arteriosus (PDA) is volume overload of the left atrium and ventricle. There is a good correlation between the size of the PDA and the changes in the preoperative ECG.[31] The ECG may be normal (20%) in those patients with a small ductus, or demonstrate left atrial enlargement and LVH in a large PDA. The QRS axis is usually normal. Isolated RVH or combined ventricular hypertrophy is usually found in young infants, associated complex cardiac lesions or in patients with pulmonary hypertension.

Successful closure of the PDA corrects the hemodynamic overload and usually leads to reversion of the abnormal preoperative ECG findings. These have been noted to occur as early as 1 mo postoperatively. In general a slight decrease in the P wave duration, PR and QT intervals is noted. The amplitude of the left ventricular potentials decrease and the abnormal ST segment and T wave changes tend to revert toward normal.[31]

VENTRICULAR SEPTAL DEFECTS

The ECG manifestations in patients with ventricular septal defects (VSD) are dependent upon the pressure, flow, and resistance relationships within the heart and great vessels. Since only those patients with moderate to large VSDs undergo surgical correction, we will confine our remarks to this group. Preoperatively left ventricular volume overload is the rule, and this results in LVH. However, if pulmonary artery and right ventricular hypertension are present, biventricular hypertrophy is observed. Additionally left atrial overloading results in left atrial hypertrophy. The mean frontal QRS axis is usually between +60° and +150° with a clockwise frontal plane loop. A counterclockwise frontal plane loop associated with a superior leftward QRS axis may be observed in those patients with VSD of the endocardial cushion variety. Low-grade atrioventricular block (first and second degree) occasionally occurs and CHB has been documented rarely.[91]

In general a good correlation has been found between the preoperative ECG and cardiac hemodynamics.[92–95] However some observers have disputed this point.[96] In spite of these conflicting reports, the following correlations are generally true: (1) if pure RVH is observed on the ECG, the VSD is associated with pulmonary vascular obstructive disease, (2) when only LVH is present there is a large pulmonary blood flow with normal right ventricular and pulmonary artery hemodynamics, and (3) biventricular hypertrophy results from the combination of a large pulmonary blood flow and an elevated pulmonary artery pressure.

The surgical approach in the correction of a VSD greatly influences the alterations observed in the postoperative ECG. The VSD may be approached either through the right atrium or right ventricle. Our initial comments will be concerned with those patients whose defect was corrected through a right atrial approach. Adequate surgical closure of a large VSD should result in a decrease in the pulmonary blood flow with a subsequent decrease in left atrial and left ventricular volume overload. It follows then, that regression of the ECG manifestations of left atrial and left ventricular hypertrophy should occur. Indeed this usually is the case. Observations in our patients who preoperatively demonstrated a large left-to-right ventricular shunt with minimal pulmonary hypertension have demonstrated a small rightward shift in the mean QRS frontal axis, and a decrease in the amplitude of the left ventricular potentials.

However many patients with VSDs are surgically corrected via a right ventriculotomy. These patients usually demonstrate a right bundle branch block (RBBB) pattern on the ECG following surgery.[97] It may appear on the ECG immediately or up to 1 yr postoperatively.[98] The appearance of this RBBB pattern makes it difficult to evaluate QRS changes in the postoperative ECG.

We feel that the most likely etiology for the postoperative RBBB pattern is disruption of the distal Purkinje system by the right vertical ventriculotomy. Numerous investigations have supported this concept.[97,99,100] Continuous ECG monitoring during surgery has revealed that the conduction defect occurred as a consequence of the right ventricular incision prior to surgical closure of the VSD.[99] Further detailed simultaneous electrocardiographic and electrophysiologic studies using epicardial electrodes during surgery have shown that the appearance of a wide slurred S wave in lead 1 with marked prolongation of the QRS complex occurred as soon as the right vertical ventriculotomy was performed. More importantly epicardial activation times of sites lateral to the ventriculotomy prolonged (30–40 msec), while those medial remained unchanged. Thus, block proximal in the right bundle could not have caused the delayed right ventricular depolarization.[100] Hefler et al. have recently further elucidated the relationship between the vertical ventriculotomy and the RBBB pattern during open heart surgery utilizing electrophysiologic techniques. By staging the ventriculotomy in small increments, incision of a precise right ventricular site, which varied in patients, could be identified as the cause of the RBBB pattern. They concluded that the ventriculotomy induced RBBB pattern was due to disruption of a distal branch or branches of the right bundle.[101]

An alternative explanation for the postoperative RBBB pattern is interruption of the proximal right bundle branch which may occur at the time of surgical closure of the septal defect. This possibility has been suggested by the observation that some patients whose VSDs are corrected via an atriotomy may develop a RBBB pattern.[102] In an attempt to understand this etiology of the RBBB pattern, knowledge of the anatomy of the ventricular conduction system and its relationship to the septal defect is important. Anatomic studies[82, 103–107] have demonstrated that a VSD involving the membranous septum and those of the endocardial cushion variety usually are located in close proximity to the specialized conduction system. In both instances the His bundle and proximal right and left bundle branch usually lie near the posterior-inferior aspect of the defect. A VSD in the more apical portion of the muscular septum is in close proximity to the peripheral ramifications of the right and left bundle branches. Recently variations in the expected location of the specialized conduction system in relation to the septal defect have been described. In an anatomic study of ten hearts having VSDs, seven had the atrioventricular bundle in the usual position. In three specimens the bundle bifurcated after deviating to the left side of the septum. Additionally in two specimens with muscular VSDs the common bundle was located on the anterosuperior portion of the defect.[108] It is not surprising then, that in the surgical correction of a VSD, trauma to the specialized ventricular conduction system has been reported. Pathologic studies have described hemorrhage, necrosis, inflammation, and interruption of the bundle of His and the right and left bundle branches.[109,110]

It has been observed that as many as 5%–14% of patients undergoing closure of a VSD will develop a RBBB pattern associated with LAD.[111,112] The most likely site of block in these cases is proximal involvement of both the right bundle branch and anterior fascicle of the left bundle branch. The anatomic proximity of these structures to the septal defect has been previously emphasized. However, direct surgical trauma to only the left anterior fascicle may have occurred, while the RBBB pattern could have been the result of a right ventriculotomy. Just as the etiology of this ECG abnormality remains controversial its prognostic significance is also unsettled. Kulbertus et al.[111] believe that a high percentage of these patients progress to chronic CHB, although other observers have not substantiated this finding.[112] Only additional years of observation will settle its true importance.

CHB is also noted postoperatively,[111,114] usually as a transient conduction abnormality in the immediate postoperative period. Its reversion to sinus rhythm occurs in the majority of cases usually within the first 6 wk.[115] On rare occasions it may develop late in the postoperative course, and may eventually revert to sinus rhythm.[116] However, if CHB persists up to 4-wk postoperatively, reversion to sinus rhythm, although possible, is rare. The occurrance of CHB is understandable in the light of the proximity of the ventricular conduction system to the defect. Early attempts to decrease the incidence of CHB involved avoidance of the posterior–inferior margin of the defect during surgical repair.[117] As in PASD electrophysiologic identification of the atrioventricular conduction system may obviate the problem.

Although the incidence is probably low, arrhythmias do occur. We have observed the development of atrial flutter 8 yr postoperatively after repair of a VSD (Fig. 6). Other chronic arrhythmias which have been reported include supraventricular tachycardia, junctional tachycardia, atrial fibrillation, and second degree atrioventricular block, prema-

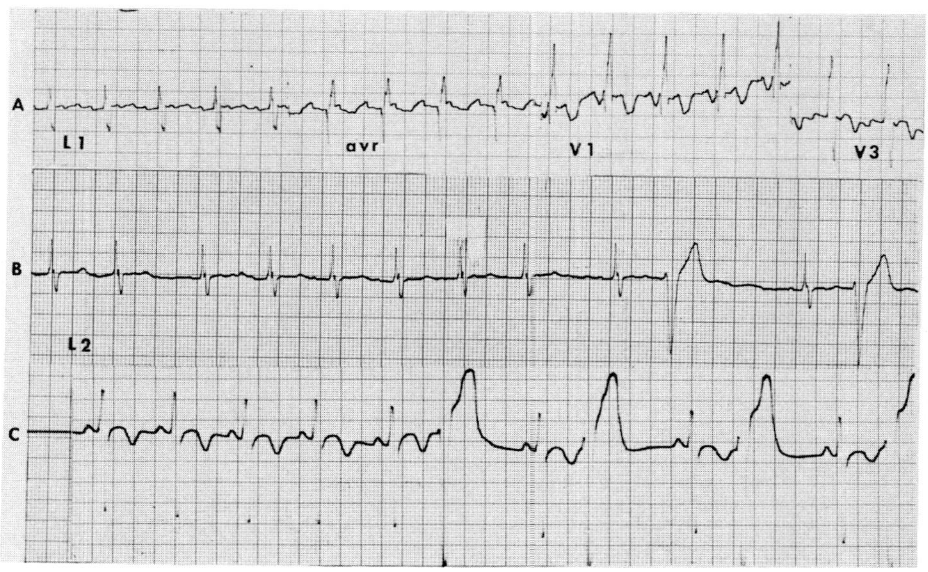

Fig. 6. Postoperative ECG tracings in a 15-yr-old girl whose ventricular septal defect was closed through an atriotomy 9 yr previously. (A) shows atrial flutter. (B) is a lead II rhythm strip demonstrating atrial fibrillation with occasional aberrantly conducted beats. (C) is a rhythm strip obtained using a 12-hr continuous ECG recording (Avionics). It demonstrates spontaneous reversion to sinus rhythm with periods of ventricular bigeminy. At postoperative catheterization, she had residual mild tricuspid insufficiency and moderate pulmonary hypertension.

ture ventricular extrasystoles, and ventricular bigeminy.[65]

TETRALOGY OF FALLOT

It is well known that RVH and right axis deviation are the major ECG manifestations in tetralogy of Fallot (TF). These are obviously the result of pulmonary outflow tract obstruction. In the usual patient with TF, because of the moderate to large VSD, right ventricular systolic pressure is never greater than systemic, and thus signs of severe RVH with strain on the ECG are rare. Various right precordial patterns have been described (Rs, rR′, qR), all of which are diagnostic of RVH when associated with an increased amplitude of the right ventricular forces for the patient's age. There is a poor correlation between the height of the R wave in V_1 and the right ventricular systolic pressure.[2] The QRS duration is usually normal, though RBBB and/or LAD have been reported.[111,118] Additional preoperative ECG features are normal sinus rhythm, occasionally with first degree heart block,[119] and an increase in the amplitude of the P wave which may occur in up to 15%–20% of patients.

Postoperatively after an excellent surgical repair[120] one would expect resolution of the abnormal preoperative ECG findings. The mean QRS frontal axis shows a leftward shift which may be oriented superiorly and to the left. No significant change is noted in the P wave amplitude. Following total correction, RBBB invariably occurs. Its etiology is thought to be similar to that already discussed with VSD. The presence of postoperative RBBB makes it difficult to evaluate QRS changes.

Most patients following surgical correction remain in sinus rhythm. We have observed occasional patients with wandering atrial pacemakers, ventricular extra systoles, recurrent ventricular tachycardia, intermittent second degree heart block, CHB, and episodes of supraventricular tachyarrhythmias (Fig. 7). The most frequently reported postoperative arrhythmia is CHB, being noted in from 1% to 18% of patients.[87,112,114,121] Detailed anatomic studies have helped to elucidate the high incidence of this postoperative complication, by demonstrating the close proximity of the atrioventricular bundle to the septal defect.[82,106] This proximity makes the conduction system vulnerable to surgical interruption during closure of the septal defect. Most patients who develop CHB do so within the immediate postoperative period. It is generally agreed that those patients who develop transient CHB in this period have a good clinical

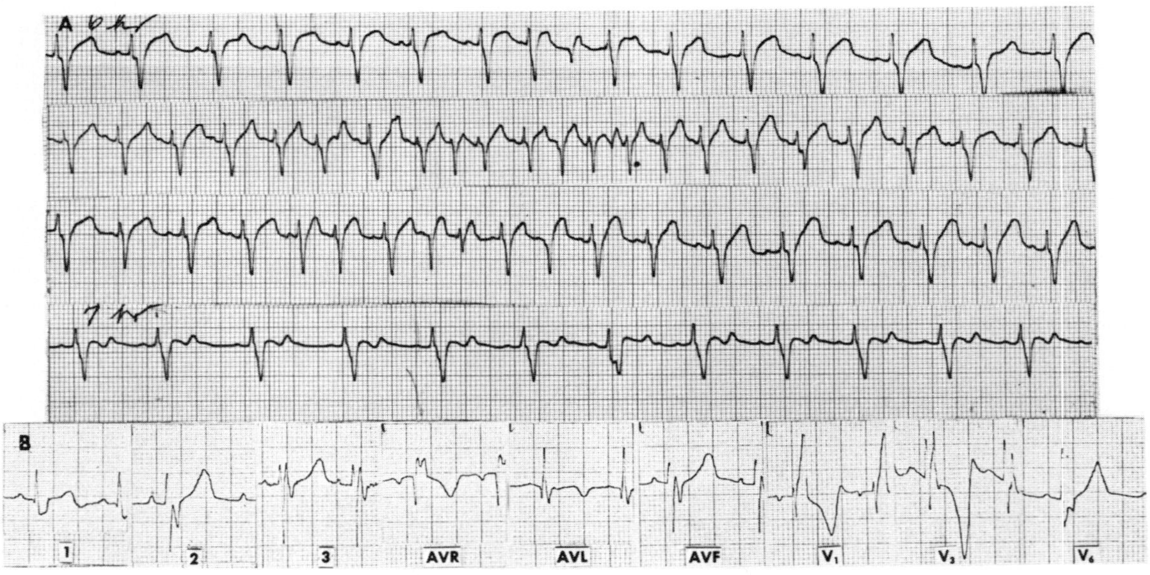

Fig. 7. These tracings were recorded from a patient who developed syncope 8 yr following total correction of tetralogy of Fallot. (A) is a continuous (Avionics) recording obtained shortly after admission to the hospital. It demonstrated a paroxysmal atrial tachyarrhythmia with a ventricular response rate of 270/min. One hr later there was spontaneous reversion to sinus rhythm at a rate of 85 beats/min. (B) is a routine ECG prior to discharge from the hospital. The only abnormalities noted are a right bundle branch block pattern (QRS duration 0.120 sec), and left axis deviation (−45°). Postoperative cardiac catheterization revealed slight residual pulmonic insufficiency and normal hemodynamics.

prognosis.[122,123] However, CHB has been reported to first appear suddenly a few years postoperatively.[124-126]

Invasive electrophysiologic studies have been carried out in a small number of patients in an attempt to determine the site of the CHB. Two patients were described by Rosen et al. who developed CHB as a consequence of the surgical procedure.[127] Both patients were found to have block distal to the His bundle potential. Additionally Anderson et al. described two patients with CHB: in one the site of the block was proximal to the His bundle potential and in the second patient it was distal.[128] Though both of these reverted to sinus rhythm in several weeks, one patient continued to demonstrate a residual conduction abnormality (Wenckebach phenomenon) distal to the His potential.

Though CHB has been reported to occur, the conduction abnormality of RBBB and LAD is much more frequent postoperatively. Slight anatomic differences in the atrioventricular conduction system in patients with TF have been noted by Lev[129] which may explain this conduction disturbance. In TF the bundle of His is positioned on the left side of the ventricular septum just below the VSD. At the level of the VSD the posterior fascicle of the left bundle branch originates. The remainder of the bundle continues to the distal portion of the defect, where bifurcation into the main right bundle branch and anterior fascicle occurs. Therefore, there is close proximity not only of the common atrioventricular bundle but also of the right bundle branch and the anterior fascicle of the left bundle branch to the septal defect. Thus, the right bundle branch and the left anterior fascicle of the left bundle branch could be easily simultaneously traumatized during surgery, while sparing the posterior fascicle of the left bundle.

Controversy surrounds the prognostic significance of the development of RBBB and LAD. Wolff et al.[130] demonstrated an 8% incidence of RBBB and LAD in patients undergoing total correction. They believe that patients with this postoperative complication not only have a greater chance of developing CHB (21% in patients with RBBB and LAD, as compared to 8% of patients with only RBBB) but also have a higher frequency of sudden death either from a conduction defect (CHB) or an arrhythmia. However, others have not found this relationship. Bocala et al.[118] found no significant dysrhythmias or sudden death in their patient population as did Godman et al.,[131] unless the patients had an associated prolonged His-Purkinje conduction time as measured by intracardiac electrograms. Continued clinical evaluation is needed to settle this controversy.

It appears then, that the RBBB pattern in surgically corrected patients with TF (or VSD) probably results from the interruption of the distal right Purkinje system induced by a vertical ventriculotomy, but in some may be due to trauma to the proximal right bundle branch. If the RBBB pattern is associated with persistent LAD, the probable site of the conduction block is proximal. However this cannot be the etiology in those patients who have ECG evidence of permanent RBBB and transient LAD.[132] In these patients a temporary insult (edema) to the left anterior fascicle resulting from surgery may have occurred; the residual RBBB representing either a proximal or distal interruption of the right conducting system.

Although there is an abundance of literature concerning the electrocardiographic manifestations following surgery for congenital heart disease, numerous questions remain as yet unsettled. The etiology of many postoperative arrhythmias and conduction disturbances is still debated. Knowledge of the frequency of the arrhythmias and the site and extent of the conduction disturbances is needed. Additionally the effect of these new and/or persistent postoperative electrocardiographic findings upon the survival of the postoperative congenital cardiac patient requires further clinical evaluation and research.

ACKNOWLEDGMENT

We are indebted to Mrs. D. Clark, Ms. J. Long, and Mrs. C. Rivas for their patience and understanding in the preparation of this manuscript.

REFERENCES

1. Perloff JK: Pediatric congenital cardiac becomes a postoperative adult: The changing population of congenital heart disease. Circulation 47:606-619, 1973

2. Nadas AS, Fyler DC: Pediatric Cardiology. Philadelphia, Saunders, 1972

3. Hugenholtz PG, Lees MM, Nadas AS: The scalar

electrocardiogram, vectorcardiogram, and exercise electrocardiogram in the assessment of congenital aortic stenosis. Circulation 26:79–91, 1962

4. Braunwald E, Goldblatt A, Aygen MM, et al: Congenital aortic stenosis: I. Clinical and hemodynamic findings in 100 patients. Circulation 27:426–450, 1963

5. Gamboa R, Hugenholtz PG, Nadas AS: Comparison of the electrocardiogram and vectorcardiogram in congenital aortic stenosis. Br Heart J 27:344–354, 1965

6. Putnam TC, Harris PD, Bernhard WF, et al: The surgical management of congenital aortic stenosis. J Thorac Cardiovasc Surg 48:540–555, 1964

7. Morrow AG, Goldblatt A, Braunwald E: Congenital aortic stenosis: II. Surgical treatment and the results of operation. Circulation 27:450–462, 1963

8. Bernhard WF, Keane JF, Fellows KE, et al: Progress and problems in the surgical management of congenital aortic stenosis. J Thorac Cardvasc Surg 66:404–419, 1973

9. Keane JF, Rosenthal A: Personal communication

10. Cutilletta AF, Radnik M, Dowell RT, et al: Regression of myocardial hypertrophy. Pediatr Res 8:348, 14, 1974

11. Shams A, Keith JD, Edibam B, et al: The rate of regression of ventricular hypertrophy in vectorcardiogram and electrocardiogram after surgery on congenital heart disease. J Electrocardiol 6:243–247, 1973

12. Ellis FH, Ongley PA, Kirklin JW: Results of surgical treatment for congenital aortic stenosis. Circulation 25:29–38, 1962

13. Bertranou E, Davignon A, Chartrand C, et al: Congenital aortic stenosis: Follow-up of surgical management. Can Med Assoc J 105:583–587, 1971

14. Morrow AG, Sharp EG, Braunwald E: Congenital aortic stenosis: Clinical and hemodynamic findings, surgical technic, and results of operation. Circulation 18: 1091–1104, 1958

15. Thomson NB, Fisher FC: Long-term postoperative follow-up in surgery for congenital aortic valvular stenosis. Circulation 32:732–739, 1965

16. Compbell M: Simple pulmonic stenosis: Pulmonary valvular stenosis with a closed ventricular septum. Br Heart J 16:273–300, 1954

17. Engle MA, Holswade GR, Goldberg HP, et al: Regression after open valvotomy of infundibular stenosis accompanying severe valvular pulmonic stenosis. Circulation 17:862, 1960

18. Bassingthwaighte JB, Parkin TW, DuShane JW, et al: The electrocardiographic and hemodynamic findings in pulmonary stenosis with intact ventricular septum. Circulation 28:893–905, 1963

19. Cagler GG, Ongley PA, Nadas AS: Relationship of systolic pressure in the right ventricle to the electrocardiogram. N Engl J Med 258:979–982, 1958

20. Celermajer JM, Izukawa T, Varghese PJ, et al: Upright T wave in V_1: A useful diagnostic sign of mild pulmonic valve stenosis in children. J Pediatr 74:413–415, 1969

21. Landtman B: Postoperative changes in the electrocardiogram in congenital heart disease: I. Pure pulmonic stenosis. Circulation 10:859–870, 1954

22. Freed MD, Rosenthal A, Bernhard WF, et al: Critical pulmonary stenosis with a diminutive right ventricle in neonates. Circulation 48:875–881, 1973

23. Campbell M, Brock R: The results of valvotomy for simple pulmonary stenosis. Br Heart J 17:229–246, 1955

24. Silverman BK, Nadas AS, Wittenborg MH, et al: Pulmonary stenosis with intact ventricular septum. Am J Med 20:53–64, 1956

25. Hanson JA, Ikkos D, Crafoord C, et al: Results of surgery for congenital pulmonary stenosis: Comparison of the transventricular and transarterial approaches. Circulation 18:588–602, 1958

26. Blount SG, McCord MC, Mueller H, et al: Isolated valvular pulmonic stenosis: Clinical and physiologic response to open valvuloplasty. Circulation 10:161–172, 1954

27. Blount SG, van Elk J, Balchum OJ, et al: Valvular pulmonary stenosis with intact ventricular septum. Circulation 15:814–826, 1957

28. Kahn M, Bleifer SB, Grishman A, et al: The vectorcardiogram and electrocardiogram before and after valvulotomy for pulmonic stenosis. Am Heart J 58:327–342, 1959

29. Kittle CF, Santos EM, Dimond EG: Persistent right bundle branch block due to pulmonic valvulotomy and infundibulectomy. Am Surg 22:80–85, 1956

30. Deverall PB, Roberts NK, Stark J: Arrhythmias in children with pulmonary stenosis. Br Heart J 32:472–476, 1970

31. Landtman B: Postoperative changes in the electrocardiogram in congenital heart disease: II. Coarctation of the aorta and patent ductus arteriosus. Circulation 10: 871–886, 1954

32. Schuster SR, Gross RE: Surgery for coarctation of the aorta: A review of 500 cases. J Thorac Cardvasc Surg 43:54–70, 1962

33. Elliott LP, Anderson RL, Tuna N, et al: Complete transposition of the great vessels: II. An electrocardiographic analysis. Circulation 27:1118–1127, 1963

34. Shaher RM, Deucher DC: The electrocardiogram in complete transposition of the great vessels. Br Heart J 28:265–275, 1966

35. Khoury GH, Shaher RM, Fowler RS, et al: Preoperative and postoperative electrocardiogram in complete transposition of the great vessels. Am Heart J 72:199–205, 1966

36. Aberdeen E: Correction of uncomplicated cases of transposition of the great arteries. Br Heart J 33 (Suppl): 66–68, 1971

37. Zuberbuhler JR, Bauersfeld SR: Unusual arrhythmias after corrective surgery for transposition of the great vessels. Am Heart J 73:752–755, 1967

38. Rodriguez-Fernandez HL, Kelly DT, Collado A, et al: Hemodynamic data and angiographic findings after Mustard repair for complete transposition of the great arteries. Circulation 46:799–808, 1972

39. Gillette PC, El-Said GM, Sivarajan N, et al: Electrophysiologic abnormalities after Mustard's operation for transposition of the great arteries. Br Heart J 36:186–191, 1974

40. Stark J, DeLeval MR, Waterston DJ, et al: Corrective surgery of transposition of the great arteries in the

first year of life. J Thorac Cardiovasc Surg 67:673–681, 1974

41. Waldhausen JA, Pierce WS, Park CO, et al: Physiologic correction of transposition of the great arteries. Circulation 43:738–746, 1970

42. Waldhausen JA, Pierce WS, Rashkind WJ, et al: Total correction of transposition of the great arteries following balloon atrioseptostomy. Circulation 41 (Suppl 2):123–129, 1970

43. Haller JA, Crisler C, Brawley R, et al: Operative correction and postoperative management of transposition of the great vessels in nine children. Ann Thorac Surg 7:212–220, 1969

44. El-Said G, Rosenberg HS, Mullins GL, et al: Dysrhythmias after Mustard's operation for transposition of the great arteries. Am J Cardiol 30:527–532, 1972

45. Isaacson R, Titus JL, Merideth RH, et al: Apparent interruption of atrial conduction pathways after surgical repair of transposition of great arteries: Am J Cardiol 30: 533–535, 1972

46. Tung KSK, James TN, Effler DB, et al: Injury to the sinus node in open heart operations. J Thorac Cardiovasc Surg 53:814–829, 1972

47. Shaher RM: Complete transposition of the great arteries. New York, Academic Press, 1973

48. Aberdeen E, Carr I: Transposition of the great arteries, in Aberdeen E, Wooler GH (eds): Modern Trends in Cardiac Surgery, vol. 2. London, Butterworth, 1968

49. Breckenridge IM, Oelert H, Stark J, et al: Mustard's operation for transposition of the great arteries. Lancet 1:1140–1142, 1972

50. Davies DH, Prior R, Blount SG Jr: Electrocardiographic changes in atrial septal defect following surgical correction. Br Heart J 22:274–280, 1960

51. Anderson PAW, Rogers MC, Canent RV Jr, et al: Atrioventricular conduction in secundum atrial septal defects. Circulation 48:27–31, 1973

52. Daicoff GR, Brandenburg RD, Kirklin JW: Results of operation for ASD in patients forty-five years of age and older. Circulation 35 (Suppl 1):143–147, 1967

53. Gault JH, Morrow AG, Gay WA Jr, et al: Atrial septal defect in patients over the age of forty years. Circulation 37:261–272, 1968

54. Hanlon CR, Barrer HB, Willman VL, et al: Atrial septal defect: Results of repair in adults. Arch Surg 99: 275–280, 1969

55. Richmond DE, Lowe JB, Barratt-Boyes BG: Results of surgical repair of atrial septal defects in the middle-aged and elderly. Thorax 24:536–542, 1969

56. Sadsena FB, Aldridge HE: Atrial septal defect in the older patient: A clinical and hemodynamic study in patients operated on after age 35. Circulation 42:1009–1020, 1970

57. Yalav E, Brown AH, Braimbridge MV: Surgery for atrial septal defect in patients over 60 years of age: Report of surgical correction in 12 patients. J Thorac Cardiovasc Surg 62:788–792, 1971

58. Dave KS, Pakrashi BC, Wooler GH, et al: Atrial septal defect in adults: Clinical and hemodynamic results of surgery. Am J Cardiol 31:7–13, 1973

59. Peterson PO: Atrial septal defect of secundum type. Acta Paediatr Scand 174 (Suppl):35–45, 1967

60. Swan H, Kortz AB, Davies DH, et al: Atrial septal defect, secundum. J Thorac Surg 37:52–80, 1959

61. Hoffman LE, Krovetz LJ, Van Mierop LHS, et al: Secundum atrial septal defects in children: A postoperative evaluation of 65 cases. Ann Thorac Surg 7:104–109, 1969

62. Cohn LH, Morrow AG, Braunwald E: Operative treatment of atrial septal defect: Clinical and hemodynamic assessments in 175 patients. Br Heart J 29:725–734, 1967

63. Neptune WB: Survey of surgical treatment of atrial septal defects. Report of the Committee in Cardiovascular Surgery, American College of Chest Physicians. Dis Chest 43:447–448, 1963

64. Linde LM, Goldberg SJ, Seigel S: The natural history of arrhythmias following septal defect repair. J Thorac Cardiovasc Surg 48:303–309, 1964

65. Sasaki R, Theilen EO, January LE, et al: Cardiac arrhythmias associated with the repair of atrial and ventricular septal defects. Circulation 18:909–915, 1958

66. Sellers RD, Ferlic RM, Sterns LP, et al: Secundum type atrial septal defects: Early and late results of surgical repair using extracoporeal circulation in 275 patients. Surgery 59:155–164, 1966

67. Popper RW, Knott JMS, Selzer A, et al: Arrhythmias after cardiac surgery: I. Uncomplicated atrial septal defect. Am Heart J 64:455–461, 1962

68. Reid JM, Stevenson JC: Cardiac arrhythmias following successful surgical closure of atrial septal defect. Br Heart J 29:742–747, 1960

69. Rosky LP, Rodman T: Medical aspects of open heart surgery. N Engl J Med 274:833–840, 1966

70. Rosenthal A: personal communication

71. Young D: Later results of closure of secundum atrial septal defect in children. Am J Cardiol 31:14–22, 1973

72. Siltanen P: Atrial septal defect of secundum type in adults. Acta Med Scand 497 (Suppl):52–67, 1968

73. Levy MJ, Cuello L, Tuna N, et al: Atrioventricularis communis. Am J Cardiol 14:587–598, 1964

74. Milnor WR, Bertrand CA: The electrocardiogram in atrial septal defect: A study of twenty-four cases with observation. Am J Med 22:223–233, 1957

75. Averill KH, Vogel JHK, Prior R, et al: Complete heart block following intracardiac surgery: Reversion to normal simus rhythm after twenty-five months. Am J Cardiol 14:556–560, 1964

76. Lee Y, Scherlis L: Atrial septal defect: Electrocardiographic, vectorcardiographic and catherization data. Circulation 25:1024–1041, 1962

77. Burch GE, DePasquale N: The spatial vectorcardiogram in proved congenital atrial septal defect. Am Heart J 58:319–326, 1959

78. Leibman J, Nadas AS: The vectorcardiogram in the differential diagnosis of atrial septal defect in children. Circulation 22:956–975, 1960

79. Chabot M, Karamehmet A, Bourassa M, et al: Vectorcardiographic evaluation of postoperative changes

in patients with interatrial septal defect: A review of 55 cases. Can Med Assoc J 93:1340–1345, 1965

80. Boineau JP, Moore EN, Patterson DF: Relationship between the ECG, ventricular activation, and the ventricular conduction system in ostium primum ASD. Circulation 48:556–564, 1973

81. Durrer D, Roos JP, Van Dam RT: The genesis of the electrocardiogram of patients with ostium primum defects (ventral atrial septal defects). Am Heart J 71:642–650, 1966

82. Lev M: Conduction system in congenital heart disease. Am J Cardiol 21:619–627, 1968

83. Feldt RH, DuShane JW, Titus JL: The atrioventricular conduction system in persistent common atrioventricular canal defect: Correlations with electrocardiogram. Circulation 42:437–444, 1970

84. Borkon AM, Varghese PJ, Pieroni DR, et al: An alternative explanation for superior axis in ostium primum ASD other than left anterior hemiblock. Pediatr Res 8 (Abstract):347, 73, 1974

85. Kaplan S: Atrial septal defects, in Watson H (ed): Paediatric Cardiology, St. Louis, CV Mosby, 1968

86. Waldo AL, Kaiser GA, Bowman FO Jr, et al: Etiology of prolongation of the PR interval in patients with an endocardial cushion defect: Further observations on internodal conduction and the polarity of the retrograde P wave. Circulation 48:19–26, 1973

87. Chen S, Arcilla RA, Moulder PV, et al: Postoperative conduction disturbances in atrial septal defect. Am J Cardiol 22:636–644, 1968

88. Fryda RJ, Kaplan S, Helmsworth JA: Postoperative complete heart block in children. Br Heart J 33:456–462, 1971

89. Gerbode R, Sanches PA, Arguero R, et al: Endocardial cushion defects. Ann Surg 166:486–495, 1967

90. Kaiser GA, Waldo AL, Beach PM, et al: Specialized cardiac conduction system: Improved electrophysiologic identification technique at surgery. Arch Surg 101:673–676, 1970

91. Lillehei CW, Sellers RD, Bonnabeau RC Jr, et al: Chronic postsurgical complete heart block: With particular reference to prognosis, management and a new P-wave pacemaker. J Thorac Cardiovasc Surg 46:436–456, 1963

92. Backman H: Influence of structural and functional features of ventricular septal defect on frontal plan QRS axis of the electrocardiogram. Br Heart J 34:274–283, 1972

93. Fyler DC, Rudolph AM, Wittenborg MH, et al: Ventricular septal defect in infants and children: Circulation 18:833–851, 1958

94. DuShane JW, Weidman WH, Brandenburg RV, et al: The electrocardiogram in children with ventricular septal defect and severe pulmonary hypertension. Circulation 22:49–54, 1960

95. Vince DJ, Keith JD: The electrocardiogram in ventricular septal defect: Circulation 23:225–240, 1961

96. Adams P Jr, Anderson RC, Lillehei CW, et al: Reversibility of pulmonary hypertension following closure of ventricular septal defect. Am J Dis Child 98:558, 1959

97. Bristow JD, Kassebaum DG, Starr A, et al: Observations on the occurrence of right bundle branch block following open repair of ventricular septal defects. Circulation 22:896–900, 1960

98. Goldberg H: Right bundle-branch block: A vectorcardiographic and electrocardiographic study of ventricular septal defect following open-heart surgery. Circulation 20:201–207, 1959

99. Coggin CJ, Wardham EE, Selvester RH: Postventriculotomy right bundle branch block: Its etiology. Circulation 22 (Abstract): 734, 1971

100. Gelband H, Waldo AL, Kaiser GA, et al: Etiology of right bundle branch block in patients undergoing total correction of tetralogy of Fallot. Circulation 44:1022–1033, 1971

101. Hefler SE, Malm JR, Bowman FO, et al: Further observations on the etiology of right bundle branch block pattern following right ventriculotomy. Proc Am Acad Ped: Sec Ped Card, 1973

102. Okoroma EO, Guller B, Maloney JD, et al: Etiology of right bundle branch block following closure of ventricular septal defect. Pediatr Res 8 (Abstract):353, 79, 1974

103. Truex RC, Bishof JK: Conduction system in human hearts with intraventricular septal defects. J Thorac Surg 35:421–439, 1958

104. Reemtsma K, Copenhaver WM, Creech O Jr: The cardiac conduction system in congenital anomalies of the heart: Studies on its embryology, anatomy, and function. Surgery 44:99–108, 1958

105. Reemtsma K, Copenhaver WM: Anatomic studies of the cardiac conduction system in congenital malformations of the heart. Circulation 17:271–276, 1958

106. Reemtsma K, Delgado JR, Creech O Jr: Heart block following intracardiac surgery: Localization of conduction tissue injury. J Thorac Cardiovasc Surg 39: 688–693, 1960

107. Titus JL, Daugherty GW, Edwards JE: Anatomy of the atrioventricular conduction system in ventricular septal defect. Circulation 28:72–81, 1963

108. Latham RA, Anderson RH: Anatomical variations in atrioventricular conduction system with reference to ventricular septal defects. Br Heart J 34:185–190, 1972

109. Titus JL, Daugherty GW, Kirklin JW, et al: Lesions of the atrioventricular conduction system after repair of ventricular septal defect: Relation to heart block. Circulation 28:82–88, 1963

110. Lev M, Fell EH, Arcilla R, et al: Surgical injury to the conduction system in ventricular septal defect. Am J Cardiol 14:464–476, 1964

111. Kulbertus HE, Coyne JJ, Hallidie-Smith KA: Conduction disturbances before and after surgical closure of ventricular septal defect. Am Heart J 77:123–131, 1969

112. Downing JW Jr, Kaplan S, Bove KE: Postsurgical left anterior hemiblock and right bundle-branch block. Br Heart J 34:263–270, 1972

113. Gerbode R, Kerth WJ, Keen G, et al: Surgical heart block. Arch Surg 86:890–896, 1963

114. Sayed HM: Complete heart block following open heart surgery. J Cardiovasc Surg 6:426–435, 1965

115. Hurwitz RA, Riemenschneider TA, Moss AJ:

Chronic postoperative heart block in children. Am J Cardiol 21:185–189, 1968

116. Murphy DA, Graham GR, Tynan M, et al: Prognosis of complete atrioventricular dissociation in children after open-heart surgery. Lancet 1:750–752, 1970

117. Kirklin JW, Harshbarger HS, Donald DE, et al: Surgical correction of ventricular septal defect: Anastomosis and technical considerations. J Thorac Surg 33:45–59, 1957

118. Bocala RR, Guller B, Danielson GK, et al: Left anterior hemiblock and complete repair of tetralogy of Fallot. Pediatr Res 8 (Abstract):347, 73, 1974

119. Moller J: Shunt operations in morbus caeruleus. Acta Paediatr 134 (Suppl):55–69, 1962

120. Malm JR, Blumenthal S, Bowman FO Jr, et al: Factors that modify hemodynamic results in total correction of tetralogy of Fallot. J Thorac Cardiovasc Surg 52: 502–513, 1966

121. Zender R, Klinner W: Total correction of tetralogy of Fallot. Dis Chest 51:311–314, 1967

122. Bristow JD, Menashe VD, Griswold HE, et al: Total correction of tetralogy of Fallot: Complications and results. Am J Cardiol 8:358–368, 1961

123. Squarcia U, Meridith J, McGoon DC, et al: Prognosis of transient atrioventricular conduction disturbances complicating open heart surgery for congenital heart defects. Am J Cardiol 28:648–652, 1971

124. Potter RT, Liu L, Maynard EP Jr: Post-surgical heart block: Report of a case with bilateral bundle-branch block and changing rhythms. Br Heart J 33:412–415, 1971

125. Chesler E, Beck W, Schrire V: Left anterior hemiblock and right bundle branch block before and after surgical repair of tetralogy of Fallot. Am Heart J 84:45–52, 1972

126. Moss AJ, Klyman G, Emmanovilides GC: Late onset complete heart block. Am J Cardiol 30:884–887, 1972

127. Rosen KM, Megta A, Rahimtoola AH, et al: Sites of congenital and surgical heart block as defined by His bundle electrocardiography. Circulation 44:833–841, 1971

128. Anderson PAW, Rogers MC, Canent RV Jr, et al: Reversible complete heart block following cardiac surgery: Analysis of His bundle electrograms. Circulation 46: 514–521, 1972

129. Lev M: The architecture of the conduction system in congenital heart disease: II. Tetralogy of Fallot. AMA Arch Path 67:114, 572–587, 1959

130. Wolff GS, Rowland TW, Ellison RC: Surgically induced right bundle branch block with left anterior hemiblock: An ominous sign in postoperative tetralogy of Fallot. Circulation 46:587–594, 1972

131. Godman MJ, Roberts NK, Izukawa T: Late postoperative conduction disturbances after repair of ventricular septal defects in tetralogy of Fallot: Analysis by His bundle recordings. Circulation 49:214–221, 1974

132. Rosenbaum MB, Corrado G, Oliveri R, et al: Right bundle branch block with left anterior hemiblock surgically induced in tetralogy of Fallot: Relation to the mechanism of electrocardiographic changes in endocardial cushion defects. Am J Cardiol 26:12–18, 1970

Assessment of the Postoperative Patient by Noninvasive Techniques

John F. Keane, Roberta Williams, Salvador Treves, and Amnon Rosenthal

THE NUMBER of children with repaired or palliated congenital cardiac lesions reaching adulthood is growing yearly. In many of these patients, a variety of cardiac abnormalities persist or new manifestations appear as a consequence of the surgical procedures. At present, cardiac catheterization remains the most accurate and reliable method for assessing the results of surgery in patients with congenital heart disease. However, a number of noninvasive laboratory studies have acquired new significance as a result of precise correlations with hemodynamic studies. When utilized in conjunction with the history and physical findings, these techniques are very helpful in the evaluation and management of the postoperative patient. The changes occurring after surgery in the most frequently obtained laboratory tests, chest x-ray and electrocardiogram, are described elsewhere. In this section, we have confined our remarks to four less commonly utilized but very useful techniques: vectorcardiogram, echocardiogram, radionuclide angiocardiography, and ear oximetry. When does one use these techniques to estimate the hemodynamic abnormality? How reliable are the techniques in the postoperative patient with a particular lesion? Answers to these questions will be provided separately for each of the techniques. In general, the best information is obtained when the equipment is well maintained and frequently calibrated, the study performed by an experienced technician and interpreted by a knowledgeable physician familiar with the usefulness and limitation of the method. Comparisons between the preoperative and postoperative data in the same patient are particularly rewarding.

From the Departments of Cardiology and Radiology, Division of Nuclear Medicine of The Children's Hospital Medical Center, and the Departments of Radiology and Pediatrics, Harvard Medical School, Boston, Mass.

Supported in part by NIH grant HL10436, Bethesda, Md and a grant-in-aid from the American Heart Association, New York, N. Y.

Reprint requests should be addressed to John F. Keane, M.D., Department of Cardiology, The Children's Hospital Medical Center, Harvard Medical School, 25 Shattuck Avenue, Boston, Mass. 02115.

VECTORCARDIOGRAPHY

The preoperative vectorcardiogram (VCG) has been shown to be of value in a variety of abnormalities, being utilized to estimate ventricular pressure, to assess ventricular cavity size, and to differentiate uncomplicated atrial and ventricular septal defects from those associated with endocardial cushion defects.[1–13] However, there are relatively few published reports concerning the changes in the VCG following surgery. A reduction in left ventricular hypertrophy was reported following aortic valvotomy[1,14,15] and a decrease in right ventricular hypertrophy following pulmonary valvotomy,[1,16,17] atrial septal defect closure[17–20] and repair of tetralogy of Fallot.[1,17] Conduction disturbances such as right bundle branch block with or without left anterior hemiblock after tetralogy of Fallot and ventricular septal defect repair, are described.[1,21–23]

The postoperative VCG changes in a number of congenital cardiac lesions will be reviewed. Repeated references will be made throughout to a recent monogram by Ellison.[1] Most authors cited have used the Frank lead system.[24]

Valvar Aortic Stenosis

The VCG, specifically the left maximum spatial vector (LMSV), has been shown to be of value in the preoperative assessment of the severity of aortic stenosis.[1–4,10] However, in our experience there is no significant correlation between the LMSV and left ventricular systolic pressure postoperatively (Fig. 1). Ellison[1] noted that while the LMSV frequently decreased, it remained unchanged in many including those without a significant residual gradient. However, among a group of patients in our institution with pre- and postoperative catheterizations and VCG's, when the LMSV decreased the left ventricular pressure was also reduced and in no patient did the LMSV decrease while left ventricular pressure increased (Fig. 2). Although the 10-msec vector decreased in the majority of patients, no significant correlation was noted between the change in magnitude and change in left ventricular pressure. Similarly, although anterior displacement of the LMSV occurred in many, no relationship was noted between

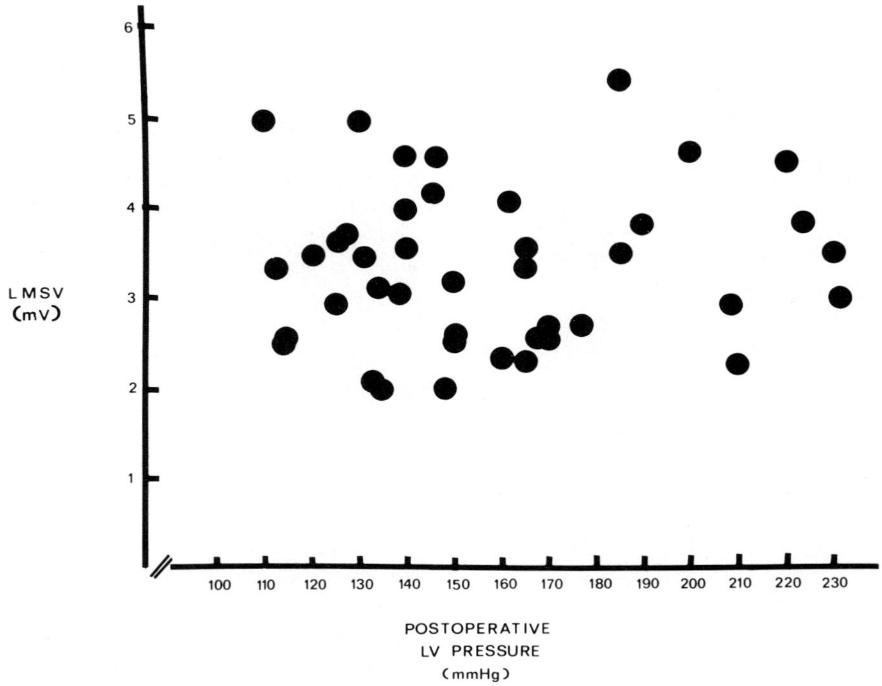

Fig. 1. **The relationship between the left maximum spatial vector (LMSV) and left ventricular (LV) pressure following aortic valvotomy in 42 patients with congenital aortic stenosis. There is no significant correlation between the LMSV and LV pressure. (mV = millivolts).**

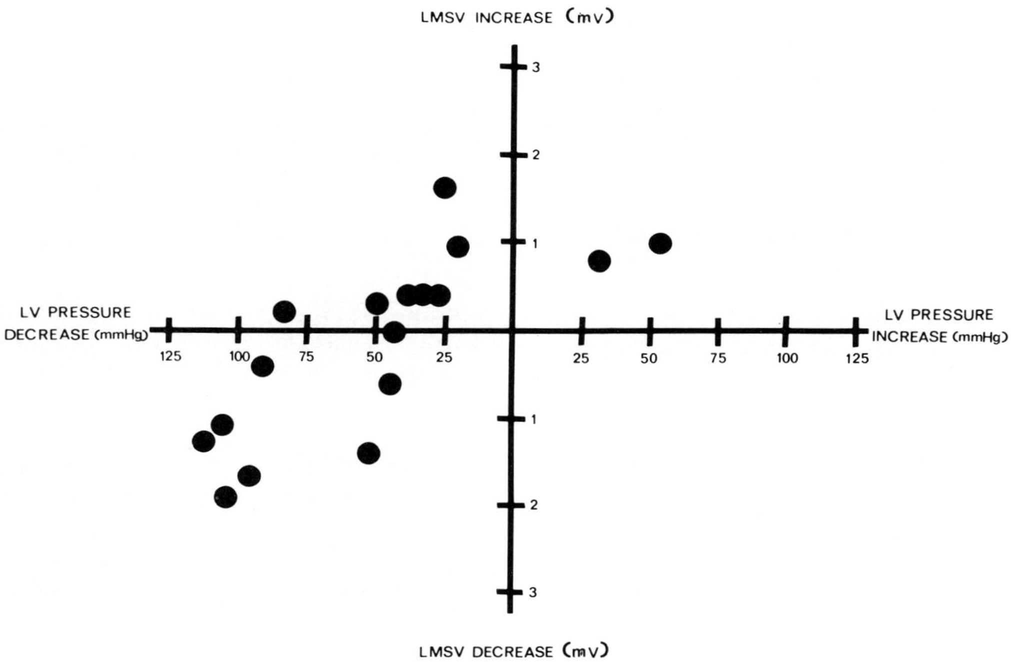

Fig. 2. **Pre- and postoperative changes in left maximum spatial vector (LMSV) related to changes in left ventricular (LV) pressure in 17 patients with aortic stenosis. In no patient did the LMSV decrease while the LV pressure increased. (mV = millivolts).**

these azimuth changes and left ventricular pressure changes. Discordant T loops were noted by Ellison[1] to persist in many, even in those with adequate relief of the obstruction and without significant aortic regurgitation.

Edibam[14] noted a reduction of left ventricular hypertrophy after surgery (6–36 mo postop) in 25 children. The patients, however, were not catheterized and reduction of left ventricular hypertrophy was interpreted on the basis of a reduction in the 40-msec and maximum QRS vectors in the horizontal plane and a more anterior displacement of this latter vector. The 10-msec vector was also noted to decrease, the significance of which was unclear. In another publication concerning 32 children[15] (6–18 mo postop), again without catheterization data, a significant reduction in LMSV was observed.

Discrete Subvalvar Aortic Stenosis

Among four patients catheterized postoperatively, the LMSV was found by Ellison[1] to remain elevated, despite adequate relief of the obstruction in two. The increased LMSV could, however, be explained by residual mitral or aortic regurgitation which was present in all patients. Initial anterior forces remained decreased and the T loops were discordant in three of the patients.

Coarctation of the Aorta

Maron[25] described a variety of electrocardiographic and VCG abnormalities after resection of coarctation (average follow-up 18.4 yr: mean age at operation, 22 yr) in 38 of 59 patients. The commonest abnormalities observed were premature ventricular beats, left anterior hemiblock, and left ventricular hypertrophy.

Valvar Pulmonary Stenosis

While the right maximum spatial vector (RMSV) correlates significantly with right ventricular pressure preoperatively,[1,3,4] Ellison[1] observed no significant correlation in the postoperative state (1-13 yr). The RMSV remained elevated in almost one-half of the 19 patients, despite adequate relief of the obstruction. Furthermore, although the horizontal loop was counterclockwise postoperatively in most patients, it remained clockwise in some despite the absence of any significant obstruction. Nevertheless, in those in whom the RMSV decreased, right ventricular pressure had also decreased.

In an earlier report involving 12 patients catheterized postoperatively (average age at operation, 26 yr), Kahn,[16] using the cube method,[26] observed that VCG changes accurately reflected changes in the right ventricular load. Incomplete regression of right ventricular hypertrophy was felt to indicate either an inadequate period of observation, incomplete surgical relief, or the presence of other hemodynamically significant defects. The VCG became normal in four patients with only small residual gradients. In these, the QRS orientation changed from right and anterior to left and posterior and the horizontal loop inscription changed from clockwise to counterclockwise. In four patients, without postoperative VCG changes, two had moderate residual obstruction while two had only trivial residual gradients; but the period of follow-up was felt inadequate. Significant regression may occur with time as shown in one patient in whom incomplete resolution at 13 mo progressed to complete resolution of right ventricular hypertrophy at 27 mo postoperatively. In two patients with trivial residual stenosis, right ventricular hypertrophy, as manifested by the horizontal loop, decreased. In the remaining patient with severe residual infundibular stenosis, the horizontal loop remained clockwise and anterior.

Among 32 children without postoperative catheterization data, Shams[15] reported a progressive decrease in RMSV without significant changes in LMSV. Similar observations were noted by Benchimol[17] in one child.

Atrial Septal Defect

In a report concerning 42 children with secundum atrial septal defects, without postoperative catheterization data, Shams[15] observed no significant change in the RMSV within 10 days; but a significant reduction in RMSV within 18 mo after surgical closure of the defect. The LMSV increased at both of these observation intervals. Using the cube system,[26] Chabot[18] reported on the postoperative VCG changes in 55 patients (age range, 4-44 yr; follow-up 2 wk-6 yr) without postoperative catheterizations. Of 49 patients with secundum defects, the ratio of right to left electromotive forces decreased by more than 20% in 42, remained unchanged in six and increased in the remaining patient. The ratio of anterior to posterior electromotive forces decreased by more than 20% in 34 patients. Among seven patients without posterior forces, anterior forces decreased in six. The horizontal loop configuration changed from figure of eight to counterclockwise in 14, from clockwise to counterclockwise in ten, from clockwise to figure of eight in six, and remained unchanged in 19 patients. Findings among six patients with ostium primum defects were similar except that the horizontal loop remained unchanged in most. Of the entire group of 55 patients, the VCG improved in 50 but became normal in only four. The VCG changes commenced within 3 mo while major changes occurred within the first year. When the preoperative conduction delay exceeded 30 msec, it persisted postoperatively.

In 1973, Hisamatsu[19] reporting on 21 patients (age range, 5–30 yr) showed that those with moderate right ventricular overload preoperatively had marked regression toward a normal pattern 1 mo postoperatively. Patients with pulmonary artery hypertension preoperatively had no horizontal loop changes 1 mo after surgery; but 1 yr later the loop, initially anterior, had become more posterior and leftward. Of 15 patients without a right ventricular conduction delay preoperatively, the ratio of left to right electromotive forces had increased at 1 yr while remaining unchanged in the six patients with a preoperative conduction delay. The ratio of posterior to anterior electromotive forces increased in both groups. One yr postoperatively, nine patients had a right ventricular conduction delay compared to six preoperatively. The T loop, abnormal at 1 mo, was normal by the end of the first year.

Among 50 children under 17 years of age with secundum atrial septal defects, all but two catheterized 6 mo–6 yr postoperatively,[20] the VCG became normal in 17 while right ventricular hypertrophy persisted in 30. The postoperative VCG was of little help in identifying the five patients who had residual shunts. Chen[27] reported VCG changes among 60 patients (45 of whom were less than 16 yr at operation), without postoperative cardiac catheterization data. Right bundle branch block disappeared in two of five patients who had this conduction abnormality preoperatively, appeared and persisted throughout the follow-up period of a few years in five, and was transiently observed in 13. In another report of seven patients (median age, 15 yr) with secundum defects, Benchimol[17] observed an increase in the left maximum vector in the horizontal plane in six patients in the early postoperative period together with an increase in the ratio of the left to right maximum vector in five. The right maximum vector and the ratio of the anterior to posterior electromotive forces decreased in three while the horizontal loop configuration remained unchanged in five patients.

Ventricular Septal Defect

Following pulmonary artery banding in 11 children with ventricular septal defect, Ellison[1] observed an increase in the RMSV in all, reflecting the increased right ventricular pressure load. There was a change to a clockwise or figure of eight pattern of the horizontal loop in 10 patients. The LMSV became anteriorly directed in all. More than 1-yr following surgical closure of the VSD in seven patients, the RMSV remained slightly increased and did not correlate significantly with right ventricular pressure. In five patients without a residual left-to-right shunt, the LMSV was normal.

Right bundle branch block and left anterior hemiblock occurs in some patients following surgical closure of a ventricular septal defect and vectorcardiographically is characterized by a counterclockwise superior rotation of the frontal plane QRS loop. This occurred in seven of 109 patients reported by Downing,[22] all of whom were asymptomatic 1–10 yr postoperatively. However, Kulbertus[23] suggested that the prognosis of this combined conduction abnormality might be unfavorable.

Patent Ductus Arteriosus

In a study of 49 children, Shams[15] observed a decrease in the LMSV within 18 mo following closure of the ductus.

Tetralogy of Fallot

In seven children with tetralogy of Fallot, Khoury[21] observed that following a systemic to pulmonary shunt procedure the QRS was less rightward, the horizontal loop more leftward and posterior and the left ventricular forces greater. Following repair, right bundle branch block (RBBB) appeared in 9 of 10 patients. Ellison[1] noted that among patients with high systemic arterial oxygen saturations, with or without systemic to pulmonary shunts, the LMSV was higher than in those with low saturations. The horizontal loop inscription was either counterclockwise or figure of eight reflecting the left ventricular volume load. Similar findings have been reported by Muster.[29] Among 10 patients catheterized after repair, Ellison[1] reported that although the majority had RBBB, the RMSV correlated well with the residual right ventricular pressure. When the right ventricular pressure was < 50 mm Hg, the RMSV had returned to normal. The horizontal loop rotation was counterclockwise in all but one.

Among three patients with repaired tetralogy of Fallot, Benchimol[17] observed that in the early postoperative period, the RMSV decreased and the LMSV increased in one while the horizontal loop rotation changed from a clockwise to a figure of eight pattern in two.

The combination of RBBB and left anterior hemiblock occurs in some patients after repair of tetralogy of Fallot and is easily identifiable by VCG (Fig. 3). In a report concerning 282 patients (age range, 18 mo–45 yr) who underwent ventricular septal defect closure (140 patients with an isolated defect, 136 with tetralogy of Fallot, and six with common atrioventricular canal), Kulbertus[25] observed episodes of complete heart block postoperatively in 24, of whom 11 died suddenly. Among these 24 patients, there were 11 who had either congenital or postsurgical RBBB and left anterior hemiblock and it was concluded that this combined conduction abnormality probably indicated a poor prognosis. In another report concerning 291 patients who underwent repair of tetralogy of Fallot, Wolff[28] noted the occurrance of this combined conduction abnormality in 24. During the period of follow-up (1–12 yr) complete heart block appeared in ten, serious ventricular arrhythmias occurred in four, and there were six deaths (three of the patients died suddenly). These complications were considerably less frequent among the postoperative patients who did not have RBBB with left anterior hemiblock.

Anomalous Origin of the Left Coronary Artery From the Pulmonary Artery

This rare lesion, seen most commonly in infancy, is characterized vectorcardiographically by a frontal plane loop which is counterclockwise and superior and a horizontal loop which is clockwise reflecting the anterolateral myocardial infarction. Ellison[1] observed that following ligation of the anomalous vessel in infancy the frontal loop usually remained unchanged. The configuration of the horizontal loop reverted to a counterclockwise pattern in patients with symptomatic and hemodynamic improvement (Fig. 4) while little change was noted in those who subsequently died. However, similar improvement in the horizontal loop was noted in two patients who survived without operation. This vectorcardiographic change was considered to indicate a more favorable prognosis. Puri[30] reported an increase in leftward and anterior forces and a slight decrease of frontal plane elevation after ligation of the anomalous vessel.

Transposition of the Great Arteries With Intact Ventricular Septum

Following creation of an atrial septal defect in seven infants with this anomaly, Ellison[1] reported a decrease in the ratio of left to right ventricular pressure which was reflected by a change in the horizontal loop from a counterclockwise to a

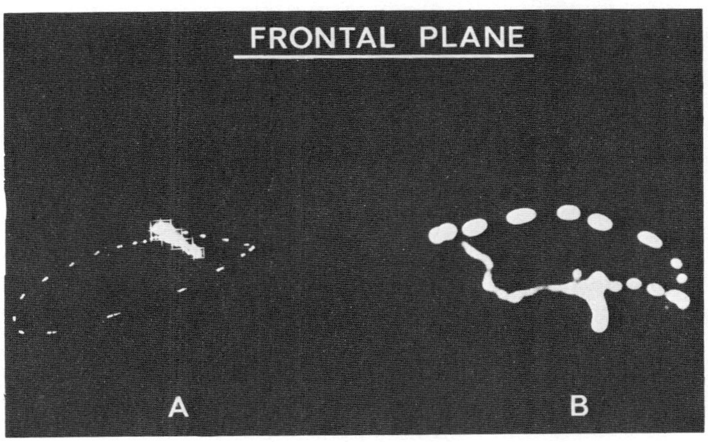

Fig. 3. Frontal plane loop in a patient with tetralogy of Fallot (blunt end of tear drop leads). (A) preoperatively, age 8 mo: showing clockwise rotation, and (B) postoperatively, age 8 yr: now counterclockwise and superior indicating left anterior hemiblock and right bundle branch block.

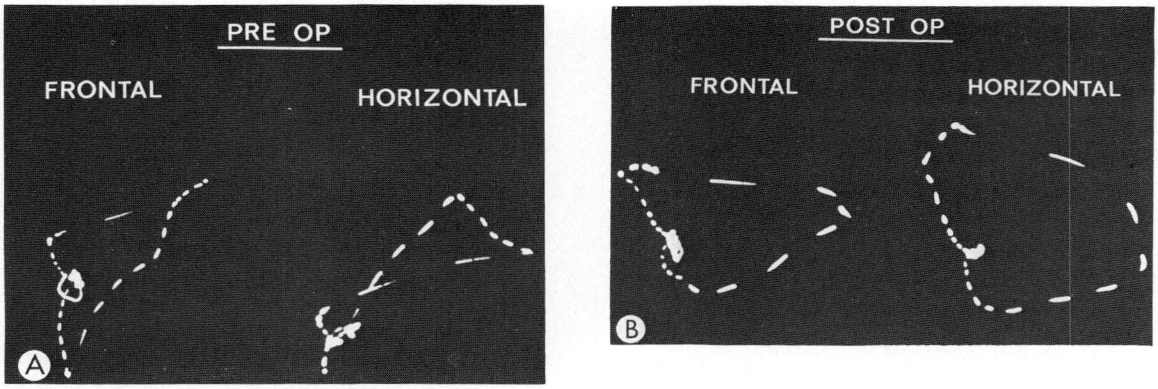

Fig. 4. Frontal and horizontal plane loops, preoperatively (preop) and postoperatively (postop) in a patient with anomalous left coronary artery originating from the pulmonary artery; the anomalous vessel was ligated at age 9 mo (blunt end of tear drop leads). (A) Preop, age 9 mo: frontal plane counterclockwise and superior (left anterior hemiblock): horizontal loop indicating loss of anterior and lateral forces due to infarction. (B) postop, age 4 yr: frontal plane rotation unchanged: horizontal loop now normal showing excellent recovery of anterior and lateral forces.

clockwise pattern in six. There is no vectorcardiographic data as yet reported in patients following the Mustard[31] procedure.

Summary

In conclusion, the postoperative VCG appears to be of value in some congenital cardiac lesions. Following aortic valvotomy, the LMSV frequently decreases. Among a small group of patients with pre- and postoperative catheterization data, none was noted to have a decrease in the LMSV while the left ventricular pressure increased. This relationship requires further investigation. There is, however, no significant correlation between the LMSV and left ventricular pressure postoperatively as there is preoperatively.

Following pulmonary valvotomy, the RMSV frequently decreases but remains elevated in many despite adequate relief of the obstruction. However, among a small group of patients catheterized postoperatively, when the RMSV decreased, the right ventricular pressure was also found to be reduced. Again, the number of patients involved was small and this, too, requires further study. While horizontal configuration returns toward a normal pattern in most, it continues to remain clockwise, suggesting significant right ventricular hypertension in some despite adequate relief of the obstruction.

Following atrial septal defect closure, there is reduction of right ventricular electromotive forces in most but the VCG rarely returns to normal. The VCG does not appear to be of value in detecting residual atrial left-to-right shunting.

There is surprisingly little data available about the VCG following ventricular septal defect closure. Now that the transatrial approach to closure seems to be increasing, changes in LMSV may be of value in long-term postoperative follow-up. One would expect the LMSV to decrease as happens in other left ventricular volume overload lesions such as patent ductus arteriosus.

Following repair of tetralogy of Fallot, the VCG is useful in identifying RBBB and left anterior hemiblock, a conduction disturbance of ominous significance. A similar abnormality occurs in some patients following ventricular septal closure.

The VCG, specifically the horizontal loop, is of value in the follow-up of patients who have undergone ligation of an anomalous left coronary artery. In patients with transposition of the great arteries and intact ventricular septum who have undergone atrial septal defect creation, the horizontal loop rotation is of value in estimating left ventricular pressure.

ECHOCARDIOGRAPHY

Echocardiography is a well established noninvasive technique utilized in the diagnosis of congenital heart disease. Its use in evaluation of the postoperative patient may be classified into two broad categories: (1) changes in the morphological features characteristic for the specific lesion (qualitative features) and (2) assessment of myocardial function (quantitative features). To date, experience with postoperative subjects has been largely limited to qualitative analysis; its quantitative use remains an untapped resource for longitudinal postoperative evaluation.

Atrial Septal Defect

The diagnostic features of right ventricular (RV) volume overload include paradoxical septal motion and increased right ventricular dimension.[32–36] In addition, Tajik[33] studied six patients 4–8 days after atrial septal defect closure and found persistent reversal of septal motion. Right ventricular dimensions were smaller than preoperative measurements but continued to be above the normal value. On the other hand, Meyer reported the appearance of normal septal motion in 12 of 18 patients studied 10 days–6 mo after atrial septal defect closure[32] (Fig. 5). Associated with this change in septal motion was a decrease in right ventricular dimension by one-third or more of the preoperative measurement. Patients whose right ventricular dimensions were not reduced by this amount retained the pattern of septal reversal. From these studies one might conclude that severe or long standing RV volume overload usually produces a change in right ventricular function resulting in persistence of the echocardiographic pattern of septal reversal and some increase in right ventricular dimension.

Mitral Stenosis

An increase in diastolic closure rate of the mitral valve after mitral commissurotomy in patients with rheumatic mitral stenosis has been described.[37,38] Lundstrom[39] described three patients with congenital mitral stenosis who had undergone valvulotomy. In each case, an increase in diastolic closure rate (E–F slope) suggested an improvement in the gradient across the mitral valve, although hemodynamic improvement was not confirmed by catheterization. Comparison of pre- and postoperative echocardiograms in a patient with parachute mitral valve is shown in Fig. 6. An increase in E–F slope of the mitral valve from 0–15 mm/sec to 50 mm/sec occurred following fenestration of the leaflet.

Left Ventricular Outflow Obstruction

Ultrasound has been used in the evaluation of medical and surgical therapy for IHSS. Shah et al.[40] reported that the anterior systolic motion of

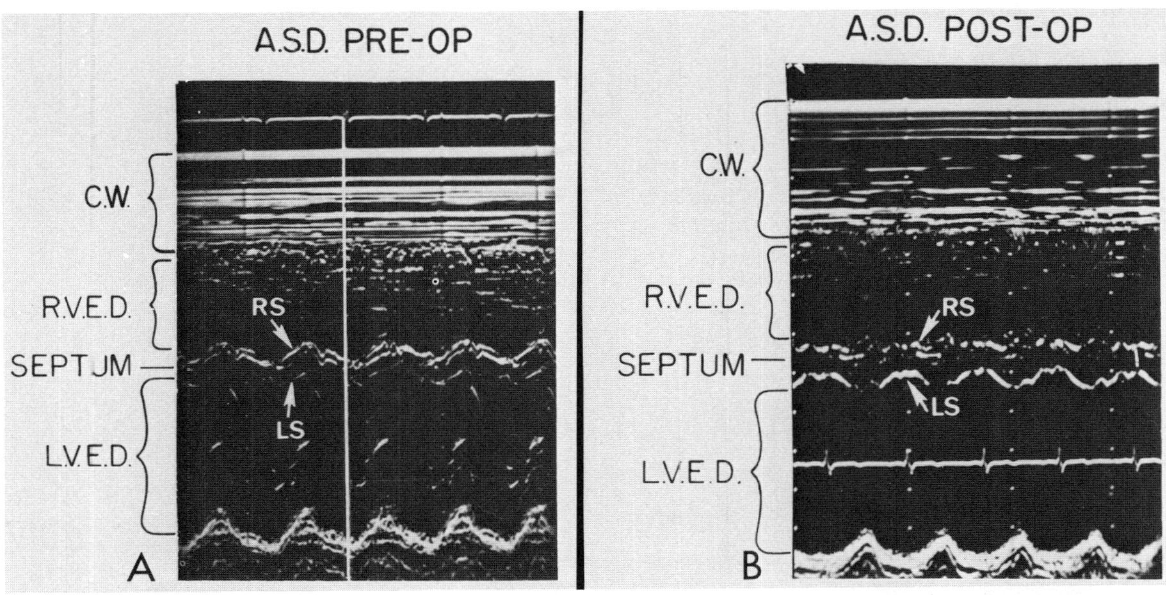

Fig. 5. (A) Preoperative and (B) postoperative echograms of a patient with secundum atrial septal defect (ASD). Preoperative echogram shows reversal of septal motion and enlarged right ventricle (3.2 cm/M^2). White line corresponds to Q wave of electrocardiogram. Postoperative echogram showing return of septal motion to normal and diminished right ventricular size (2.5 cm/sq/m). CW = chest wall; RVED = right ventricular end-diastolic dimension; RS = right septum; LS = left septum; LVED = left ventricular end-diastolic dimension. (By permission.[32])

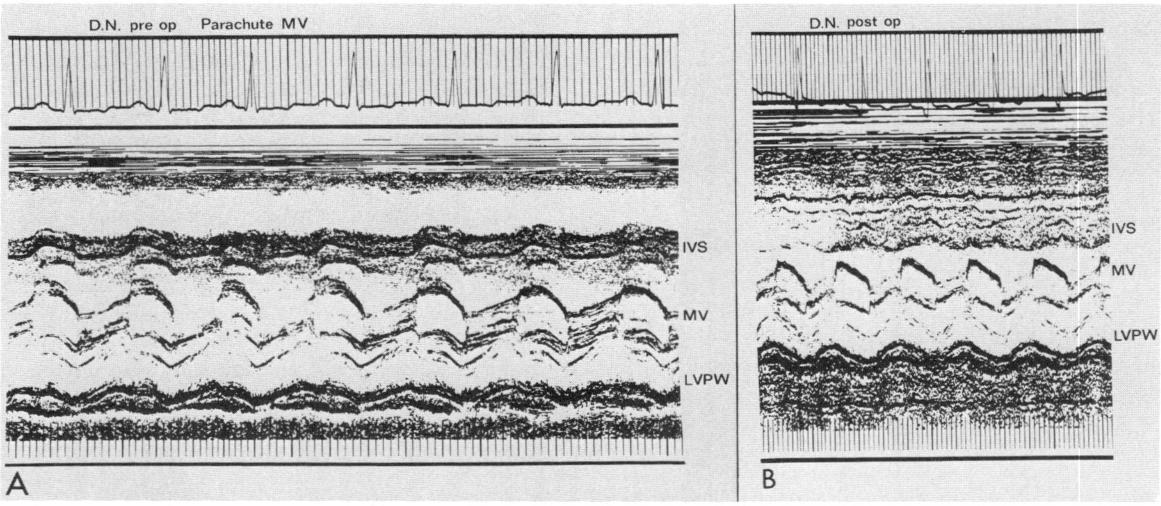

Fig. 6. (A) Preoperative echogram in a patient with a large diastolic pressure gradient across a parachute mitral valve (MV). The mitral valve is shown within the left ventricle bounded by the interventricular septum (IVS) anteriorly and the left ventricular posterior wall (LVPW) posteriorly. Multiple echos of the MV are seen during systole. With diastole, the anterior leaflet moves with an excursion of 1.4 cm which is modestly limited. The diastolic closure rate is 0–15 mm/sec depending on the points selected for measurement. Note that the 'posterior' leaflet of the MV moves posteriorly in early diastole, unlike patients with rheumatic or other forms of congenital mitral stenosis. (B) Postoperatively diastolic excursion of the MV remains 1.4 cm, but the diastolic closure rate has increased to 50 mm/sec, suggesting a decrease in gradient across the valve following fenestration of the valve leaflet anteriorly.

the anterior leaflet of the mitral valve, characteristic of left ventricular outflow obstruction in patients with IHSS, was abolished after surgical palliation in 11/14 patients (Fig. 7). The three patients with incomplete relief of obstruction continued to show an anterior systolic motion of the mitral valve

Popp et al.[41] examined two patients before and after resection of discrete fibromuscular subaortic stenosis. The postoperative echocardiogram of one patient showed a slight increase in the width of the left ventricular outflow tract associated with a thinning of the basal portion of the interventricular septum compared with the preoperative tracing. No change in left ventricular outflow dimension could be demonstrated following excision of a fibromuscular ring in the other patient.

In our laboratory, we have seen this same variability in the postoperative tracings following resection of both discrete and long segment left ventricular outflow obstruction in four patients with normally related great arteries and five patients with transposition of the great arteries. In Fig. 8 the pre- and postoperative scans in a patient

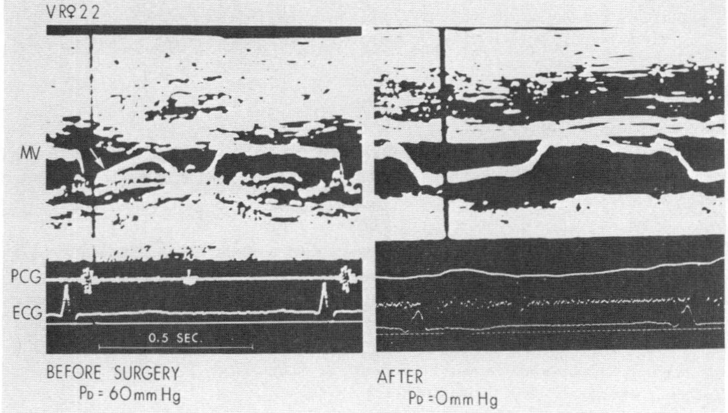

Fig. 7. Echocardiogram of mitral valve (MV) in a patient with idiopathic hypertrophic subaortic stenosis recorded before and after surgery. It shows the presence of significant abnormality before surgery (left panel arrow), which disappeared after surgery (right panel). Resting pressure gradient (P_D) across the left ventricular outflow was reduced from 60 mm Hg–0 (by permission[40]).

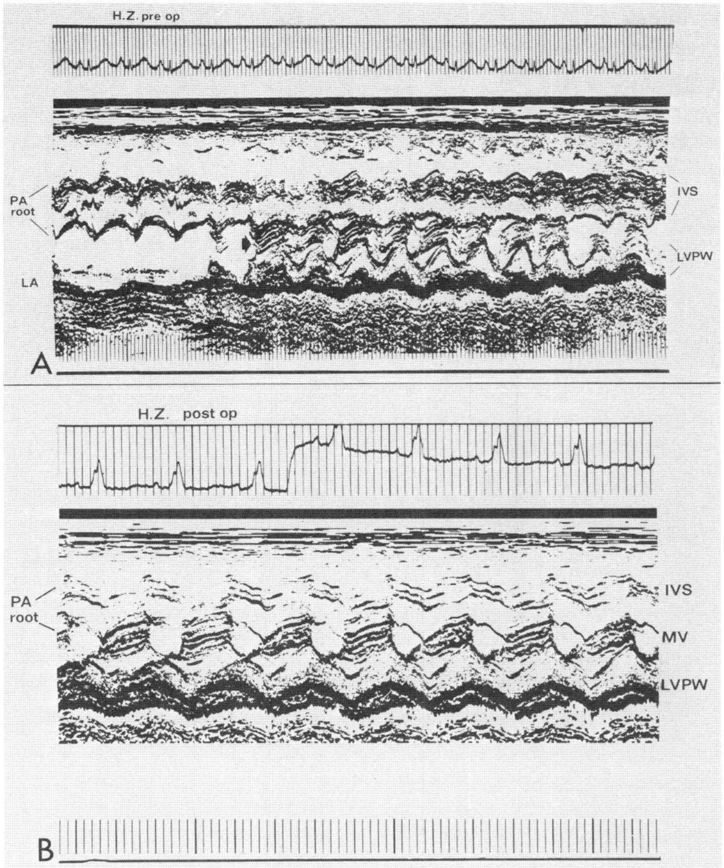

Fig. 8. (A) Preoperative scan in a patient with D-transposition of the great arteries, pulmonary stenosis and intact ventricular septum. A 105-mm Hg gradient across the subpulmonary area was produced by hypertrophy of the interventricular septum (IVS) which encroached on the subpulmonary area. On the left side of the illustration, the pulmonary artery (PA) root is seen containing echos from the pulmonary valve cusps. The transducer was swung inferiorly and to the left until the beam crossed the left ventricular cavity. MV echos (solid arrow) are crowded anteriorly by the left septal surface which is actually at the same level as the posterior border of the PA root. Septal thickness is 0.8 cm while left ventricular posterior wall (LVPW) thickness is 0.5 cm, suggesting asymmetrical septal hypertrophy. Abnormal movement of the mitral valve may be obscured by the severe encroachment of the left septal surface. (B) After surgical excision of a large portion of hypertrophied muscle from the subpulmonary area, thickness of the IVS is now equal to that of the LVPW.

with striking subpulmonary obstruction associated with D-transposition of the great arteries and intact ventricular septum are shown. Following resection of a large amount of hypertrophied septal muscle which bulged into the outflow tract, an increase in width of the subpulmonary area as well as thinning of echos from the interventricular septum in the subpulmonary area was demonstrated. One explanation for the occasional lack of change in left ventricular outflow dimension postoperatively is that the geometry of the left ventricular outflow tract after asymmetric surgical resection does not lend itself to a one dimensional measurement especially if the width of the transducer beam is sufficient to cause overlapping of adjacent structures.

Left Ventricular Function

Echocardiographic determination of left ventricular function although well described[42–51] has not yet been applied to the serial evaluation of postoperative patients. Jarmakani and Graham have described changes in left ventricular volumes, determined by angiography following repair of ventricular septal defect[52] tetralogy of Fallot,[53] and transposition of the great arteries.[54] Echocardiography provides a unique noninvasive means for determining volume changes, ejection fraction, velocity of fiber shortening, and other function studies, at frequent intervals, during both the early and late postoperative periods.

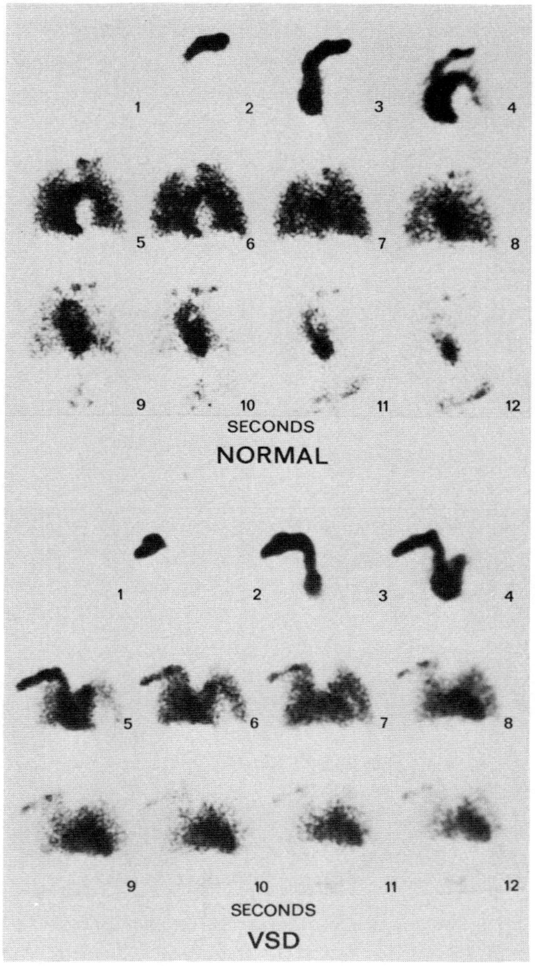

Fig. 9. Top: Normal radionuclide angiocardiogram in the left anterior oblique projection. Frames at 2, 3, and 4 sec show radioactivity within the superior vena cava, right atrium, right ventricle, and pulmonary artery. The lung fields appear in frames at 5 and 6 seconds followed by appearance of radioactivity within the left atrium on frames at 7 and 8 sec. The left ventricle and the aorta are seen on frames at 8, 9, 10, and 11 sec. Note the rapid disappearance of radioactivity from the lungs and right heart. Bottom: Radionuclide angiocardiography (anterior projection) in a patient with a left-to-right shunt through a ventricular septal defect (VSD). The right innominate vein, superior vena cava, right atrium, right ventricle and pulmonary artery are seen on sequence in frames at 2, 3, and 4 sec. Pulmonary radioactivity is apparent first at 5 sec and persists for an abnormally long period of time due to early pulmonary recirculation. Note also the failure to clearly visualize the left heart and the aorta and the persistence of radioactivity with the right heart.

RADIONUCLIDE ANGIOCARDIOGRAPHY (RAC)

The relatively recent availability of gamma scintillation cameras with on-line computer systems and short lived radionuclides, particularly technetium-99^{m} represented a major advance in the diagnosis of cardiovascular lesions by external detection.[55-63] Radionuclide angiocardiography is simple to perform and requires an intravenous injection of radionuclide solution. It has many advantages. The volume of injectate is small (0.1–0.5 ml) and, therefore, no hemodynamic disturbance is produced. The radionuclide solution lacks any pharmacologic effect and the patient's radiation absorbed dose with radiotechnetium is low and within the levels of routine radiographic procedures.[59]

Technetium-99^{m} has a physical half-life of 6 hr and decays with emission of a 140 KeV gamma ray without beta emission. Repeated studies are easily tolerated by the patients and, for the reasons listed above, with no significant risk. A normal radionuclide angiogram with injection in an antecubital vein is shown in Fig. 9, top. It can be seen that the radioindicator circulates through the superior vena cava, right atrium, right ventricle, pulmonary artery, lungs, left atrium, left ventricle, and aorta and provides information on the relative size of the cardiovascular structures. Normal and abnormal circulatory patterns can be detected by visual inspection (qualitative RAC).[57-60] In addition, with the aid of on-line digital computers that can acquire, store, display, and analyze dynamic scintigraphic information, a number of physiologic parameters such as circulation time, cardiac output, ejection fraction, forward stroke volume, shunt flow, and mean pulmonary blood volume

Table 1. Postoperative Evaluation of Patients With Congenital Heart Disease by Radionuclide Angiocardiography

(1) Detection and localization of residual left-to-right and right-to-left shunts.[59]
(2) Assessment of palliative shunts: Waterston, Potts, Blalock, and Glenn.[71]
(3) Evaluation of reconstructive surgery: Repair of D-transposition of the great arteries (Mustard), repair of tetralogy of Fallot, arterial grafts, and pulmonary artery reconstruction in pulmonary artery sling.
(4) Determination of left ventricular ejection fraction, cardiac output, shunt quantitation, circulation time, and stroke volume.

can be evaluated (quantitative RAC).[61–67] Since radionuclide angiocardiography is a relatively new technique many of its possible clinical applications have not yet been found. In our experience it has been helpful in the postoperative assessment of patients with congenital heart disease (Table 1).

Detection and Localization of Residual Left-to-Right Shunts and Right-to-Left Shunts

Left-to-right shunts can be detected by visual analysis of time-activity curves obtained over the lung fields.[59,62,68,69] A normal pulmonary tracing reveals a rapid upslope, a peak, a less rapid downslope, a valley, and a second (recirculation) peak. Inspection of the pulmonary curve in left-to-right shunting reveals recirculation peaks and an overall delay in the downslope due to early pulmonary recirculation (Fig. 10). The radionuclide angiocardiogram in left-to-right shunting reveals persistance of radioactivity within the lungs and poor visualization of the left heart and aorta (Fig. 9, bottom). More recently[70] it has been possible to localize intracardiac shunts by analysis of time-activity histograms generated from the right heart chambers and the lungs. Following intracardiac repair of communications between the left and right sides of the heart (e.g., ventricular septal defect) there may be a hemodynamically significant residual defect. The presence and size of a residual shunt through such a defect can be accurately diagnosed by radionuclide angiocardiography.

Right-to-left shunts are detected on radionuclide angiogram by early visualization of the left heart chambers and the aorta before the radionuclide appears over the lungs.[59,71] However, systemic arterial oxygen saturation determinations are adequate for assessing the functional size of right-to-left shunts and radionuclide methods are not very useful for this purpose except in special circumstances. The site of right-to-left shunts can be assessed by radionuclide angiocardiography if attention is focused in the cardiac chambers and the aorta.[59,71]

Assessment of Palliative Shunts

Patency of a Glenn anastomosis (superior vena cava to right pulmonary artery) can be assessed by visual evaluation of the radionuclide angiogram.[71] If the injection is done in an arm vein the radioactivity can be seen as it circulates from the

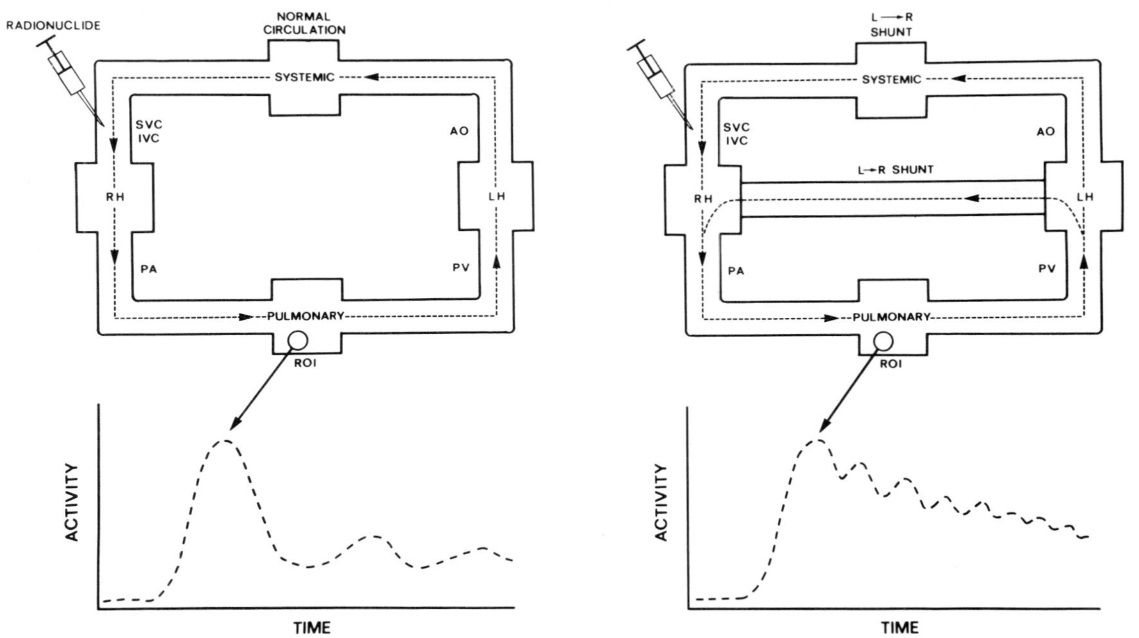

Fig. 10. Left: Pulmonary time-activity histogram. The tracing in the normal child shows a rapid upslope, a peak and a rapid downslope, followed by a recirculation peak. Right: The pulmonary time-activity histogram in left-to-right shunting shows various peaks superimposed on delayed downslope reflecting early pulmonary recirculation. SVC = superior vena cava; IVC = inferior vena cava; RH = right heart; LH = left heart; PA = pulmonary artery; Ao = aorta, PV = pulmonary vein; ROI = region of interest.

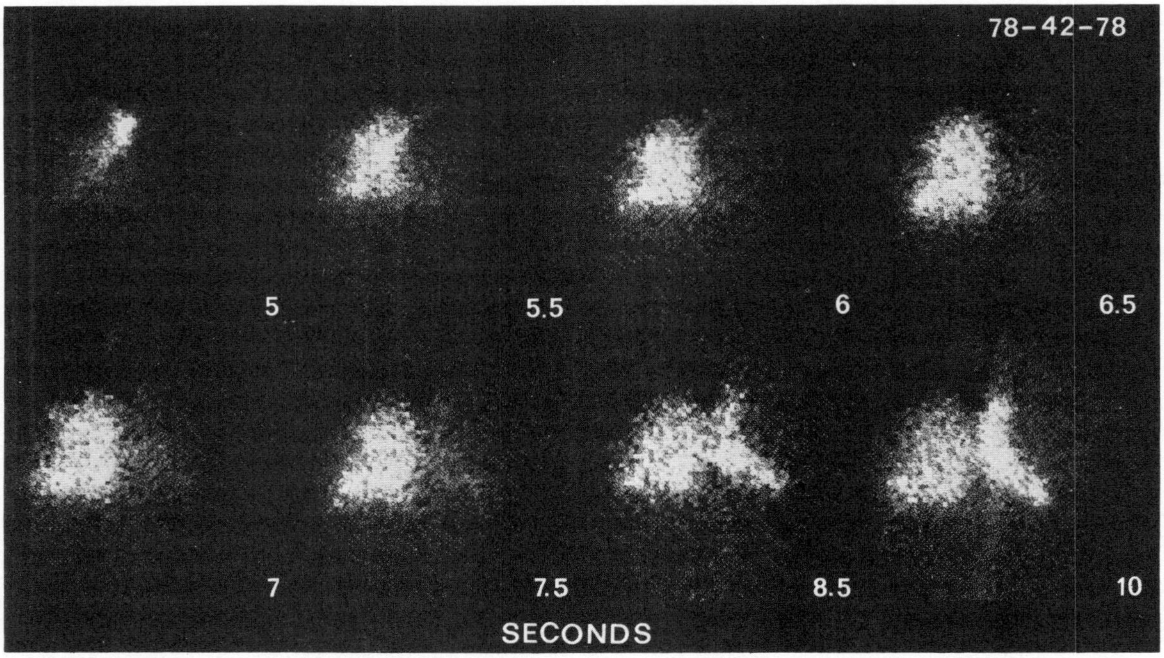

Fig. 11. Glenn anastomosis (superior vena cava to right pulmonary artery). The radioisotope circulates into the right lung first (5–6 sec), then returns to the left side of the heart and the aorta (6.5–10 sec) (with permission[71]).

superior vena cava into the right lung followed by transit of the radiocompound into the left atrium, left ventricle and the aorta (Fig. 11). In the case of a patent systemic to pulmonary shunt (Blalock-Taussig anastomosis, Potts anastomosis and Waterston anastomosis) a greater amount of early pulmonary recirculation due to the shunt is detected over the lung field on the side of the anastomosis (Fig. 12).[62,67,71]

Evaluation of Reconstructive Surgery

The results of the Mustard procedure for physiologic correction of transposition of the great vessels, can be readily evaluated (Fig. 13).[59,71] If residual shunting between the systemic and pulmonary circuits exists, the angiocardiogram will reveal evidence of intracardiac mixing and the chambers of the heart and great arteries would not be easily distinguishable. Similarly, after repair of tetralogy of Fallot, return to a normal angiographic pattern is seen if the operation is successful. If, however, residual shunting is present there will be evidence of early pulmonary recirculation and poor visualization of the left heart and the aorta in case of left-to-right shunt.

There are a wide variety of vascular anomalies that can be anatomically reconstructed to correct abnormal circulatory physiology. Occasionally such a reconstruction fails due to thrombosis at the anastomatic site. Examples of such a lesion is pulmonary artery sling or pulmonary artery graft. Radionuclide angiocardiography can help to assess the status of the anastomosis.

Determination of Left Ventricular Ejection Fraction, Cardiac Output, Shunt Quantitation, Circulation Times, and Forward Stroke Volume

Quantitative evaluation of data acquired during radionuclide angiocardiography can provide accurate information on the above parameters.

Quantitation of left-to-right shunts. The development of a method for analysis of pulmonary time-activity histograms[71] has provided a means for accurate detection and quantitation of left-to-right shunts. It is based on a gamma variate model fit to pulmonary time-activity histograms and provides pulmonary-to-systemic flow ratios (Qp : Qs) directly. This technique has been found to correlate quite well with Qp : Qs between 1.2 : 1 and 3.0 : 1, (Fig. 14). This method can be used in patients with atrial septal defect (ASD) and ventricular septal defect (VSD) and to a more limited degree in patients with aortopulmonary

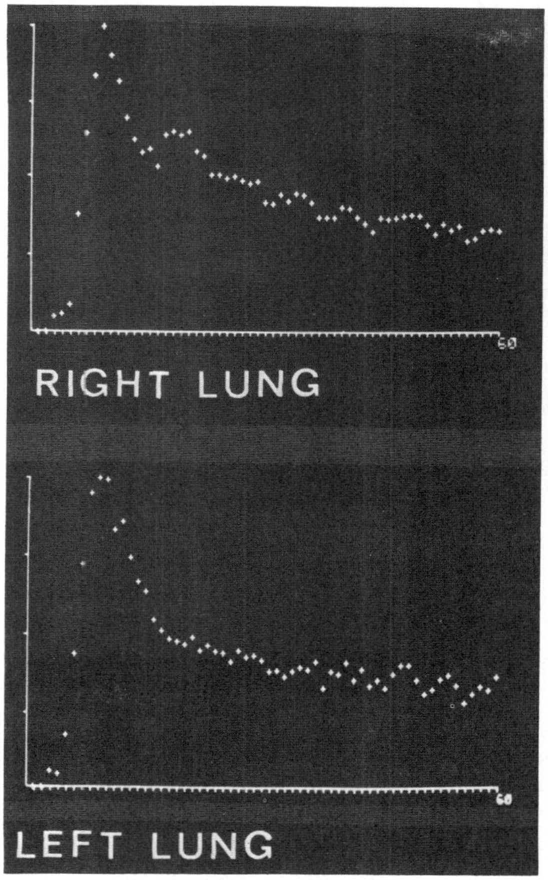

Fig. 12. Right Blalock-Taussig anastomosis. Time-activity histograms from both lung fields reveal increased recirculation over the right lung due to the patent shunt.

connections such as patent ductus arteriosus (PDA).[71]

Left ventricular ejection fraction. A number of radionuclide methods have been proposed. These can be divided into two groups: (1) those that evaluate the heart activity during equilibration of an intravascular indicator;[72] (2) those that rely on the analysis of the heart activity during a single pass of the radioindicator following intravenous injection.[66,73]

The first method is performed using technetium-99^m labeled human serum albumin and electrocardiographic gating of the gamma scintillation camera. Recording modalities vary from worker to worker. Some record two images: one at end-diastole and another at end-systole. Each image is composed of 300-500 heart beats. This is done to achieve high counting statistics. These can be evaluated: (1) visually for areas of dyskinesis; (2) graphically using an area/length method to calculate volumes and ejection fraction or; (3) numerically by calculating the changes in intracardiac radioactivity during end-systole and end-diastole. Other workers use biplane techniques and acquire information during the entire heart cycle thus obtaining several intermediate images between end-diastole and end-systole. These methods provide scintigraphs of high counting statistics. One of the problems with this technique is the uncertainty in finding the mitral valve plane. The other modalities rely on rapid recording of the intracavity changes of radioactivity levels during the first transit of an intravenously injected radioindicator (usually technetium-99^m). All information can be acquired at a rate of 100 observations/sec with the ability to divide the study into a varied number of frames/sec (10-20 frames/sec). This information can also be evaluated visually and numerically. Scintigraphs obtained in this fashion usually contain a relatively low density of counts and are not suitable, at present, for careful anatomic evaluation. It is possible, however, to obtain rapid, accurate, and reliable ejection fraction estimates by numerical analysis of time-activity curves generated from the left ventricle.

Circulation time. The circulation time between regions within the cardiovascular system such as superior vena cava to right heart, right heart to lungs, lungs to left ventricle, etc. can be measured accurately and objectively by recording the activity as a function of time over these structures.

Cardiac output. An estimate of cardiac output can be obtained by analysis of the tracing obtained over the heart or one of its chambers following intravenous injection of an intravascular radioindicator such as technetium-99^m labeled human serum albumin. A blood sample is necessary to determine the blood volume. The calculation of cardiac output is based on the dye dilution principle.[63-66,74,75]

EAR OXIMETRY

The ear oximeter is a photoelectric device utilized to measure arterial oxygen saturation in the intact ear. It is based on the differences in light absorption by oxygenated and reduced hemoglobin of red light at 640 mμ and on their similarity in absorption of infrared light at 800 mμ. The oximeter can measure arterial oxygen saturation changes in response to varying situations and

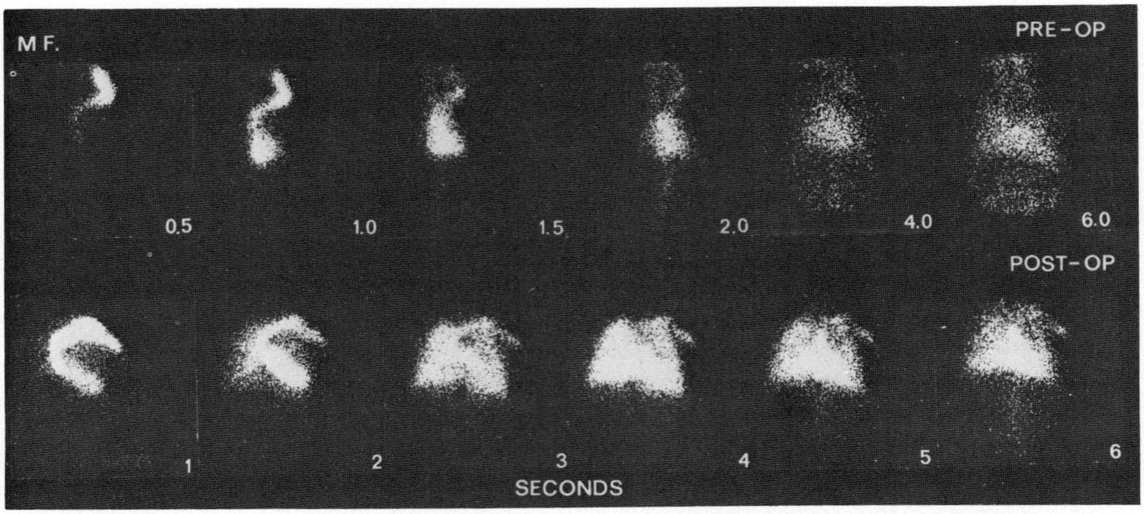

Fig. 13. Transposition of great arteries with intact ventricular septum before and after Mustard procedure in a 6-mo old boy. In the preoperative study radioactivity appears early in the ascending aorta and arch at 1.5 sec and in the descending aorta at 2.0 sec. The radionuclide appears in the lungs only after its appearance in the aorta. In the postoperative study, the left ventricle fills from the 'atrial baffle' at 1 and 2 sec. The right ventricle is not seen at 1, 2, and 3 sec. After the radioactivity appears in the lungs, the common atrium, right ventricle, and ascending aorta are seen at 5 and 6 sec. Radioactivity in the aorta appears rapidly in the preoperative study, but appears 3-sec later in the postoperative study (with permission[59]).

can also be utilized to measure a dye dilution curve.[76,77] Its use is not intended as a substitute for arterial blood gas or capillary blood pO_2 determination in the management of a critically ill patient. It does, however, provide a reasonable alternative in the management of the ambulatory patient. Precision of the instrument is not very high and the accuracy varies with the range of saturation measured. When compared to manometric analysis of blood, variability in the low range of saturations is 3.5%–5.2% versus 2.6% in normal subjects.[76,78] Fig. 15 illustrates the relationship between simultaneously measured arterial oxygen saturation by a reflection oximeter (arterial

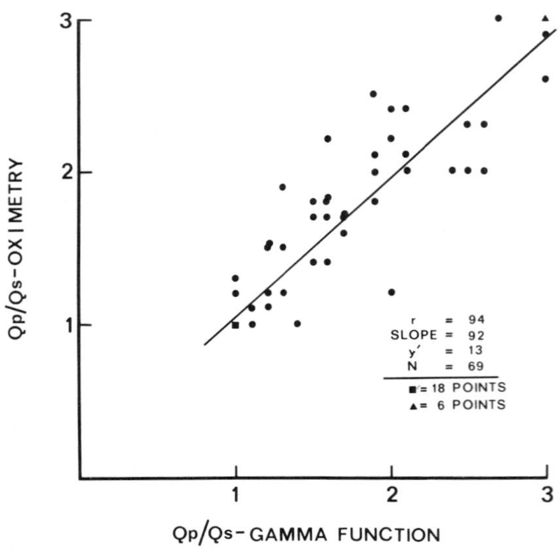

Fig. 14. Pulmonary to systemic flow ratios (Qp : Qs) calculated by oximetry and by the radionuclide method in 69 patients with and without left-to-right shunts.

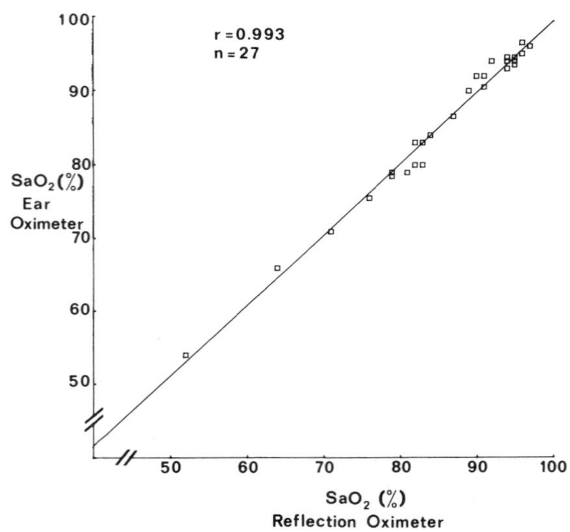

Fig. 15. Simultaneous measurements of systemic arterial oxygen saturation by ear oximeter and a reflection oximeter during cardiac catheterization.

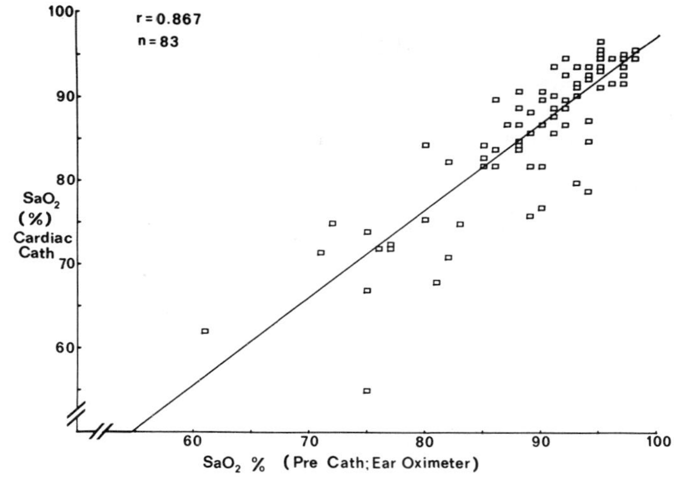

Fig. 16. Systemic arterial oxygen saturation measured by an ear oximeter, while patient is ambulatory, approximately 24 hr prior to catheterization compared to systemic arterial saturation obtained at catheterization by using a reflective oximeter.

blood) and ear oximeter. In Fig. 16 the resting oxygen saturations obtained in ambulatory patients by ear oximeter (24 hr before cardiac catheterization) are compared with arterial saturations taken during catheterization. Although considerable scatter is present, particularly at the lower range of values, the ear oximeter performance is sufficiently accurate for practical clinical purposes.

The oximeter has been widely used in outpatient care facilities and in the follow-up of infants and children with cyanotic congenital heart disease. If the instrument is adequately cared for and periodically calibrated it can be a useful adjunct in the pre- and postoperative management of patients with cyanotic CHD. In the preoperative patient, the oximeter may aid in the diagnosis of congenital heart disease or estimation of its severity.[77] Periodic determinations at rest and exercise are helpful in the evaluation of subjective symptoms or the need for surgery. Fig. 17 illustrates the progressive decrease in oxygen saturations in an infant with tetralogy of Fallot. Congestive heart failure disappeared as the infant developed increasing right ventricular outflow obstruction. This resulted in an increased right-to-left shunt and a fall in arterial oxygen saturation. Following repair of the lesion, oxygen saturation became normal.

In the postoperative ambulatory patient, ear oximetry permits a noninvasive assessment of the effect of surgery on peripheral systemic oxygen saturation. Surgical procedures whose effectiveness can be assessed by ear oximetry are outlined in Table 2. Serial measurements of saturation by ear oximetry in postoperative patients will, for example, aid in recognizing the patients with ventricular septal defect and pulmonary artery band who are developing a right-to-left shunt or those with tetralogy of Fallot whose systemic to pulmonary shunt has diminished in size or become too small to meet their need. Persistence of mild systemic arterial unsaturation in patients with D-transposition of the great arteries after the Mustard procedure is the result of incorporation of the coronary sinus into the physiologic left atrium. Incomplete surgical relief of right ventricular outflow obstruction in severe pulmonary stenosis (in

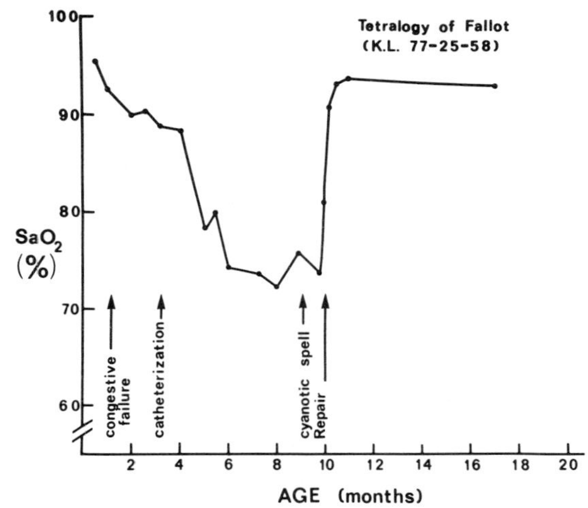

Fig. 17. Serial measurements of arterial oxygen saturations by an ear oximeter in an infant with tetralogy of Fallot. Progressive narrowing of the right ventricular infundibulum resulted in diminished pulmonary blood flow and increased right-to-left shunting. Cyanosis increased and the infant developed a spell. Surgical repair of the tetralogy of Fallot resulted in a return to normal arterial saturation.

Table 2. Postoperative Situations in Which the Ear Oximeter is Clinically Useful

Palliative Surgery	Corrective Surgery (Physiologic or Anatomic)
(1) Systemic to pulmonary arterial anastomoses (Blalock-Taussig, Potts, and Waterston shunt).	(1) Repair of tetralogy of Fallot or double outlet right ventricle with pulmonary stenosis
(2) Systemic venous to pulmonary arterial anastomosis (Glenn shunt).	(2) Mustard procedure for D-transposition of the great arteries.
(3) Atrial septal defect creation (D-transposition of the great arteries).[81]	(3) Pulmonary valvotomy (in the presence of a patent foramen ovale or atrial septal defect).[79]
(4) Palliative Mustard procedure (in patients with D-transposition of the great arteries, ventricular septal defect, and severe pulmonary vascular obstructive disease in whom the ventricular septal defect is not closed).[82]	(4) Fontan operation for tricuspid atresia.
(5) Pulmonary artery banding (ventricular septal defect and single ventricle).	

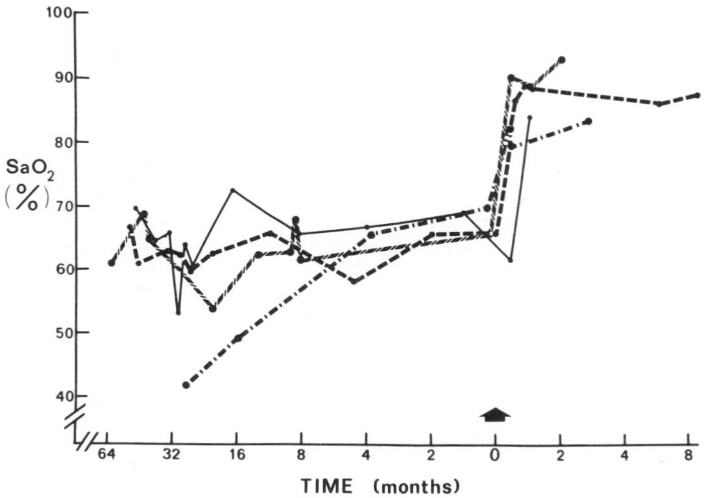

Fig. 18. Rise in systemic arterial oxygen saturation monitored by an ear oximeter in four patients with D-transposition of the great arteries, ventricular septal defect, and severe pulmonary venous obstruction after a palliative Mustard procedure (placement of an intraatrial baffle without closure of the ventricular septal defect). Surgery is indicated by the arrow.

the presence of an atrial septal defect or patent foramen ovale) may also be associated with persistant postoperative right-to-left shunting. Arterial oxygen saturation in infants with critical pulmonary stenosis and diminutive right ventricle may not reach normal levels until many months after surgery.[79] The changes in arterial oxygen saturation following a palliative Mustard procedure are illustrated in Fig. 17.

The magnitude of the right-to-left shunt may become more apparent on exercise.[76,77] In addition to the resting state, oximetry values should; therefore, also be obtained after standardized exercise. In conjunction with a hemoglobin or hematocrit determination[80] the appropriate oxygen content for the patient may thus be estimated. If the results are interpreted in conjunction with the clinical findings, the ear oximeter becomes a valuable noninvasive tool in the care of the postoperative ambulatory patient with cyanotic congenital heart disease.

REFERENCES

1. Ellison RC, Restieaux NJ: Vectorcardiography in Congenital Heart Disease. Philadelphia, Saunders, 1972

2. Hugenholtz PG, Ellison RC, Miettinen OS: Spatial voltages in the assessment of left ventricular hypertrophy (Frank System). J Electrocardiol 1:77, 1968

3. Hugenholtz PG, Gamboa R: Effect of chronically increased ventricular pressure on electrical forces of the heart. A correlation between hemodynamic and vectorcardiographic data (Frank System) in 90 patients with aortic or pulmonic stenosis. Circulation 30:511, 1964

4. Ellison RC, Restieaux NJ: Quantitation of ventricular hypertrophy and hemodynamic load with vectorcardiogram. Prog Cardiovas Dis 14:559, 1972

5. Abramson H, Burton CR: The spatial vectorcardiogram in proven atrial septal defect. Br Heart J 24:103, 1963

6. Lee Y-C, Sclerlis L: Atrial septal defect. Electrocardiographic, vectorcardiographic and catheterization data. Circulation 25:1024, 1962

7. Liebman J, Nadas AS: The vectorcardiogram in the

differential diagnosis of atrial septal defect in children. Circulation 22:956, 1960

8. Burchell HB, DuShane JW, Brandenburg RO: The electrocardiogram of patients with atrioventricular conduction defects (defects of the atrioventricular canal). Am J Cardiol 6:575, 1960

9. Khoury GH, Shaher RM, Fowler RS: The vectorcardiogram in complete transposition of the great vessels. Analysis of 50 cases. Circulation 35:178, 1967

10. Ellison RC, Restieaux NJ, Hugenholtz PG: Use of the orthogonal electrocardiogram in the assessment of ventricular hypertrophy in children, in Vectorcardiography 2. Amersterdam, North-Holland, 1971, p 580

11. Restieaux NJ, Ellison RC, Albers WH, Nadas AS: The Frank electrocardiogram in complete transposition of the great arteries: Its use in assessment of left ventricular pressure. Am Heart J 83:219, 1972

12. Restieaux NJ, Ellison RC, Nadas AS: Assessment of left ventricular pressure in transposition of the great arteries by the Frank electrocardiogram. Am J Cardiol 25:124, 1970

13. Mair DD, McCarthy FJ, Weidman WH, et al: The vectorcardiogram in complete transposition of the great arteries: Correlation with anatomic and hemodynamic findings and calculated left ventricular mass. J Electrocardiol 3:217, 1970

14. Edibam BC, Fowler RS, Keith JD: Postoperative vectorcardiographic changes in cases of congenital aortic stenosis. Indian Pediatr 12:799, 1971

15. Shams A, Keith JD, Edibam BC, et al: The rate of regression of ventricular hypertrophy in vectorcardiogram and electrocardiogram after surgery on congenital heart disease. J Electrocardiol 6:243, 1973

16. Kahn M, Bleifer SB, Grishman A, et al: The vectorcardiogram and electrocardiogram before and after valvotomy for pulmonic stenosis. Am Heart J 58:327, 1959

17. Benchimol A, Tio S: Early involutionary vectorcardiographic signs of right ventricular hypertrophy. Am Heart J 80:19, 1970

18. Chabot M, Karamehmet A, Bourbassa M, et al: Vectorcardiographic evaluation of postoperative changes in patients with interatrial septal defect. Can Med Assoc J 93:1340, 1965

19. Hisamatsu M: Studies on the vectorcardiographic changes following surgical correction of atrial septal defect of the secundum type. Jap Circ J 37, 1973

20. Hoffman LE, Krovetz J, Van Mierop LHS, et al: Secundum atrial septal defects in children. Ann Thorac Surg 7:104, 1969

21. Khoury GH, DuShane JW, Ongley PA: The preoperative and postoperative vectorcardiogram in tetralogy of Fallot. Circulation 31:85, 1965

22. Downing JW Jr, Kaplan S, Bove KE: Post surgical left anterior hemiblock and right bundle branch block. Br Heart J 34:263, 1972

23. Kulbertus HE, Coyne JJ, Hallidie-Smith KA: Conduction disturbances before and after surgical closure of ventricular septal defect. Am Heart J 77:123, 1969

24. Frank E: An accurate, clinically practical system for spatial vectorcardiography. Circulation 13:737, 1956

25. Maron BJ, Humphries JO, Rowe RD, et al: Prognosis of surgically corrected coarctation of the aorta: A 20-year postoperative appraisal. Circulation 47:119, 1973

26. Grishman A, Borun ER, Jaffe HL: Spatial vectorcardiography: Technique for the simultaneous recording of the frontal, saggital, and horizontal projections. Am Heart J 41:483, 1951

27. Chen S, Aralla RA, Moulder PV, et al: Postoperative conduction disturbances in atrial septal defect. Am J Cardiol 22:636, 1968

28. Wolff GS, Rowland TW, Ellison RC: Surgically induced right bundle branch block with left anterior hemiblock—an ominous sign in postoperative tetralogy of Fallot. Circulation 46:587, 1972

29. Muster AJ, Paul MH: Combined ventricular hypertrophy. A vectorcardiographic study in tetralogy of Fallot with systemic pulmonary anastomosis. Circulation 32: 265, 1965

30. Puri PS, Rowe RD, Neill CA: Varying vectorcardiographic patterns in anomalous left coronary artery arising from the pulmonary artery. Am Heart J 71:616, 1966

31. Mustard WT: Successful two-stage correction of transposition of the great vessels. Surgery 55:469, 1964

32. Meyer RA, Swartz DA, Benzing G III, et al: Ventricular septum in right ventricular volume overload. Am J Cardiol 30:349, 1972

33. Tajik AJ, Gau GT, Ritter DG, et al: Echocardiographic pattern of right ventricular volume overload in children. Circulation 36:36, 1972

34. Diamond MA, Dillon JC, Haine CL, et al: Echocardiographic features of atrial septal defect. Circulation 43:129, 1971

35. Meyer RA, Kaplan S: Noninvasive techniques in pediatric cardiovascular disease. Prog Cardiovasc Dis 15:341-367, 1973

36. Ultan LB, Segal BL, Likoff W: Echocardiography in congenital heart disease. Am J Cardiol 19:74, 1967

37. Johnson ML, Holmes JH, Spangler RD, et al: Usefulness of echocardiography in patients undergoing mitral valve surgery. J Thorac Cardiovasc Surg 64:922, 1972

38. Effert S: Pre- and postoperative evaluation of mitral stenosis. Am J Cardiol 19:59, 1967

39. Lundstrom NR: Echocardiography in the diagnosis of congenital mitral stenosis and in evaluation of the results of mitral valvulotomy. Circulation 36:44, 1972

40. Shah PM, Gramiak R, Adelman AG, et al: Echocardiographic assessment of the effects of surgery and propranolol on the dynamics of outflow obstruction in hypertrophic subaortic stenosis. Circulation 35:516, 1972

41. Popp RL, Silverman JF, French JW, et al: Echocardiographic findings in discrete subvalvular aortic stenosis. Circulation 49:226, 1974

42. Troy BL, Pombo JF, Rackley CE: Ultrasonic measurements of left ventricular thickness and mass. Circulation (Suppl III) 42 1970

43. Feigenbaum H, Wolfe SB, Popp RL, et al: Correlation of ultrasound with angiography in measuring left ventricular diastolic volume. Am J Cardiol 23:111, 1969

44. Popp RL, Harrison DC: Ultrasonic cardiac echography for determining subvalvular and valvular regurgitation. Circulation 41:493, 1970

45. Murray JA, Johnston W, Reid JM: Echocardio-

graphic determination of left ventricular performance. Ann Intern Med 72:777, 1970

46. Fortuin NJ, Sherman ME, Hood WP Jr, et al: Evaluation of left ventricular function by echocardiography. Circulation (Suppl III) 42:120, 1970

47. Feigenbaum H, Nassei WK, Rosse E, et al: Left ventricular stroke volume measured by ultrasound. Circulation (Suppl III) 4079, 1969

48. Pombo J, Russell RO Jr, Rackley CB, et al: Comparison of SV and CO determination by ultrasound and dye dilution in acute myocardial infarction. Am J Cardiol 27:630, 1971

49. Feigenbaum H, Zaky A, Nasser WK: Use of ultrasound to measure left ventricular SV. Circulation 35: 1092, 1967

50. Popp RL, Wolfe SB, Hirata T, et al: Estimation of right and left ventricular size by ultrasound. Am J Cardiol 24:523, 1969

51. Pombo JF, Troy BL, Russell RO Jr: Left ventricular volumes and ejection fraction by echocardiography. Circulation 43:480, 1971

52. Jarmakani JM, Graham TP Jr, Canent RV: Left ventricular contractile state in children with successfully corrected ventricular septal defect. Circulation (Suppl) 45:102, 1972

53. Jarmakani JM, Graham TP Jr, Canent RV, et al: Left heart function in children with tetralogy of Fallot before and after palliative or corrective surgery. Circulation 46:478, 1972

54. Graham TP Jr, Jarmakani JM, Canent RV Jr, et al: Quantification of left heart volume and systolic output in transposition of the great arteries. Circulation 44:899, 1971

55. Rosenthall L: Applications of the gamma-ray scintillation camera to dynamic studies in man. Radiology 86:634, 1966

56. Anger HO, VanDyke DC, Gottschalk A, et al: The scintillation camera in diagnosis and research. Nucleonics 23:57, 1965

57. Kriss JP, Yeh SH, Farrer PA, et al: Radioisotope angiocardiography. J Nucl Med 7:367, 1966

58. Kriss JP, Enright LP, Hayden WG, et al: Radioisotopic angiocardiography: Findings in congenital heart disease. J Nucl Med 13:31, 1972

59. Treves S, Maltz DL, Adelstein SJ: Intracardiac shunts, in James AE, Wagner HN Jr, Cooke RE (eds): Pediatric Nuclear Medicine. Philadelphia, Saunders, p 231–246, 1974

60. Hurley PJ, Strauss HW, Wagner HN Jr; Radionuclide Angiography and cine-angiography in screening patients for cardiac disease. J Nucl Med 11:633, 1970

61. Treves S, Lange RC, Freeman GS: Study of cardiopulmonary hemodynamics using a gamma camera and a computer. J Nucl Med 11369, 1970

62. Alazraki NP, Ashburn WL, Hagan A, et al: Detection of left-to-right cardiac shunts with the scintillation camera pulmonary dilution curve. J Nucl Med 13:142, 1972

63. Van Dyke D, Anger HO, Sullivan RW, et al: Cardiac evaluation from radioisotope dynamics. J Nucl Med 13: 585, 1972

64. Stewart GN: The output of the heart in dogs. Am J Physiol 57:27, 1921

65. Donato L, Giuntini C, Lewis ML, et al: Quantitative radiocardiography. I. Theoretical considerations. Circulation 26:174, 1962

66. Weber PM, Dos Remedios LV, Jasko IA: Quantitative radioisotopic angiocardiography. J Nucl Med 13:815, 1972

67. Maltz DL, Treves S: Quantitative radionuclide angiocardiography: Determination of Qp : Qs in children. Circulation 47:1049, 1973

68. Prinzmetal M, Corday E, Bergman HC, et al: Radiocardiography: New method for studying blood flow through chambers of the heart in human beings. Science 108:340, 1948

69. Folse R, Braunwald E: Pulmonary vascular dilution curves recorded by external detection in the diagnosis of left-to-right shunts. Br Heart J 24:166, 1962

70. McIlmoyle G, Ahnberg D, LaFarge G, et al: Localization of left-to-right shunts by radionuclide angiocardiography (RAC). Symposium on Dynamic Studies with Radioisotopes in Clinical Medicine and Research, International Atomic Energy Agency, Knoxville, 1974

71. Treves S, Maltz DL: Radionuclide angiocardiography. Postgrad Med 56:99–107, 1974

72. Zaret BL, Strauss HW, Hurley PJ, et al: A noninvasive scintiphotographic method for detecting regional ventricular dysfunction in man. N Engl J Med 284:1165, 1971

73. Ashburn WL, Kostuk WJ, Karliner JS, et al: Left ventricular volume and ejection fraction determination by radionuclide angiography. Sem Nucl Med 3:165, 1973

74. Hamilton WF, Moore JW, Kinsman JM, et al: Simultaneous determination of the pulmonary and systemic circulation times in man and of a figure related to the cardiac output. Am J Physiol 84:338, 1928

75. Yoder RD, Swan EA: Cardiac output: Comparison of Stewart-Hamilton and gamma-function techniques. J Appl Physiol 31:318, 1971

76. Burchell HB, Wood EH: Symposium on In Vivo photometry of blood in human beings. Mayo Clin Proc 25:377, 1950

77. Woolf CR, Paul W, Gunton RW: The diagnostic use of an ear oximeter in congenital heart disease. Br Heart J 20:311, 1958

78. Montgomery GE, Wood EH, Burchell HB, et al: Continuous observations of the arterial oxygen saturation at rest and during exercise in congenital heart disease. Am Heart J 36:668, 1948

79. Freed MD, Rosenthal A, Bernhard WF, et al: Critical pulmonary stenosis with a diminutive right ventricle in neonates. Circulation 48:875, 1973

80. Rosenthal A, Button LN, Nathan DG, et al: Blood volume changes in cyanotic congenital heart disease. Am J Cardiol 27:162, 1971

81. Rosenthal A, Freed MD, Litwin SB, et al: Atrial septectomy in patients with D-transposition of the great arteries, ventricular septal defect and severe pulmonary vascular obstructive disease. Circulation (Suppl) 50:35, 1974

82. Sloss L, Bernhard WF, Nadas AS: Mustard's operation for palliation of transposition of the great arteries with ventricular septal defect and pulmonary vascular obstructive disease. Circulation (in press)

Myocardial Performance After Anatomic or Physiologic Corrective Surgery

Thomas P. Graham, Jr.

ALTHOUGH MAJOR ADVANCES in surgery for congenital heart disease over the past 20 yr have left only a very few congenital cardiac defects nonamenable to some type of either palliative or "corrective" procedure, there is limited information available regarding myocardial performance following successful surgery. In the past several years, increasingly encouraging results have been obtained with surgical repair of both simple and complex defects in infancy, but data comparing myocardial function following infant surgery versus surgery after infancy is virtually nonexistent at this time. Possibly because of the marked clinical improvement in many patients following successful repair of complex congenital defects, quantitative assessment of myocardial function frequently has been neglected.

The purpose of this review is to attempt to summarize results obtained on evaluation of myocardial performance following successful repair of the more common congenital heart lesions and to indicate areas in which new information would be of vital interest in the continuing reevaluation of current therapy for congenital heart disease.

VOLUME OVERLOAD

Left Ventricle–Ventricular Septal Defect

Ventricular septal defect (VSD) is the most common congenital heart lesion causing left ventricular (LV) volume overload. Jarmakani et al. studied 23 patients from 1 to 5 yr (*x* 2.4 yr) following successful VSD closure and found evidence for residual dilatation, hypertrophy, and depressed contractile function. Age at surgery in these patients averaged 4.8 yr, and there were no residual ventricular defects in 16 patients and small shunts detectable by hydrogen electrode studies only in seven patients. All patients with both pre and postoperative studies showed a decrease in LV end-diastolic volume (EDV) either in absolute terms or in ml/BSA, but the postoperative volumes remained increased by an average value of 18% ($p < 0.01$, Fig. 1). In addition, LV ejection fraction (EF) was decreased in the postoperative group averaging 0.54 versus a normal value of 0.63 ($p < 0.01$, Fig. 2). The ejection fraction decreased from the preoperative value in eight of 11 patients following corrective surgery. This finding suggests that one may be unmasking abnormal left ventricular function by reverting from a subnormal afterload preoperatively in which the LV can "unload" by means of a large VSD and low pulmonary resistance to a normal afterload following successful surgery. In the face of a normal afterload following correction, the left ventricle cannot eject a normal percentage of its end-diastolic volume.

These patients also showed evidence for residual left ventricular hypertrophy with LV wall mass averaging 34% above normal in the postoperative group. There was no significant correlation between postoperative LV mass and age at time of surgery, time lapse between surgery and restudy, preoperative right ventricular pressure, or preoperative LV mass.

These studies led to further investigations of LV function following successful VSD surgery using pressure-velocity indices of LV contractile state.[2] Two groups of patients were studied: group I included nine patients with isolated VSD and preoperative left-to-right shunts $\geq 40\%$ of pulmonary flow (*x* 55%) and group II included nine patients with VSD plus pulmonary stenosis or pulmonary banding and preoperative left-to-right shunts $\leq 40\%$ (*x* 24%). Contractile state was clearly depressed following surgery in the high flow patients (group I) but was normal in patients with only slightly increased pulmonary flow (group II). Thus, VSD patients with a large left-to-right shunt demonstrate depressed LV function following successful VSD closure both in terms of pump function

From the Departments of Pediatrics and Pediatric Cardiology, Vanderbilt University Medical Center, Nashville, Tenn.

Supported in part by NIH grant HL-14454-03 and a grant from the Tennessee Heart Association, Nashville, Tenn.

Reprint requests should be addressed to Thomas P. Graham, Jr., M.D., Professor of Pediatrics, Director of Pediatric Cardiology, Vanderbilt University Medical Center, Nashville, Tenn. 37232.

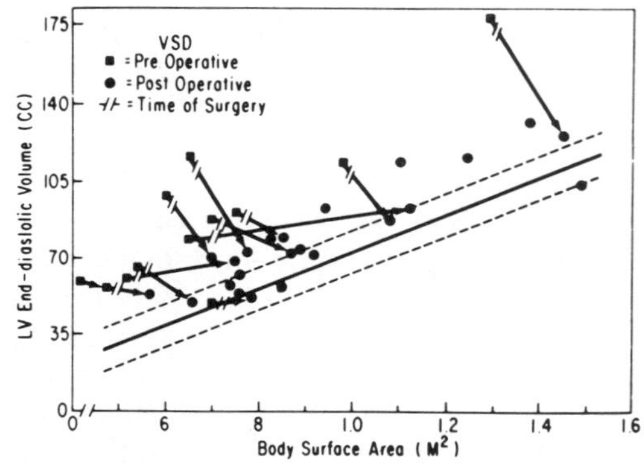

Fig. 1. Left ventricular end-diastolic volume as a function of body surface area for 23 patients after successful closure of ventricular septal defect (by permission).[1] Eleven patients had preoperative values which are indicated. The solid line indicates the regression of normal subjects, and the dashed line the standard error of the estimate.

(depressed ejection fraction) as well as by estimates of cardiac muscle function.

Maron and co-workers[3] recently have reported abnormal responses to intense upright exercise in five of 11 asymptomatic patients studied from 3 to 15 yr after successful VSD surgery (Fig. 3). Age at surgery averaged 15 yr in the entire group of patients, and all five patients with an abnormal exercise response was operated upon after 10 yr of age. In addition, the magnitude of the abnormality was directly related to age at operation. Lueker et al.[4] also have shown abnormalities in the cardiac output response to exercise in four of 16 postoperative VSD patients and borderline responses in

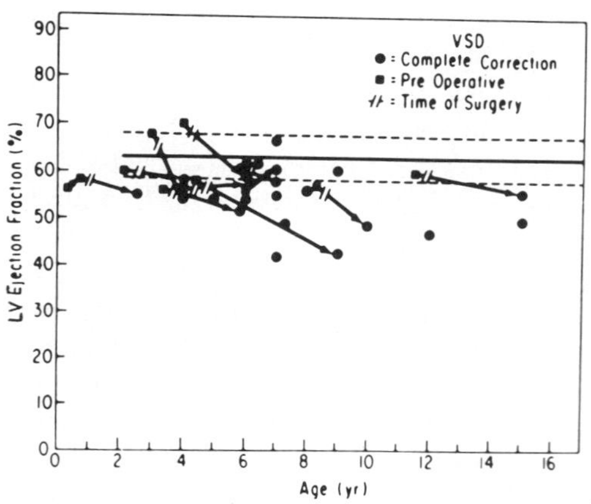

Fig. 2. Left ventricular ejection fraction as a function of age for 23 patients after successful closure of ventricular septal defect (by permission).[1] The solid line indicates the mean normal value and the dashed line the standard error of the estimate.

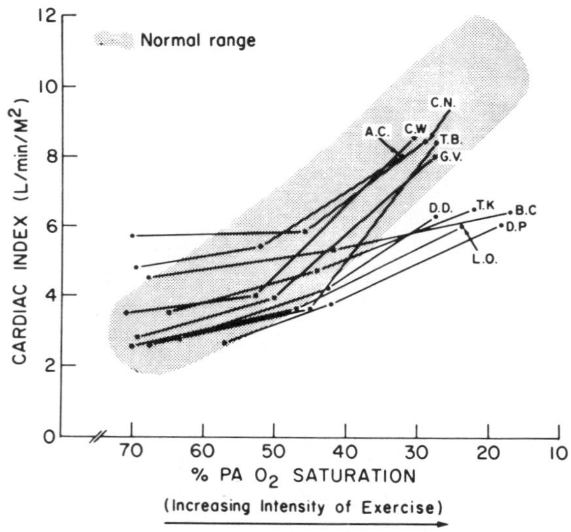

Fig. 3. Relation between cardiac index and pulmonary arterial oxygen saturation at rest in the sitting position, and during mild and intense levels of upright exercise. Shaded area depicts the range of performance in a group of normal subjects (by permission).[3]

five additional patients. It would be of considerable interest to correlate in the same patients exercise studies with direct cardiac catheterization studies of both right and left ventricular performance as well as pulmonary vascular resistance in an attempt to more definitively determine the cause of the abnormal response to exercise. In

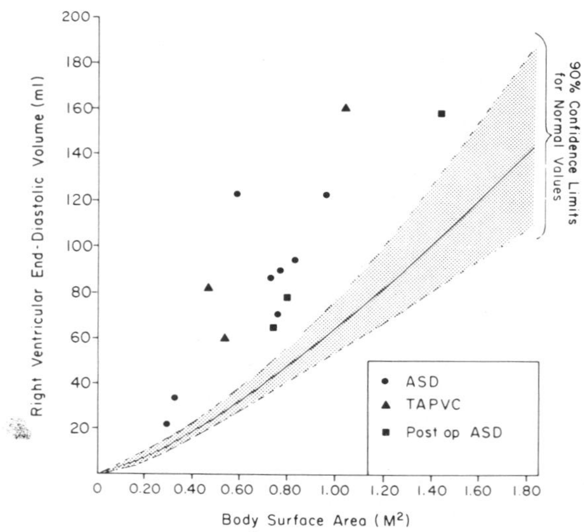

Fig. 4. Right ventricular end-diastolic volume in patients with atrial septal defect or total anomalous pulmonary venous connection plotted as a function of body surface area. Three patients are shown following ASD repair (by permission).[5]

addition, the possible relationship of postoperative cardiovascular abnormalities to age at surgery is of vital importance in continuing to evaluate current therapy.

Right Ventricle–Atrial Septal Defect and Total Anomalous Pulmonary Venous Return

Very little data are available on right ventricular (RV) function following correction of a large right heart volume overload. We have studied three patients 1-2 yr following successful secundum atrial septal defect (ASD) repair and found residual increase in RVEDV (Fig. 4) in all three and depressed ejection fraction in one.[5] Thus, both right and left heart volume overload can be associated with residual abnormalities of ventricular size and function despite successful corrective surgery.

Exercise studies by several different groups have shown abnormalities in patients following repair of atrial defects.[4,6,7] These abnormalities have been more common in patients whose surgery was performed as adolescents or adults. Epstein and co-workers[8] found an abnormal cardiac index response to intense upright exercise in seven of 12 asymptomatic patients studied 6-15 mo following successful closure of secundum ASD's, Fig. 5. These patients ranged in age from 14 to 56 yr at the time of the postoperative study, and there was not a significantly different exercise response in the younger versus the older patients. No data were available on patients with surgery prior to 11 yr of age.

These abnormal exercise responses do not distinguish between a primary right heart versus a left heart abnormality. We have studied left heart volume characteristics in 35 patients with secundum or sinus venosus ASD's and 15 patients with total anomalous pulmonary venous connection (TAPVC).[9] In these patients, the large left-to-right shunt bypasses the left ventricle and the potential for "underloading" the chamber is present. Figure 6 shows LVEDV as a function of age for the ASD group and includes two postoperative studies. Preoperatively LVEDV was significantly decreased averaging 87% of normal. Following surgery, there was an increase in LVEDV in both patients studied. Similar findings were obtained for LV systolic output in the ASD group.

Only five of 15 preoperative patients with TAPVC showed decreases in LVEDV and the average value for this group was not decreased

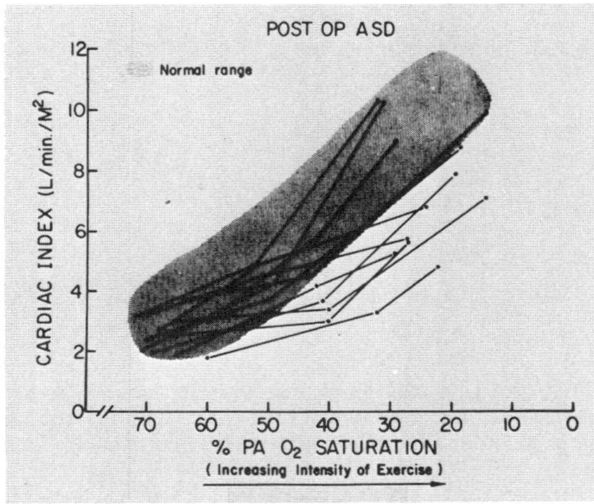

Fig. 5. Relation between cardiac index and pulmonary arterial O_2 saturation at rest and during mild and intense levels of exercise in patients following closure of ASD (by permission).[8]

(Fig. 7). Two patients studied following surgery showed increases in LVEDV. Left ventricular output was mildly depressed in the TAPVC group and increased following surgery. The LV ejection fraction was normal in both groups.

Thus, in patients with a large right heart volume overload, mild abnormalities of LVEDV and LV output can be present in a number of patients prior to surgery. These mild abnormalities have not been associated with what we felt was clinically significant LV dysfunction following surgery. It is apparent that a more extensive analysis of both right and left heart function following repair of large right heart volume overload lesions would be of considerable value.

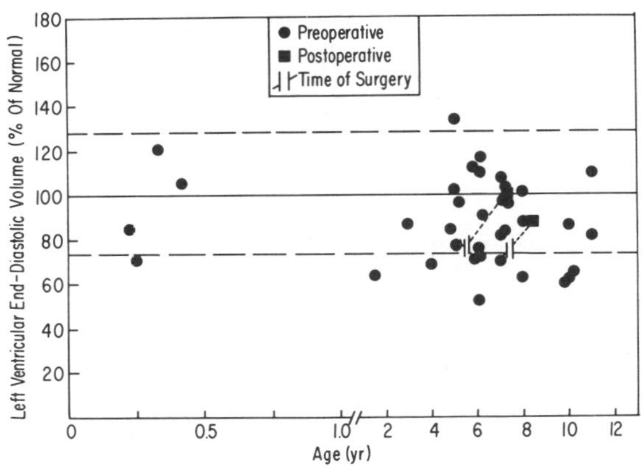

Fig. 6. Left ventricular end-diastolic volume as a percentage of predicted normal for patients with large atrial septal defects: left-to-right shunts ≥ 50% (by permission).[9]

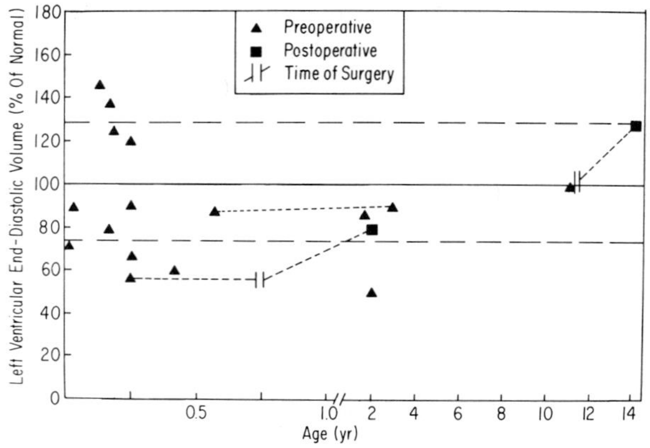

Fig. 7. Left ventricular end-diastolic volume as percentage of predicted normal for patients with total anomalous pulmonary venous connection (by permission).[9]

In patients with TAPVC, there has been virtually a uniform decrease in left atrial (LA) maximal volume to approximately 50% of normal.[9] In one patient studied following successful correction, LA volume had increased to a normal value. We feel that an important factor in LA volume becoming normal following surgery is the current practice of shifting the septum over so that the new left atrium incorporates part of the anatomical right atrium. This technique allows the left atrium to enlarge postoperatively without excessive elevation of pressure and is one factor which probably has resulted in the improving surgical mortality for this lesion.

PRESSURE OVERLOAD

Left Ventricle–Aortic Stenosis

The majority of children beyond infancy with left ventricular overload secondary to aortic stenosis do not have clinical evidence for impaired ventricular performance. Left ventricular volume studies in these patients have shown that end-diastolic volume is either normal or decreased while wall mass is increased and ejection fraction is increased.[10–11] Thus, despite an increase in resistance to ventricular ejection which would be expected, in the acute situation, to depress the ejection fraction, these patients have an elevation of this variable and in terms of pump function might be classified as supernormal. This supernormal pump function, however, might be achieved by hypertrophy of ventricular fibers although measurements of contractile state of the myocardium might be subnormal. In an attempt to investigate this possibility, a group of preoperative patients with significant left ventricular pressure overload were studied. In these patients, pressure-velocity curves were obtained with high-fidelity left ventricular pressure measurements.[12] These data are shown in Fig. 8. Only four of the 15 patients have definite depressions of LV contractile state. These studies indicate that modest depressions of contractility may be present with pressure-induced hypertrophy in childhood. At this time, there are no data on ventricular performance following successful surgery in these patients.

There is a good deal of literature regarding depression of contractile state in myocardium of dogs, cats, and rats following pressure-induced hypertrophy.[13–18] In addition, investigations in adults with aortic stenosis[19–21] have shown that

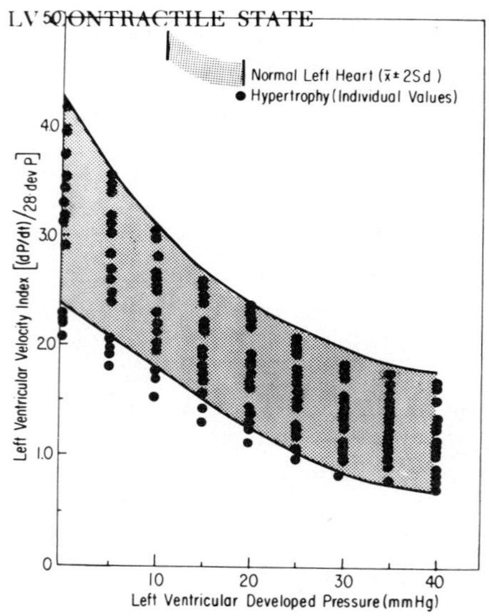

Fig. 8. Pressure-velocity indices for the hypertrophy group plotted against the normal "pressure-velocity curve." All data calculated with regression equations derived with the use of developed pressure > 10 mm Hg (by permission).[12]

the majority of patients with long-standing hypertrophy do have a depression of contractile state when measured by pressure-velocity indices similar to those shown in Fig. 8. It is of interest that Simon et al.[19] were able to show that at comparable levels of hypertrophy secondary to moderately severe aortic stenosis, the contractile state was compromised more in the older adult patients. Thus, long-standing pressure-induced myocardial hypertrophy can be associated with alterations in contractile state. There are no studies currently available comparing pre- and postoperative measurements of left ventricular contractility in patients with aortic stenosis. The information which is lacking at this point is the time range over which possible irreversible alterations in contractile state take place in order to provide more meaningful information regarding optimal surgical management. An answer to this question will require a long-term committment to pre- and postoperative evaluation of a large number of patients with successful surgery for aortic stenosis.

Right Ventricle–Pulmonary Stenosis and Pulmonary Atresia

There are very little data available on right ventricular performance with a chronic pressure overload secondary to pulmonary stenosis. There have been various reports that overall cardiovascular function may not be normal when surgery for pulmonary stenosis is performed in adult life. Hoffman[22] has reviewed these data as well as 39 reports of diffuse right ventricular myocardial fibrosis in patients who died from pulmonic stenosis. These fibrotic changes are most likely secondary to relative myocardial ischemia as suggested by Hoffman. When this condition is studied preoperatively in children, right ventricular end-diastolic volumes and ejection fractions are within the normal range.[5] At present, there are no right ventricular volume data following relief of long-standing pulmonary stenosis.

Pulmonary atresia with intact ventricular septum is a condition causing intrauterine right ventricular pressure overload. We have studied eight preoperative and five postoperative patients with this condition.[23] Preoperative studies in the majority of patients show a diminutive right ventricle with severe depression of the ejection fraction (Figs. 9 and 10). However, if severe tricuspid insufficiency is associated with this condition, the right ventricle is large and the ejection fraction is normal probably as a result of the ventricle being able to "unload" during systole.

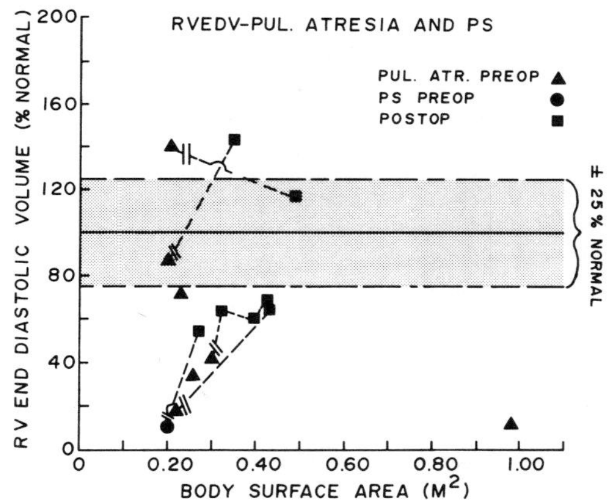

Fig. 9. RVEDV as a percentage of normal versus B.S.A. in patients with pulmonary atresia (PAt) or critical pulmonary stenosis (PS) with intact ventricular septum (by permission).[23]

In three patients studied before and after successful valvulotomy for pulmonary atresia or critical pulmonary stenosis, there have been significant increases in right ventricular end-diastolic volume with the values approaching the normal range (Fig. 9) and increases in the ejection fraction to values which are well within the normal range (Fig. 10). Thus, despite a severe intrauterine pressure overload, these ventricles can eject a normal amount of the end-diastolic volume after relief of the obstruction. However, these patients do show significant elevations of right ventricular end-diastolic pressure in association with subnormal

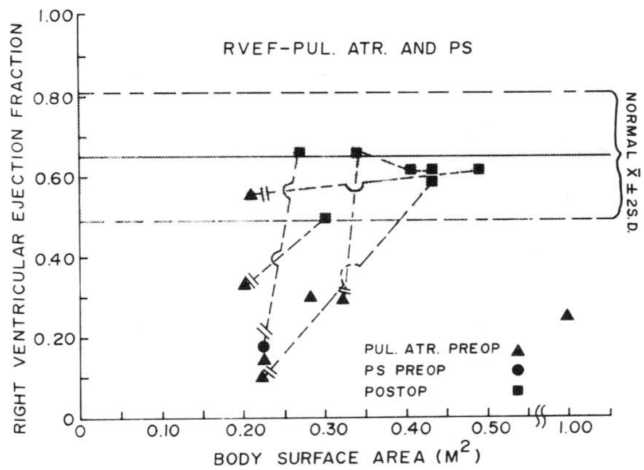

Fig. 10. RV ejection fraction as a function of B.S.A. in patients with PAt or PS and intact ventricular septum (by permission).[23]

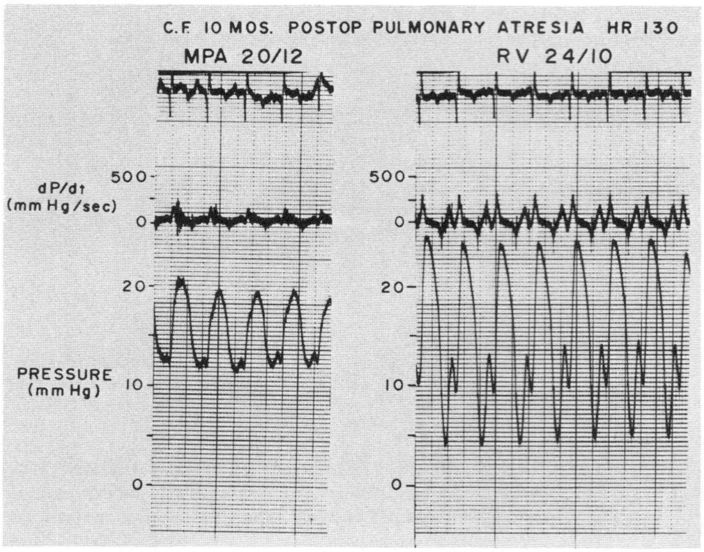

Fig. 11. Right ventricular and pulmonary artery pressures recorded with a micromanometer in an infant studied 10.5 mo following valvulotomy for pulmonary atresia with intact ventricular septum.

volumes following successful valvulotomy. In Fig. 11, pulmonary artery and right ventricular pressures are shown in a 10.5-mo old infant who had successful valvulotomy performed at age 1 day. Despite virtually complete relief of the pressure overload, RV end-diastolic pressure is significantly elevated with a prominent "a" wave and there was a 35% right-to-left atrial shunt. Almost identical findings were present in a 7-wk old infant with successful valvulotomy for critical pulmonary stenosis at age 2 days. These findings indicate impaired right ventricular distensibility and suggest an intrauterine alteration of the myocardium which persists despite successful relief of the pressure overload.

Impaired right ventricular distensibility and a residual right-to-left atrial shunt following relief of severe pulmonary stenosis or atresia has been reported previously both in children and adults.[24–27] Freed et al.[27] showed in eight infants operated upon in infancy for critical pulmonary stenosis that ear oximetry measurements increased to $\geqslant 90\%$ within a year following valvulotomy. In the patients who show persistent right-to-left atrial shunting despite adequate relief of RV outflow obstruction, there are at present no guidelines to indicate optimal therapy in regard to ASD closure, ductal ligation, and/or surgical shunt closure.

COMPLEX CYANOTIC CONDITIONS

Tetralogy of Fallot

Left ventricular volume studies have been performed by Jarmakani and co-workers[28] in patients with tetralogy of Fallot before and after corrective or palliative surgery. With tetralogy and a moderately severe decrease in pulmonary blood flow, the inflow into the left ventricle may be decreased with resultant mild to moderate degrees of left ventricular hypoplasia. Left ventricular end-diastolic volume was decreased in cyanotic patients who were 2 yr of age or older and averaged only 79% of normal.[28] These findings indicate an effect of age as well as pulmonary flow on LVEDV with a decrease in this variable present only with older patients who had definite cyanosis.

Figure 12 shows LVEDV as a function of age before and after corrective surgery for tetralogy. There are 24 postoperative patients ages 6–16 yr ($x = 11 \pm 0.7$ yr) who were studied an average of 2.5 yr following correction. Twenty of the 24 postoperative tetralogy patients have end-diastolic volumes above normal. The mean value for LVEDV following surgery was significantly increased and averaged 117% of normal.

Fig. 13 shows the ejection fraction in the entire group of 58 tetralogy patients. This variable was significantly decreased in all groups and averaged 0.50 following complete correction. In contrast Sunderland et al.[29] have shown normal values for LV ejection fraction in 17 postoperative tetralogy patients who had corrective surgery performed before 24 mo of age and were studied at least 12 mo following correction. As these authors point out, these data indicate that early correction may avoid, halt, or reverse abnormalities of LV function which continue to be present in the older

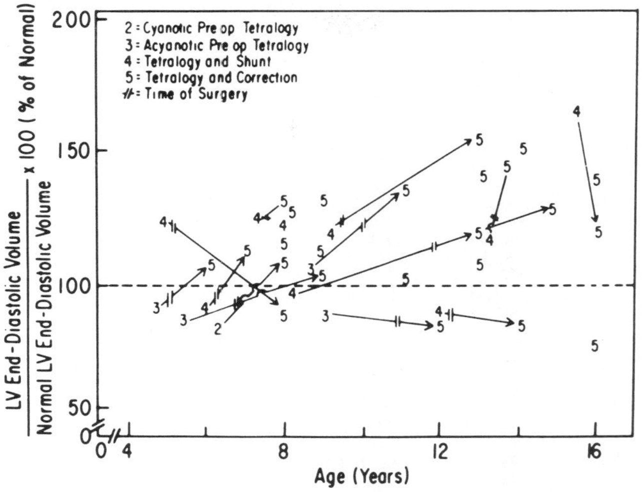

Fig. 12. Left ventricular end-diastolic volume (percentage of normal) before and after corrective surgery for tetralogy as a function of age (by permission).[28]

child following total correction.[28] More data are needed to attempt to clarify this most important concept.

In summary, mild to moderate impairment of left ventricular function can be shown in tetralogy patients who are corrected in late childhood.[28] Krymskii[30] has described focal fibrosis of the left ventricle and diffuse fibrosis of the right ventricle in tetralogy of Fallot patients. Thus, there may be an anatomical correlate for the left ventricular dysfunction which has been described. It is well known that tetralogy patients frequently require cardiac glycosides as well as salt restriction and diuretics for a period of time following successful surgery. Whether or not these findings are all secondary to right ventricular dysfunction is not known at this time. Studies on both right and left ventricular function in these patients would be of obvious value.

Epstein et al.[8] have shown an abnormally low cardiac index response to intense upright exercise in nine out of ten postoperative tetralogy patients ages 12–36 yr who were studied from 6 mo to 4 yr following surgery (Fig. 14). In six of these patients with RV systolic pressure measurements, this variable increased from an average of 34.7 ± 3.0 at rest to 80.2 ± 9.1 mm Hg during intense exercise. This increase in RV pressure was primarily due to an increase in an RV outflow tract gradient from 17.0 ± 2.5 at rest to 41.8 ± 9.5 mm Hg with exercise. Thus, the overall cardiovascular response to exercise was impaired in these patients who were

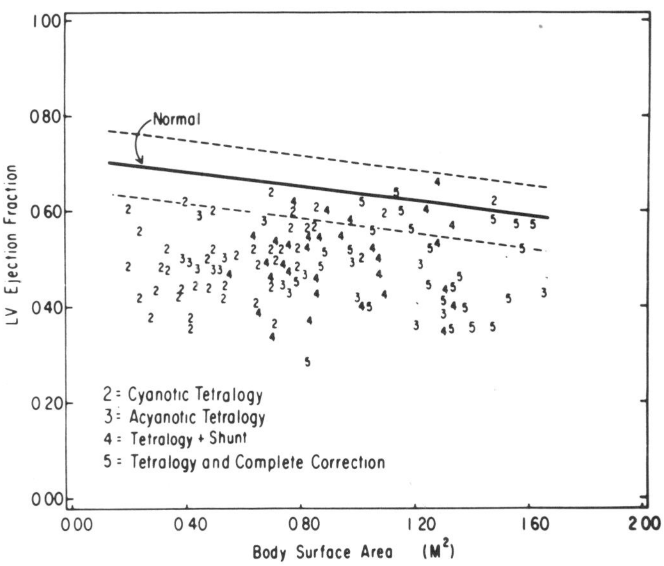

Fig. 13. Left ventricular ejection fraction as a function of B.S.A. for all tetralogy patients (by permission).[28]

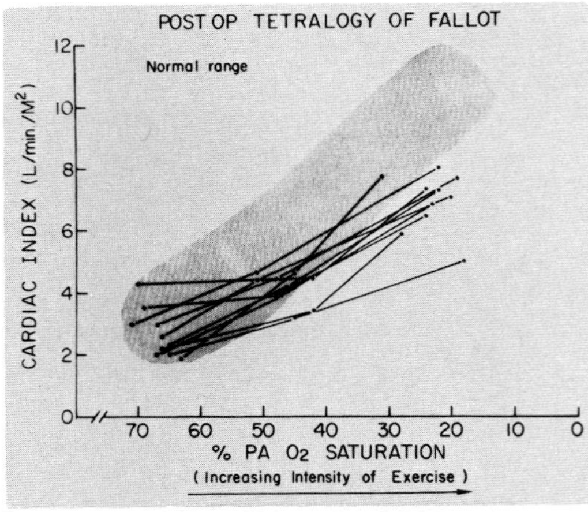

Fig. 14. Relation between cardiac index and pulmonary arterial (PA) O_2 saturation at sitting rest and during mild and intense treadmill exercise in patients following repair of tetralogy of Fallot (by permission).[8] Shaded area depicts the range of performance in a group of normal subjects.

corrected in late childhood or as adults. Multiple factors which contribute to this abnormal exercise response include right and left heart performance as well as exercise-induced RV outflow tract obstruction.

Transposition of the Great Arteries (TGA)

The majority of infants with TGA who are above 6 mo of age show increases in left ventricular end-diastolic volume and left ventricular output.[31-32] In general, these values are higher with an associated ventricular septal defect or patent ductus arteriosus, and in the presence of pulmonary stenosis, these variables can be normal. There are very few data on postoperative left ventricular volume studies in these patients. We have studied four patients following a successful Mustard procedure, and these data are shown in Fig. 15. Left ventricular volume and systolic output decreased to normal or near normal levels in these patients who were "corrected" between 2 and 3 yr of age. Further studies are needed in order to document whether or not left ventricular performance remains normal following surgery and whether or not this variable is normal when surgery is performed at an earlier or a later age.

Right ventricular volumes are elevated in the majority of patients with transposition of the great arteries who are above the neonatal age period.[33-34] We have been unpleasantly surprised at the number of patients who have a low right ventricular ejection fraction despite showing no clinical evidence of heart failure. Postoperative studies have indicated that many of these patients will continue to have elevations of RV end-diastolic volume and depressions of the ejection fraction following surgery.[34] A great deal more information is needed in order to determine if these abnormalities will persist and if they are related to preexisting degree of cyanosis, age at surgery, or other yet unknown factors.

Myocardial Disease—Anomalous Origin of the Left Coronary Artery From the Pulmonary Artery (ALCA)

This is the one form of myocardial disease of congenital origin in which surgical intervention can be of value. There remain conflicting opinions as to proper management of infants and children with this condition. It has been suggested that patients with ejection fractions less than 0.35 should be treated medically because of their very poor prognosis.[35] Wagner et al.[36] studied one infant who had ligation of an anomalous left coronary at the age of 5 wk. Ventricular volume studies at age 21 mo showed a left ventricular end-diastolic volume of 230 ml/M^2 or 329% of normal

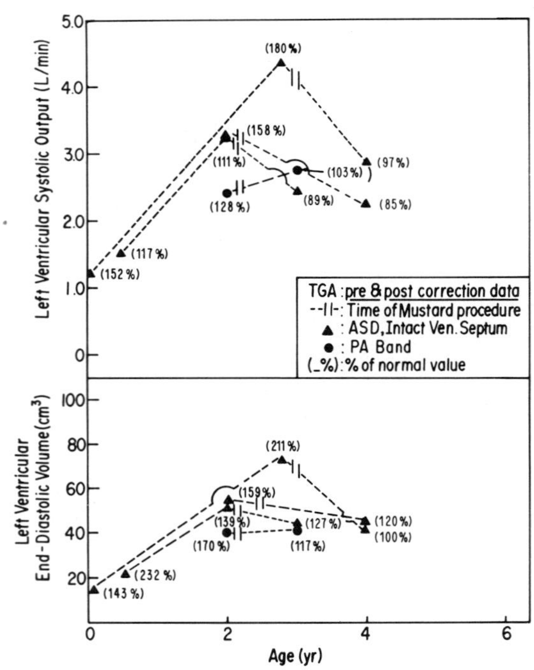

Fig. 15. Left ventricular volume data before and after corrective surgery by the Mustard procedure (by permission).[31]

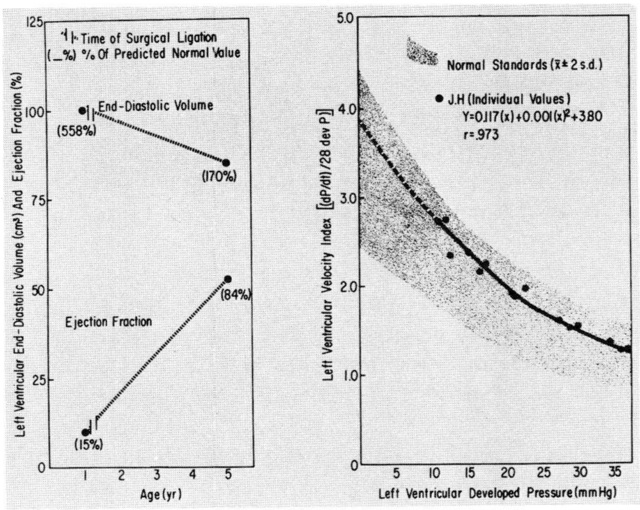

Fig. 16. Evaluation of ventricular function in a patient with an anomalous coronary artery arising from the pulmonary artery. There is a large decrease in end-diastolic volume and a highly significant increase in ejection fraction following surgery. In addition, the left ventricular pressure-velocity curve evaluated 4 yr following surgery is within the normal range (by permission).[37]

and an ejection fraction of 0.19. Preoperative volume studies were not performed. Despite this evidence for severe LV dysfunction, this infant was doing well clinically with normal growth and development.

We have had the opportunity to study one patient before and following successful surgery. This patient was seen first at 11 mo with chronic heart failure and electrocardiographic evidence of an antero-lateral myocardial infarction. Cardiac catheterization revealed an anomalous left coronary artery rising from the pulmonary artery. There was severe myocardial dysfunction with the left ventricular end-diastolic volume 558% of normal and ejection fraction 0.10. He underwent surgical ligation of the anomalous coronary artery at its site of origin and improved markedly. He was restudied at 5 yr at which time his LV had amazingly enough decreased in absolute as well as relative values to 170% of normal and his ejection fraction had increased to 0.52 despite an akinetic segment of the LV free wall (Fig. 16).[37] In addition, his postoperative study did show a normal pressure velocity index of myocardial function. Thus, this child demonstrates an excellent hemodynamic and clinical result can occur with surgical ligation of the anomalous left coronary. Even a severe depression of the ejection fraction should not rule out this form of therapy in infancy.

Tyrrell and Bharadwaj[38] have reported pre- and postoperative volume studies in a $3\frac{1}{2}$-yr old girl with aortocoronary vein bypass for ALCA. Preoperative studies showed LVEDV to be 140 ml/M^2 (approximately twice normal) with an ejection fraction of 0.39. Postoperative studies 14 days following surgery revealed LVEDV to be 129 ml/M^2 with a normal ejection fraction of 0.62. This mode of therapy is undoubtedly the treatment of choice for patients requiring treatment after infancy when the coronary vessels are large enough to perform the anastomosis.

SUMMARY

Data on ventricular performance following "corrective" surgery for congenital heart disease at the present time are limited in number and scope. In isolated right and left heart pressure and volume overload lesions, information is available indicating suboptimal cardiac performance in many patients following successful corrective surgery. Patients with complex cyanotic lesions such as tetralogy of Fallot or transposition of the great arteries also have evidence for impaired myocardial function following "corrective" procedures. Histologic data show focal and diffuse myocardial fibrosis in most patients with long-standing hypertrophy. This fibrosis is probably a result of a discrepancy between myocardial oxygen demands and supply in patients with hypertrophy, and it may be the anatomical correlate of abnormal myocardial performance. Despite laboratory evidence for mild to moderate degrees of mechanical cardiac dysfunction, most patients are asymptomatic, lead useful lives, and are able to tolerate at least moderate levels of exercise without difficulty. Many questions which are of vital importance to the patient, the cardiologist, the primary physician, and the surgeon remain unanswered. What is the time reference over which irreversible changes in myocardial structure and function takes place for each congenital heart lesion? For what lesions will infant surgery prevent important residual cardiac dysfunction? What are the long-term effects of outflow tract patches, ventriculotomy, pulmonary insufficiency, and residual pulmonary or aortic stenosis on cardiovascular function? Does hypothermia and total circulatory arrest ever permanently affect cardiac function? What are the time limits for anoxic arrest to prevent residual cardiac dysfunction in severe pressure overload lesions? Are mild degrees of abnormal pump function (ejection fraction 0.45–0.55) clinically important as regards morbidity, longevity, and "quality" of life for patients following surgery for congenital heart disease? These are only a few of the general questions for which very little data are available to attempt to answer. Obviously, each specific lesion and procedure will require study in an attempt to provide specific answers regarding optimal therapy. It is apparent that close liaisons must be formed and maintained between physicians who care primarily for children with heart disease and adult cardiologists in order to provide adequate longitudinal studies to evaluate current therapy for all patients with congenital heart disease.

ACKNOWLEDGMENTS

I would like to acknowledge the research groups with whom I have worked at Vanderbilt University and Duke University, and particularly express my gratitude to my colleagues, Dr. Jay Jarmakani, Dr. Gerald Atwood, Dr. Madison Spach, and Dr. Ramon Canent. Much of the data reviewed in this manuscript has been published previously by these investigators. I would also like to thank Miss Odessa Gatlin for her long hours and hard work in preparing this manuscript.

REFERENCES

1. Jarmakani JM, Graham TP Jr, Canent RV, et al: The effect of corrective surgery on left heart volume and mass in children with ventricular septal defect. Am J Cardiol 27:254–258, 1971

2. Jarmakani JM, Graham TP Jr, Canent RV: Left ventricular contractile state in children with successfully corrected ventricular septal defect. Circulation 45/46(I): 102–110, 1972

3. Maron BJ, Redwood DR, Hirshfeld JW, et al: Postoperative assessment of patients with ventricular septal defect and pulmonary hypertension. Circulation 48:864–874, 1973

4. Lueker RD, Vogel JHK, Blount SG: Cardiovascular abnormalities following surgery for left-to-right shunts. Circulation 40:785–801, 1969

5. Graham TP Jr, Jarmakani JM, Atwood GF, et al: Right ventricular volume determinations in children. Circulation 47:144–153, 1973

6. Petersson PO: Atrial septal defect of secundum type: A clinical study before and after operation with special reference to hemodynamic function (thesis). Acta Paediatr Scand (Suppl) 174:5–95, 1967

7. Tikoff G, Keith TB, Nelson RM, et al: Clinical and hemodynamic observations after surgical closure of large atrial septal defect complicated by heart failure. Am J Cardiol 23:810–817, 1969

8. Epstein SE, Beiser GD, Goldstein RE, et al: Hemodynamic abnormalities in response to mild and intense upright exercise following operative correction of an atrial septal defect of tetralogy of Fallot. Circulation 47:1065–1075, 1973

9. Graham TP Jr, Jarmakani JM, Canent RV: Left heart volume characteristics with a right ventricular volume overload. Circulation 45:389–396, 1972

10. Miller GAH, Swan HJC: Effect of chronic pressure and volume overload on left heart volumes in subjects with congenital heart disease. Circulation 30:205–216, 1964.

11. Graham TP Jr, Lewis BW, Jarmakani MM, et al: Left heart volume and mass quantification in children with left ventricular pressure overload. Circulation 41: 203–212, 1970

12. Graham TP Jr, Jarmakani JM, Canent RV, et al: Evaluation of left ventricular contractile state in childhood. Circulation 44:1043–1052, 1971

13. Meerson FZ, Pshennikova MG: Effect of myocardial hypertrophy on cardiac contractility. Byull Eksp Biol Med 59:T957–T959, 1965

14. Spann JF, Buccino RA, Sonnenblick EH, et al: Contractile state of cardiac muscle obtained from cats with experimentally produced ventricular hypertrophy and heart failure. Circ Res 21:341–354, 1967

15. Krayenbuhl HP, Pierce EC, Agishi T: Left ventricular dynamics in the dog under chronic pressure load from coarctation of the aorta. Arch Kreislaufforsch 56:1–25, 1968

16. Bing OHS, Matsushita S, Fanburg BL, et al: Mechanical properties of rat cardiac muscle during experimental hypertrophy. Circ Res 28:234–245, 1971

17. Kaufman RL, Hamburger H, Wirth H: Disorder in excitation-contraction coupling of cardiac muscle from cats with experimentally produced right ventricular hypertrophy. Circ Res 28:346–357, 1971

18. Cooper G, Satava RM, Harrison CE, et al: Mechanism for the abnormal energetics of pressure-induced hypertrophy of cat myocardium. Circ Res 33:213–223, 1973

19. Simon H, Krayenbuehl HP, Rutishauser W, et al: The contractile state of the hypertrophied left ventricular myocardium in aortic stenosis. Am Heart J 79:587–602, 1970

20. Mason DT, Spann JF, Zelis R: Comparison of the contractile state of the normal, hypertrophied, and failing heart in man, in Alpert N (ed): Cardiac hypertrophy. New York, Academic Press, 1970

21. Levine HJ, McIntyre KM, Lipana JG, et al: Force-

velocity relations in failing and nonfailing hearts of subjects with aortic stenosis. Am J Med Sci 259:79–89, 1970

22. Hoffman JIE: The natural history of congenital isolated pulmonic and aortic stenosis. Annu Rev Med 20:15–28, 1969

23. Graham TP Jr, Bender HW, Atwood GF, et al: Increase in right ventricular volume following valvulotomy for pulmonary atresia or stenosis with intact ventricular septum. Circulation (II) 49–50, 69–79, 1974

24. Oakley CM, Brainbridge MV, Bentall HH, et al: Reversed interatrial shunt following complete relief of pulmonary valve stenosis. Br Heart J 26:662–670, 1964

25. Moller JH, Girod D, Amplatz K, Varco R: Pulmonary valvulotomy in pulmonary atresia with hypoplastic right ventricle. Surgery 68:630–634, 1970

26. DeCastro CM, Nelson WP, Jones RC, et al: Pulmonary stenosis: Cyanosis, interatrial communication, and inadequate right ventricular distensibility following pulmonary valvulotomy. Am J Cardiol 26:540–543, 1970

27. Freed MD, Rosenthal A, Bernhard WF, et al: Critical pulmonary stenosis with a diminutive right ventricle in neonate. Circulation 48:875–881, 1973

28. Jarmakani JM, Graham TP Jr, Canent RV, et al: Left heart function in children with tetralogy of Fallot before and after palliative or corrective surgery. Circulation 46:478–490, 1972

29. Sunderland CO, Matarazzo RG, Lies MH, et al: Total correction of tetralogy of Fallot in infancy: Postoperative hemodynamic evaluation. Circulation 48:398–405, 1973

30. Krymskii LD: Pathological anatomy of the tetralogy, pentalogy, and trilogy of Fallot. Arkh Patol 24: T1160–T1168, 1962

31. Graham TP Jr, Jarmakani JM, Canent RV, et al: P quantification of left heart volume and systolic output in transposition of the great arteries. Circulation 44:889–909, 1971

32. Keane JF, Ellison C, Rudd M, et al: Pulmonary blood flow and left ventricular volumes in transposition of the great arteries and intact ventricular septum. Br Heart J 35:521–526, 1973

33. Atwood GF, Graham TP Jr, Nelson JH: Right heart volume characteristics in transposition of the great arteries. Circulation, May 1975

34. Jarmakani JM, Canent RV: Pre and postoperative right ventricular function in children with transposition of the great arteries. Circulation (Suppl II) 49–50, 39, 1974

35. Menke JA, Shaker RM, Wolff GS: Ejection fraction in anomalous origin of the coronary artery from the pulmonary artery. Am Heart J 84:325–329, 1972

36. Wagner HR, Nadas AS, Hugenholtz PG: Anomalous left coronary artery originating from the pulmonary artery. Pediatrics 40:320–328, 1967

37. Graham TP Jr, Jarmakani JM: Evaluation of ventricular function in infants and children. Pediatr Clin North Am 18:1109–1132, 1971

38. Tyrrell MJ, Bharadwaj B: Anomalous origin of the left coronary artery: The effects of aortocoronary bypass on left ventricular function. Can Med Assoc J 107:118–122, 1972

Pulmonary Hemodynamics After Repair of Left-to-Right Shunt Lesions Associated With Pulmonary Artery Hypertension

Victor Whitman and Nancy G. Ellis

THE PROGNOSIS of patients with congenital heart disease and pulmonary hypertension is at least partially related to the reversibility of pulmonary hypertension after surgery. In normal individuals, the great compliance of the normal pulmonary vascular tree permits pulmonary blood flow to increase several fold (e.g., during exercise) with only a slight increase in pulmonary arterial pressure.[1] In congenital heart lesions with left-to-right shunts, pulmonary artery pressure is often elevated out of proportion to the increased blood flow, indicating that some other factor or factors must be influencing pulmonary artery pressure in these individuals. The principal pathophysiologic mechanisms here are anatomic pulmonary vascular disease, which may or may not be reversible depending on its severity, and reactive pulmonary vasoconstriction. Pulmonary vasoconstriction is known to occur in response to hypoxemia, acidosis, and elevated pulmonary venous pressure. Increased pulmonary venous pressure is most often seen in patients with decreased left ventricular compliance; but may also be related to increased pulmonary venous blood flow. The relative contributions of vasoconstrictive and anatomic factors to pulmonary hypertension associated with increased pulmonary vascular resistance in a given individual are rarely, if ever, definable. The term "hyperdynamic pulmonary hypertension" is somewhat of a misnomer since some degree of increased pulmonary vascular resistance exists in most patients with pulmonary hypertension and increased pulmonary blood flow.

The spectrum of increased pulmonary vascular resistance extends from the slight increase in the individual with greatly increased pulmonary blood flow to the individual with pulmonary vascular resistance at or above systemic level. Correlations of hemodynamic data with pathologic specimens have shown increasing severity of pulmonary arteriolar lesions with increasing pulmonary vascular resistance. However, correlation of pathologic findings with reversibility after surgery are well established only for mild anatomic changes.[2-4]

The criteria of operability and optimum age for surgery of patients with left-to-right shunt lesions have varied widely among institutions and surgeons. In particular, opinions of the optimum age for surgery have changed with improvements in surgical techniques. In general, the principal contraindication to surgery has been the presence of Eisenmenger's syndrome: pulmonary hypertension with pulmonary vascular resistance at or above systemic level, and right-to-left or bidirectional shunting through the channel or channels which originally conducted a left-to-right shunt.[5] In such patients, surgical closure of a defect does not lessen right ventricular work. Indeed, it may increase right ventricular work in patients with ventricular septal defect (VSD) or patent ductus arteriosus (PDA) by removing the right ventricular "pop-off valve" into the systemic arterial circulation. In addition, the right ventricle may be unable to eject an adequate cardiac output in the presence of greatly increased pulmonary vascular resistance. Eisenmenger's syndrome is rare and becoming rarer as diagnostic techniques improve and physicians' sophistication increases. However, pulmonary hypertension of various degrees in children with left-to-right shunt lesions continues to be a fairly common clinical problem. Pulmonary hypertension associated with left-to-right shunt in childhood is almost exclusively seen in patients with isolated VSD, VSD with PDA, PDA alone, or aortopulmonary window, or other complex lesions associated with VSD or absent interventricular septum. This paper reviews the published data on pulmonary hemodynamics following surgery in patients with left-to-right shunt lesions and pulmonary hypertension. The reported postoperative catheterization data deal almost exclusively with patients operated on for isolated VSD, VSD with PDA, PDA alone, or aortopulmonary window. The studies are presented in chronologic order. Surgical mortality is not considered.

From the Division of Cardiology, Hershey Medical Center, Hershey, Pa., and the Department of Pediatrics, University Hospitals of Cleveland, Cleveland, Ohio.

Reprint requests should be addressed to Victor Whitman, M.D., Assistant Professor of Pediatrics, Division of Cardiology, Hershey Medical Center, Hershey, Pa. 17033.

TECHNICAL CONSIDERATIONS IN EVALUATING PUBLISHED RESULTS

It will be seen that various authors use different paramenters to describe pulmonary hemodynamics, so that comparable data are not available for all patients. Pulmonary vascular resistance values, in particular, are often difficult to interpret. Vascular resistance in dyne-sec-cm^{-5} is readily converted to units (mm Hg-$liter^{-1}$-min) by division by 80.[6] In this article, all resistance values will be reported in units. The number value of pulmonary vascular resistance (Rp) varies depending upon whether it is calculated from pulmonary blood flow (Qp) expressed as an absolute number (L/min) or indexed for body surface area (L/min/M^2). For individuals with body surface areas less than one square meter, and especially for infants, the absolute number value of Rp may be much less than the indexed value, rendering comparisons among individuals of different body sizes inaccurate. The same holds for repeated measurements on the same individual of more than a few months elapse between studies, as body surface area may change significantly, particularly in infants.

Calculation of pulmonary and systemic blood flows by the Fick principle may be inaccurate when oxygen consumption is assumed rather than measured. This inaccuracy may be minimized by calculating the ratio of pulmonary to systemic resistance (Rp:Rs). Errors in calculated blood flows affect both circuits equally and are eliminated where the ratio is used. Use of the Rp:Rs ratio rather than the number value of Rp also eliminates the indexing problem, so that individuals of different sizes may be compared directly. Normal pulmonary vascular resistance is 1-3 units/M^2 and normal systemic vascular resistance is 10-20 units/M^2,[7] the normal value of the Rp:Rs ratio is, therefore, 0.1-0.15.

The normal limits of pulmonary artery pressure are well established.[1] However, conditions at catheterization (general anesthesia, heavy sedation, and oxygen administration) may affect pulmonary artery pressure measurements. This may be particularly important in the older literature, as general anesthesia or heavy sedation were frequently used for cardiac catheterization at that time, and unsuspected hypoventilation might cause spurious elevation of pulmonary artery pressure and pulmonary vascular resistance.

LITERATURE REVIEW

Adams et al.[8] reported pre- and postoperative data from 57 patients who were restudied an average of 1.8 yr after VSD closure. Patients were divided into three groups according to the postoperative systolic pulmonary artery pressure (SPAP). Patients in group 1 (postoperative SPAP $\geqslant$ 40 mm Hg) were 9 mo-9 yr of age (median = 5 yr). Mean preoperative SPAP was 88 mm Hg (range 30-95) and mean preoperative pulmonary vascular resistance 11 units (range 3-23.1). Mean postoperative SPAP was 51 mm Hg (range 40-88). SPAP fell in all but three patients in whom significant rises were recorded. Postoperatively, pulmonary vascular resistance was unchanged in three, decreased in four, and increased above the preoperative value in 12. None were normal. There were 18 patients in group 2 (postoperative SPAP 28-40 mm Hg) ages 9 mo-14 yr (median = 5 yr). Mean preoperative SPAP was 87 mm Hg (range 40-115) similar to group 1. The mean preoperative pulmonary vascular resistance of group 2 (6.4 units; range 1.6-19.4) was, however, significantly less than in group 1 and the mean preoperative pulmonary blood flow significantly greater. Postoperatively SPAP's in group 2 all decreased and eight were normal. The mean postoperative SPAP was 32 mm Hg. Pulmonary vascular resistance was unchanged in ten patients; one showed a small decrease in resistance and nine showed small increases.

Group 3 (postoperative SPAP $\leqslant$ 28 mm Hg) comprised 19 patients aged 6 mo-8 yr (median was slightly greater than 1 yr). Mean preoperative SPAP was 40 mm Hg (range 20-90) and mean preoperative pulmonary vascular resistance was 1.4 units (range 1.3-22.5). All postoperative SPAP's were less than 30 mm Hg. Changes in pulmonary vascular resistance were very small; five showed slight increases, four were slightly decreased, and the remainder were unchanged. Seven were within the normal range and none was more than three times normal. The authors concluded that closure of the VSD had not lessened pulmonary vascular pathology, and that the observed decreases in pulmonary artery pressures were due almost entirely to the reduction in pulmonary blood flow.

Braunwald et al.[9] reported on 20 patients following surgery for VSD, PDA, and aortopulmonary window, whose preoperative SPAP's were at least 50 mm Hg with mean pulmonary artery pressures

(MPAP) at least 30 mm Hg. The interval between surgery and recatheterization was 12 mo or less in 21 patients, and between 24 and 38 mo in eight patients. Two patients with isolated VSD were 4 yr old and six were 12–28 yr of age. All eight had lower MPAP postoperatively; however, the MPAP remained above normal in six (24–42 mm Hg), including the 4 yr olds. Changes in the ratio of pulmonary vascular resistance to systemic vascular resistance (Rp:Rs) were small or absent, and the ratio remained abnormal in all (0.17–0.48).

Twelve patients with PDA or aortopulmonary window (three, 2 yr of age or younger; seven, ages 7–15 yr, and two adults) showed less pulmonary hypertension postoperatively. Only two maintained MPAP > 20 mm Hg (27 and 64) and these two had had preoperative mean pressures of 66 and 100 mm Hg, respectively. When the patient whose MPAP was 64 mm Hg 12 mo after surgery was restudied 26 mo later, the MPAP had fallen further to 44 mm Hg. Rp/Rs was measured in ten patients and returned to normal in nine.

Leachman[10] reported four patients with isolated VSD aged 3½–7 yr who were selected because they had some degree of bidirectional shunting and normal left atrial pressures. Preoperative MPAP's were at least 60 mm Hg in all and Rp/Rs ranged from 0.39 to 0.85. At repeat catheterization 1 yr after surgery, MPAP and Rp/Rs decreased in all patients; but none were normal. The authors point out that the postoperative findings are consistent with pressure changes due solely to elimination of the left-to-right shunt without any change in pulmonary vascular resistance.

Hallman et al.[11] reported results of catheterizations performed 1 yr after surgery in 56 of 241 patients with VSD and preoperative pulmonary hypertension, defined as pulmonary artery systolic pressure greater than 50% of systemic artery systolic pressure (SPAP/SSAP > 0.5). The majority of the 241 patients (90%) were below 16 yr of age at the time of surgery, and 30% were < 2 yr old. Of the ten patients with mild preoperative pulmonary hypertension (SPAP/SSAP 0.5–0.64), eight had postoperative ratios < 0.5 and two were unchanged. Of ten patients with preoperative SPAP/SSAP ratios of 0.65–0.80, the ratio was < 0.5 postoperatively in nine and remained in the 0.5–0.64 range in one. Of 36 patients with severe pulmonary hypertension preoperatively (SPAP/SSAP > 0.8), 21 patients had postoperative ratios < 0.5, five had ratios of 0.5–0.64, one had a ratio between 0.64 and 0.8, and nine continued to have ratios > 0.8. Five of these had persistent shunts; two were reoperated, and five died with chronic congestive failure 1–7 yr after surgery.

Lillehei et al.[12,13] restudied 40 postoperative patients with VSD selected because preoperative catheterization showed systolic pulmonary artery pressure (SPAP) of 80 mm Hg or greater, with predominant left-to-right shunt. Six patients had additional PDA. Five patients were 2 yr old or younger, 27 were 3–10 yr old, and eight were 11–16 yr of age at the time of surgery. Follow-up catheterizations were done between 5 mo and 5 yr postoperatively (mean 17 mo). Almost every patient exhibited a significant decrease in his SPAP but only nine returned to normal (≤ 30 mm Hg); two maintained SPAP > 80. Pulmonary vascular resistance declined only slightly in this group of patients and the authors felt that the greatest improvements occurred in the younger patients. There were ten patients whose preoperative pulmonary vascular resistance exceeded 12.5 units. Postoperatively, resistance returned to normal in one, fell significantly but not to normal in six and rose significantly in three, one of whom died 26 mo after surgery with severe pulmonary vascular disease. Six patients underwent at least two postoperative catheterizations. SPAP declined further in four, was unchanged in one, and rose in comparison to the first postoperative study in one. In four of these patients, pulmonary vascular resistance was higher postoperatively than preoperatively. Second postoperative catheterizations showed decreased resistance in three while resistance rose in the fourth.

Cartmill et al.[14] studied 42 patients following VSD closure whose preoperative systolic pulmonary artery pressure to systolic systemic artery pressure ratio (SPAP/SSAP) was > 0.75. The ages of these patients are not stated. Postoperative catheterizations were performed in most patients at least 1 yr postoperatively (range 6 mo–6 yr). Twelve of 42 patients had preoperative Rp/Rs ratios < 0.45. The ratio declined in four to an average value of 0.17, was unchanged in six, and rose in two (0.5 and 0.78). There were 26 patients whose Rp:Rs ratios were between 0.45 and 0.75; 15 had a fall to an average level of 0.28, six showed no change, and in five the ratio rose to an average of 0.9. There were four patients whose Rp:Rs ratios exceeded 0.75; the ratio declined in two (0.26 and 0.28) and showed no change in two. The average age of seven patients whose resistance ratios increased postoperatively was, 7 yr, of 14 patients whose Rp:Rs did not change, 13 yr, and of 21 patients whose resistance ratio declined significantly after surgery, 5 yr. The authors found that of their patients with VSD and significant pulmonary hypertension (SPAP/SSAP > 0.75), those with Rp:Rs < 0.45 had a 7% incidence of severe pulmonary vascular disease postoperatively, while those with Rp:Rs between 0.45 and 0.75 had a 16% incidence of severe pulmonary vascular disease postoperatively.

Grosse-Brockhoff and Loogen[15] studied 65 patients after VSD closure. All were over 2 yr of age; most (57) were 5-20 yr of age, and five were adults. The first postoperative catheterization was 6-8 wk after surgery and a second catheterization was done a year or more later. All patients had MPAP > 20 mm Hg preoperatively. Most showed decreased MPAP postoperatively, and one-third reached normal values. All patients with normal postoperative values had preoperative MPAP < 50 mm Hg. In 43 patients, MPAP fell but remained above 20 mm Hg; in 21 of these, MPAP was above 30 mm Hg. MPAP remained unchanged in five patients and rose in two patients in the 11-20-yr old group. Subsequent postoperative catheterization either showed no changes or slight lowering of the MPAP; two individuals whose values had initially fallen to 40 and 62 mm Hg later showed increases to 50 and 90 mm Hg, respectively. These two patients and one other whose MPAP rose postoperatively, had preoperative pulmonary vascular resistances greater than 10 units. One must note that many of Grosse-Brackhoff's patients, unlike most others reviewed, had only mild or moderate elevations of pulmonary artery pressure.

Sterns et al.[16] reported pre- and postoperative hemodynamic data from 22 patients aged 5-30 mo at the time of VSD closure. Preoperatively, three infants had SPAP > 80 mm Hg (group A); ten had SPAP between 50 and 80 mm Hg (group B), and nine had SPAP < 50 mm Hg (group C). Follow-up catheterizations were done 5 mo-9½ yr after surgery; the average MPAP in group A patients fell from 87 to 18 mm Hg and mean total pulmonary resistance from 15.8 to 5.9 units. In group B mean MPAP fell from 57 to 28 mm Hg, and mean total resistance fell from 15.5 to 10.6 units. In group C, mean MPAP fell from 37 to 24 mm Hg and mean total resistance rose slightly from 8 to 8.3 units.

Hallidie-Smith et al.[17] reported pre- and postoperative data on 25 patients with VSD and pulmonary vascular disease. These patients all had SPAP $\leqslant 10$ mm Hg below systemic, pulmonary vascular resistance 8 units or more and ratio of pulmonary to systemic blood flow (Qp/Qs) was 2.5-1 or less. Preoperative Rp:Rs ratios were 0.38-0.88. No patient was accepted for surgery who had dominant right-to-left shunting at catheterization or who was clinically cyanotic at rest. Patients were 3-12 yr old at the time of surgery and follow-up catheterizations were at least 1 yr after surgery.

At the first postoperative catheterization the systolic pulmonary artery pressure (SPAP) was normal ($\leqslant 30$ mm Hg) in two patients, 31-49 mm Hg in 17, 50-59 mm Hg in seven, and > 59 mm Hg in four. Of the ten patients who underwent two postoperative catheterizations, the SPAP of two additional patients became normal; other changes were random and slight. Preoperatively, pulmonary vascular resistance was mildly elevated (Rp/Rs = 0.25-0.45) in five, moderately elevated (0.46-0.75) in 16, and markedly elevated (> 0.76) in four. The ratio Rp:Rs fell in all patients except two; in one it rose from 0.55 to 0.66 and subsequently fell to 0.54; in the other there was no change at the first postoperative catheterization but a fall at the second recatheterization from 0.5 to 0.3. Postoperatively, the resistance ratio was below 0.25 in seven and one had a resistance ratio of 0.18, near normal. Twelve patients had mild pulmonary vascular disease (Rp:Rs 0.25-0.45) and six had moderate disease (Rp:Rs 0.45-0.75). At subsequent recatheterizations of ten patients the Rp:Rs ratio showed slight random changes in nine and a decline in one, as noted above.

Gotsman et al.[18] restudied 21 patients with VSD and pulmonary hypertension 1 yr after surgical closure of the defects. Patients were about 5 yr old at the time of surgery unless they had severe symptoms, in which case surgery was performed when they reached about 10 kg in weight. There were nine patients whose preoperative ratio of systolic pulmonary artery pressure to systolic systemic artery pressure (SPAP/SSAP) was 0.4-0.8. Postoperatively, SPAP/SSAP fell in all except one patient with pulmonary stenosis, in whom it was unchanged. Five had ratios 0.25 or less. Preoperative Rp/Rs ratios were < 0.20 in all patients. Postoperatively, the Rp/Rs was unchanged in eight and rose to 0.23 in one.

There were 11 patients whose preoperative SPAP/SSAP ratios were 0.8 or more (mean 0.85) with large left-to-right shunts (mean 61% of pulmonary blood flow). Postoperatively SPAP/SSAP fell in all and was <0.25 in three. Preoperative Rp:Rs ratios were 0.1–0.55 (mean 0.27). Postoperative resistance ratios were unchanged in four, decreased in four, and increased significantly in three, including one whose resistance ratio was normal preoperatively.

Wagner et al.[19] recatheterized nine patients after surgical closure of ventricular septal defects associated with pulmonary hypertension (SPAP/SSAP >0.8). In this series, patients were recatheterized only if they were doing poorly clinically, or had evidence of persistent significant shunts; hence this group represents a deliberate selection of patients with unsatisfactory or questionable results. Patients were 2–22 yr of age at the time of surgery. The recatheterized group all had preoperative mean pulmonary artery pressures of 50 mm Hg or more (range 50–80). Postoperatively MPAP fell to normal in two, decreased but not to normal in four, (one of whom had a persistent defect) and rose in three (one of whom had a persistent defect). The ratio Rp/Rs was normal preoperatively in two and remained normal postoperatively. Preoperative Rp/Rs in the other seven ranged from 0.18 to 0.56. Rp/Rs fell from 0.56 to 0.4 in one patient with a persistent defect. Rp:Rs increased in five patients to 0.23 in 1.5 and was unchanged in one. Three patients whose Rp/Rs ratio increased postoperatively developed systemic or suprasystemic pulmonary vascular resistance.

Castaneda et al.[20] reported catheterization findings in 22 patients studied 1 yr after VSD closure. Patients' ages at the time of surgery ranged from 1 to 17 yr (mean 5.5 yr). The mean pulmonary ranged from 52 to 90 mm Hg (mean 79 mm Hg) and preoperative pulmonary vascular resistances were 11.25–31.3 units (mean 18.3 units). Postoperatively, SPAP and pulmonary vascular resistance decreased in all patients. Postoperative MPAP ranged from 16 to 60 mm Hg (mean 31 mm Hg) and in six patients it was within the normal range. The mean postoperative pulmonary vascular resistance was 6 units (range 1.9–10 units). Twelve patients maintained pulmonary vascular resistance values of at least 6 units. The only patients whose pulmonary vascular resistance values returned to normal* were six who were <4 yr of age at the time of surgery. A seventh patient in this age group did not return to normal. No patient's pulmonary vascular resistance increased postoperatively.

Ibach et al.[25] reported hemodynamic findings in 71 patients who were recatheterized between 1 and 2 yr following VSD closure. They were part of a total surgical group of 102 patients with a mean age at surgery of 5.7 yr (range 6 mo-13 yr). Twenty-six patients had preoperative ratios of mean pulmonary artery pressure to mean systemic artery pressure (MPAP/MSAP) <0.25; the postoperative ratios remained <0.25 in all. Thirty-six patients had preoperative MPAP/MSAP ratios 0.25–0.75; postoperatively the ratio decreased to <0.25 in 31, and remained above 0.25 in five. Seven patients had preoperative ratios >0.75. Postoperatively two were unchanged, one decreased to 0.26, and four decreased to <0.25.

Friedli et al.[26] reported postoperative hemodynamic data from 25 patients with VSD whose preoperative Rp/Rs ratios were 0.25 or above and whose pulmonary vascular resistance was in excess of 5 units/M^2. Mean age at surgery was 4.8 yr (range 11 mo–17 yr). Catheterizations were done 1–11 yr after operation. Postoperative catheterizations showed that MPAP had fallen significantly in 23 patients, and had risen slightly in two. The MPAP was normal in seven patients, greater than 30 mm Hg in ten, and above 40 mm Hg in six. Among patients operated on after 2 yr of age, six of eight patients with mild elevations of the resistance ratio (Rp/Rs 0.25–0.33) had decreased Rp/Rs postoperatively; the ratio increased in two. Of ten patients whose preoperative Rp/Rs ratios were >0.33, only two showed decreased resistance ratios postoperatively. One was essentially unchanged, and seven rose, three to systemic level. Three patients in this group died of pulmonary vascular disease 1–7 yr postoperatively. Two other patients not catheterized preoperatively but who were thought to have moderately elevated pulmonary vascular resistance on clinical grounds, had progressive pulmonary vascular disease after surgery, and one died.

*The authors use the data of Lucas et al.[21] to describe the normal fall in pulmonary vascular resistance with age. Other authors[22,24] describe a more rapid fall.[22–24]

There were three survivors of surgery who had had normal pulmonary vascular resistance with large pulmonary blood flows in the first year of life and who developed increased resistance in the second year. Surgery was done before 2 yr of age. The resistance ratio fell in all three and was near normal 6–10 yr postoperatively.

CONCLUSIONS

Most of the studies reviewed are not directly comparable with one another. Some groups chose to report only patients with increased pulmonary vascular resistance preoperatively[17,26] while others chose levels of pulmonary hypertension ranging from the upper limit of normal[15] to near systemic level.[10,14,20] Those who report their total surgical experience indicate that these patients are a small fraction (10%–25%) of all patients operated for VSD. In some cases, particularly those reported by Hallidie-Smith et al.[17] and Ross et al.[27] one questions whether heavy sedation or general anesthesia at catheterization produced conditions under which pulmonary artery pressures were spuriously elevated. Hypoxemia and respiratory acidosis which may exist under these conditions are factors causing pulmonary arteriolar constriction. In addition, some anesthetic agents depress myocardial contractility. Despite these difficulties, general findings among different groups are quite similar, and several conclusions may be drawn.

As would be expected, pulmonary artery pressure usually declines when pulmonary blood flow declines after surgery. However, in patients with VSD and at least moderate pulmonary hypertension, pulmonary artery pressure was unlikely to return to normal. Residual pulmonary hypertension was noted to occur more often in older patients and those few patients whose pulmonary artery pressure rose postoperatively were in the older age group. Second postoperative studies generally showed a continuation of the trend seen at the first postoperative study or no change. However, there were a few patients whose pulmonary pressure rose again after an initial fall.

Changes in pulmonary vascular resistance are less dramatic. In general, it did not change or became lower, but very rarely returned to normal. Cartmill et al.[14] noted a striking age difference between patients whose resistance ratio remained unchanged (mean age 13 yr) and those whose resistance ratio declined (mean age 5 yr); other groups made similar observations. In almost every series there were a few patients whose pulmonary vascular resistance increased postoperatively and some of these developed resistance at systemic level. In Cartmill's series, increased pulmonary vascular resistance postoperatively seemed related more to preoperative resistance than to age; this was generally true in other series but there does not seem to be any one factor (age, preoperative resistance, or volume of left-to-right shunt) which alone will predict the individual whose resistance will increase postoperatively. Second postoperative catheterizations generally either showed no changes as compared to the first postoperative catheterization or a continuation of the trend seen at the first postoperative study.

The existence of any pulmonary hypertension in the presence of normal pulmonary blood flow is indicative of significant changes in the pulmonary vasculature, since it implies loss of the normal pulmonary vascular compliance (provided conditions that cause vasoconstriction are eliminated). It would appear that the majority of patients with VSD and significant pulmonary hypertension who have even mild elevations of pulmonary vascular resistance preoperatively continue to have elevated resistance postoperatively. The significance of mildly elevated pulmonary vascular resistance over a 40–50-yr period is unknown at present and further follow-up studies of the patients in the series reviewed here will be very informative.

In the absence of data about the prognosis of mild and moderate pulmonary vascular disease after VSD closure, it would seem advisable to operate on individuals with VSD and moderate pulmonary hypertension before there is any increase in pulmonary vascular resistance, probably before age two. Catheterization of individuals with pulmonary hypertension should be done in such a way as to exclude vasoconstrictive factors such as hypoxemia and acidosis. Long-term follow-up will be necessary to define the ultimate prognosis of individuals with pulmonary hypertension after closure of ventricular septal defects.

REFERENCES

1. Fowler NO: The normal pulmonary arterial pressure-flow relationships during exercise. Am J Med 47:1–5, 1969

2. Wagenwoort CA, Newfeld HN, DuShane JW: The pulmonary arterial tree in ventricular septal defect. Circulation 23:740–748, 1961

3. Wagenwoort CA, Nauta J, van der Schaab PJ: Effect of flow and pressure on pulmonary vessels. Circulation 35 1028–1037, 1967
4. Heath D, Edwards JE: The pathology of hypertensive pulmonary vascular disease. Circulation 18:533–547, 1958
5. Brammel HL, Vogel JHK, Pryor R: The Eisenmenger syndrome: A clinical and physiological reappraisal. Am J Cardiol 28:679–691, 1971
6. Yang SS, et al: From Cardiac Catheterization Data to Hemodynamic Parameters. Philadelphia, Davis, 1972, p 242
7. Nadas AS, Fyler DC: Pediatric Cardiology. Philadelphia, Saunders, 1972, p 137
8. Adams P, et al: Physiologic changes after closure of ventricular septal defects. Lancet 81:497–501, 1961
9. Braunwald NS, Braunwald E, Morrow AG: The effects of surgical abolition of left to right shunts on the pulmonary vascular dynamics of patients with pulmonary hypertension. Circulation 26:1270–1278, 1962
10. Leachman RD: Observations on the pulmonary vascular resistance following surgical closure of high-resistance ventricular septal defects. Cardiovas Res Center Bull 2:23–25, 1963
11. Hallman GL, Cooley DA, Wolfe RR: Surgical treatment of ventricular septal defect associated with pulmonary hypertension. J Thorac Cardiovasc Surg 48:588–600, 1964
12. Lillehei CW, Levy MJ, Adams P: High pressure ventricular septal defects. JAMA 188:949–952, 1964
13. Lillehei CW, Anderson RC, Eliot RS: Pre and postoperative cardiac catheterization in 200 patients undergoing closure of ventricular septal defects. Surgery 63: 69–76, 1968
14. Cartmill TB, DuShane JW, McGoon DC: Results of repair of ventricular septal defect. J Thorac Cardiovasc Surg 52:486–499, 1966
15. Grosse-Brockhoff F, Loogen F: Ventricular septal defect. Circulation 37, 38 (Suppl) V:13–21, 1968
16. Sterns LP, Indoglia RA, Lillehei CW: Clinical and hemodynamic results of ventricular septal defect closure in infancy. Can J Surg 11:431–434, 1968
17. Hallidie-Smith KA, Hollman A, Cleland WP: Effects of surgical closure of ventricular septal defects upon pulmonary vascular disease. Br Heart J 31:246–260, 1969
18. Gotsman MS, Beck W, Barnard CN: Hemodynamic studies after repair of ventricular septal defect. Br Heart J 31:63–71, 1969
19. Wagner RB, Ankeney JL, Liebman J: Correlation of mean pulmonary arterial pressure with results of surgery for non-restrictive ventricular septal defects. J Thorac Cardiovasc Surg 60:510–515, 1970
20. Castaneda AR, Zamora R, Nicoloff DM: High-pressure, high-resistance ventricular septal defect: Surgical results of closure through right atrium. Am Thorac Surg 12:29–36, 1971
21. Lucas RV: Maturation of the pulmonary vascular bed. Am J Dis Child 101:467–475, 1961
22. Adams FH, Lind J: Physiologic studies on the cardiovascular status of normal newborn infants, (with special reference to the ductus arteriosis). Pediatrics 19:431–437, 1957
23. Rowe RD, Jonus LS: The normal pulmonary arterial pressure during the first year of life. J. Pediatr 51:1–4, 1957
24. Emmanouilides GC, Moss AJ, Duffie ER: Pulmonary arterial pressure changes in human newborn infants from birth to three days of age. J Pediatr 65:327–333, 1964
25. Ibach JR, Bartley TD, Daicoff GR: Correction of ventricular septal defect in childhood. Am Thorac Surg 11:499–507, 1971
26. Friedli B, Langford Kidd BS, Mustard WT: Ventricular septal defect with increased pulmonary vascular resistance: Late results of surgical closure. Am J Cardiol 33:403–409, 1974
27. Ross J, Morrow AG, Braunwald E: Regression of severe pulmonary hypertension after repair of a defect of the ventricular septum in a patient with a bidirectional shunt. N Engl J Med 270:946–948, 1964

Growth and Development After Cardiovascular Surgery in Infants and Children

Amnon Rosenthal and Aldo R. Castaneda

GROWTH DISTURBANCE is a major consequence of congenital heart disease in infancy and childhood. The severity of growth retardation is generally dependent on the anatomic lesion and its functional effects. Most children with mild defects grow normally. In addition to the symptoms and limitations imposed by the cardiovascular malformation, the child with delayed physical development may not only lag in height and weight maturation but also in motor skills and in the development of intelligence.[1] The child with retarded development will not do as well in athletics or school and may be kept back a year or placed in a class more appropriate to his chronological age. Children with growth failure tend to be treated as younger than age, are teased by peers, and become socially isolated. As a consequence, they often feel rejected and may become either very passive or aggressive.

The goal of surgery in infants and children with congenital heart disease is not only the saving of life but also the prevention of the adverse effects of congenital heart disease on growth, and intellectual and psychologic development. Growth assessment may provide the parents and the postoperative child with a reassurance they need about the individual's health. The purpose of this report is to examine to what extent palliative and corrective surgery has influenced subsequent growth.

METHODOLOGY

Growth in children is commonly assessed by the use of height and weight curves or charts. Using data from a large group of normal children, graphs are constructed which show the relationship of height and weight to chronological age (Fig. 1). Because of individual variations in growth, a considerable scatter exists for any given age. This is designated by percentile lines on the chart. Thus, in Fig. 1, 3% of the group of children had measurements which were on or below the line marked 3. The 16th percentile reflects one standard deviation and the third percentile line, two standard deviations from the mean.

Longitudinal measurements taken on any individual can be plotted against chronological age to indicate progress of growth. A child growing normally tends to maintain his relative position with respect to his age group. Height and weight often differ in their actual percentile positions but tend to maintain the same general relationship from period to period during childhood, with some greater variation during adolescence.[2] The growth charts do not indicate or define the optimum but are helpful in evaluating the effects of treatment on growth. It is generally felt that if the measurement is above the 97th percentile or below the third percentile, or if the rate of growth has changed more than 20 percentile points, the doctor should seek to determine a cause for the deviation.[3] Children with congenital heart disease whose height and weight measurements fall near or below the third percentile or in whom weight falls in a widely lower percentile group than height may be considered to have a growth abnormality.

EVALUATION OF PUBLISHED DATA

Conflicting data and confusion regarding the effects of cardiac surgery on growth stems from a number of factors. There is lack of uniform criteria for defining growth failure and reporting results. The criteria for defining growth failure are often vague and not sufficiently stringent with some studies including patients below the 16th percentile[4] or 10th percentile[5] and others below the third percentile[6] (two standard deviations) or one percentile (three standard deviations).[7] Standards for normal growth used for comparison have included the Iowa grid,[8] Wetzel grid,[9] Gray and Ayers[10] or Reed-Stuart[11] norms. Analysis of the anthropomorphic data obtained has usually been by standard deviation or percentile deviation from normal. Most reported studies are retrospective and limited to the evaluation of growth by weight

---

From the Departments of Cardiology, Pediatrics, and Surgery, The Children's Hospital Medical Center, Harvard Medical School, Boston, Mass.

Reprint requests should be addressed to Amnon Rosenthal, M.D., Senior Associate in Cardiology, The Children's Hospital Medical Center, 300 Longwood Avenue, Boston, Mass. 02115

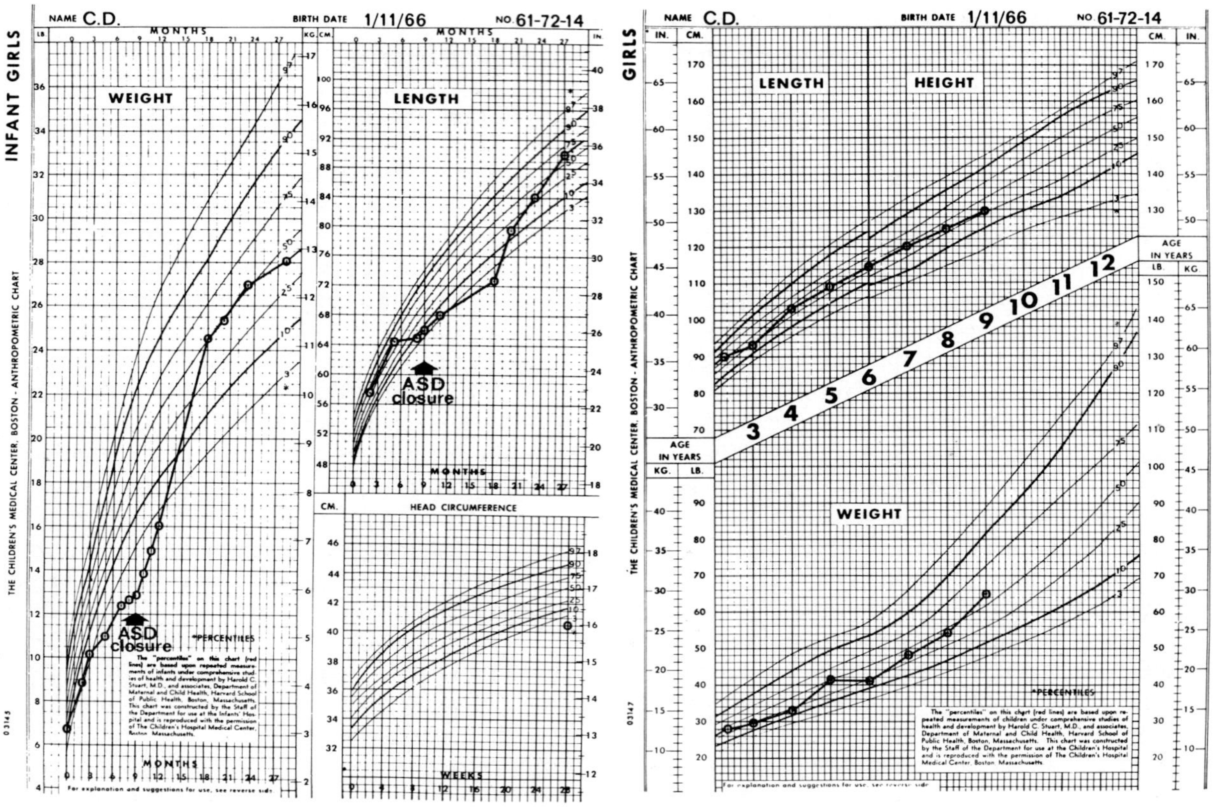

Fig. 1. Growth pattern before and after surgical closure of an atrial-septal defect (ASD) primum in a 9-mo-old infant with intractable congestive heart failure. Note the marked improvement in weight and height maturation with an initial catch-up period and subsequent 'normal' growth. The child has residual mitral regurgitation due to a cleft mitral valve.

and height or by weight alone.[12–14] In only a few are other measures of growth such as bone age,[15] head or chest circumference,[16] triceps and subscapular skin fold[10] considered. The small number of patients or the hetrogeniety of the population in many studies is inadequate to form definite conclusions. Patients with associated gross congenital abnormalities may be excluded but those with intrauterine growth failure included.[17,18] Cardiac diagnostic categories are sometimes combined.[15]

Age at operation may be expected to have a significant effect on subsequent growth. Once maturation and growth have come to an end when the epiphyses close, little changes can be achieved. Many reports, however, include large numbers of adolescents or postadolescents,[19] while others exclude the infant population.[20] The reported duration of follow-up before growth assessment has varied widely from a mean of 1 yr to $3\frac{1}{2}$ yr[17] or a minimum of 6 mo[13] to 2 yr postoperatively.[5] Only a few of the studies address themselves to such important considerations as parental or sibling growth, accurate pre- and postoperative hemodynamic data, or the effect of corrective surgery performed during infancy.[13,16] There are practically no histologic, cellular, physiologic, or metabolic studies comparing pre- and postoperative growth.

PREOPERATIVE GROWTH ASSESSMENT

Mehrizi et al.[19] observed that 27% of 390 patients with congenital heart disease were below the third percentile for both height and weight. Retarded growth was present in 18% of acyanotic patients and 40% in those with cyanotic heart disease.

In general, delay in weight maturation is considerably greater than linear growth.[8,21] Boys are more retarded in growth than girls,[8,15,19,21] especially in the second decade.[15] Not only growth retardation but also mortality is higher among male infants in all types of congenital heart disease.[22] Girls, in general, are more resistent than boys to adverse influences. The striking effect of the atomic bombing in Japan on the growth of boys versus girls illustrates this point well.[23]

The severity of growth inhibition is dependent on the type of cardiac lesion and its hemodynamic effects. In patients with atrial-septal defect secundum, ventricular-septal defect, and patent ductus arteriosus, retardation for weight is greater than height; whereas, in cyanotic congenital heart disease, height and weight tend to parallel each other.[19] Patients with pulmonary stenosis and coarctation on the whole have normal growth but a delay in linear growth relative to weight has been observed.[19] The discrepancy between weight gain and linear growth is most striking in infants with congestive heart failure or large left-to-right shunt and is related to the hemodynamic abnormality.

When bone age (i.e., skeletal maturity) has been measured, the skeletal retardation was associated with a retardation in height and weight but was not necessarily parallel to it.[15,24,25] Delay in skeletal maturation is related to the severity of the hypoxemia[24] in cyanotic heart disease but can also be demonstrated in infants with congestive heart failure.[25]

FACTORS AFFECTING GROWTH PRIOR TO SURGERY

The failure to grow of infants and children with congenital heart disease is due to multiple and complex factors in addition to the important hemodynamic consequences of the cardiac malformation (Table 1). The interference with growth is usually most severe in infants with congestive heart failure associated with patent ductus arteriosus,[6] ventricular-septal defect,[18] D-transposition of the great arteries, or coarctation.[21] The mechanisms of growth retardation are poorly understood and require further elucidation.

Insufficient nutrients and caloric intake may well be the most important factor in retarding growth. Anorexia may be the result of cardiac decompensation, fatigue due to excessive respiratory work, recurrent infection, or psychologic factors. Food intake may be insufficient because of psychologic factors that may prevail in the presence of chronic or life-threatening disease.[1,26] An excellent response to forced feeding has been reported[26] but is usually of limited value. Moreover, patients with congenital heart disease and growth impairment are in positive nitrogen balance while on normal diets.[27]

Table 1. Factors Which May Produce Growth Retardation in Infants and Children with Congenital Heart Disease

1. Severe hemodynamic abnormality (particularly congestive heart failure)
2. Recurrent respiratory infections
3. Hypoxemia
4. Intrauterine growth retardation
5. Hypermetabolism
6. Emotional disturbance[58]
7. Physical incapacity
8. Insufficient nutrient intake
9. Malabsorption[56] or protein loss
10. Associated extracardiac anomalies
11. Congenital heart disease as a part of recognizable syndromes

A quantitative study of organ structure and cellular dimension of infants who died with congenital heart disease suggests that malnutrition may play a role in retarded growth with congenital heart disease.[28] Brain weights of infants with congenital heart disease are approximately two standard deviations below mean value for control. Malnutrition during the period of rapid growth may result in permanent anatomic and functional impairment. Since 50% of normal postnatal brain growth occurs in the first year of postnatal life and 20% during the second year, early corrective surgery may be preferable if optimal neurologic development is to be achieved.

Hypermetabolism, proposed as a cause for failure to thrive in infants with congenital heart disease,[29] may possibly be the effect rather than the cause of the growth inhibition.[26] Folic acid, a necessary vitamin for normal growth, may be deficient in children with congenital heart disease but has not been shown to be related to growth impairment in these patients.[30] Acidosis, if severe and associated with a disturbance of cation balance, may also contribute to interference with growth.[31,32] Total body potassium is significantly reduced for body length.[31]

The role of hypoxemia as a primary cause for growth retardation is unclear. Some studies have shown significant differences in growth between cyanotic and acyanotic children with congenital heart disease,[8,19,33] while others have not.[9,17] Patients with cyanotic congenital heart disease without associated congestive heart failure (e.g.,

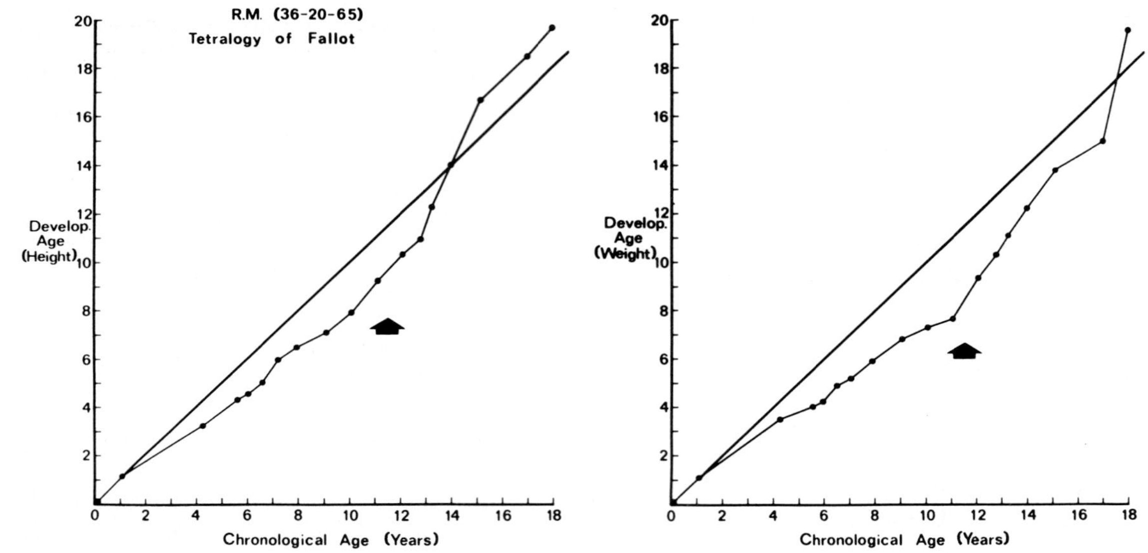

Fig. 2. Chronological and developmental height and weight age in a child with tetralogy of Fallot, before and after successful surgical repair (arrow). During childhood, a gradual decline in systemic arterial oxygen saturation (85% at 4 yr, 77% at 10 yr of age) was associated with progressive symptomatology and growth retardation. After surgical repair at age 11 yr, there is a prolonged catch-up period and a return to the growth pattern present before the appearance of cyanosis.

tetralogy of Fallot) are only moderately underdeveloped (Fig. 2); whereas those with associated congestive heart failure (e.g., D-transposition of the great arteries) are usually more severely affected (Fig. 3). Delayed skeletal maturation[24] and growth in adolescents with cyanotic congenital heart disease[34] has been related directly to the severity of the hypoxemia. The apparent disparity between the severity of hypoxemia and the severity of growth retardation may be due to the fact that a critical low level of P_{O_2} may be required for a given period of time before sufficient interference with growth is observed.[24] Animal studies have shown that muscle-cell multiplication is arrested[35] and the utilization of nutrients is affected by hypoxemia.[36] Newborn animals raised in an hypoxic environment exhibit marked growth and skeletal retardation.[37] Similar findings have been observed in residents living at high altitudes.[28]

Prenatal factors such as intrauterine infection, chromosomal or other hereditary and nonhereditary syndromes causing growth failure are frequent among infants and children with cardiovascular malformations[39] and may account for a large number of infants with growth retardation. Extracardiac anomalies associated with cardiovascular disease[40] may themselves interfere with proper growth in the postnatal period.

The delay in adolescence in patients with congenital heart disease[8,19,33] suggests possible endocrine involvement. Pubescence in very cyanotic children may be very delayed and not begin until an height age of 12–13 yr is achieved. It is more closely related to height age than chronological age.[8] Normal adrenal and thyroid function has been demonstrated in a small group of infants with congenital heart disease and severe growth retardation.[41]

EFFECTS OF CARDIAC SURGERY

Surgery, corrective or palliative, is currently available for most children with congenital heart disease and growth retardation. Correction of the hemodynamic abnormality usually results in an acceleration of growth rate, catch-up growth, and subsequent return to normal dimensions.

If the growth retardation is secondary to the cardiac malformation, surgical correction of the hemodynamic disturbance will result in acceleration in growth and maturation, after which the growth rate will usually parallel the normal (Figs. 1, 2, and 3). Homeorrhesis, however, may not compensate for the loss of growth. Prolonged duration of failure to thrive or failure to correct the cause in the first few years may lead to significant subsequent growth retardation.[42] The greatest acceleration in height and weight maturation after

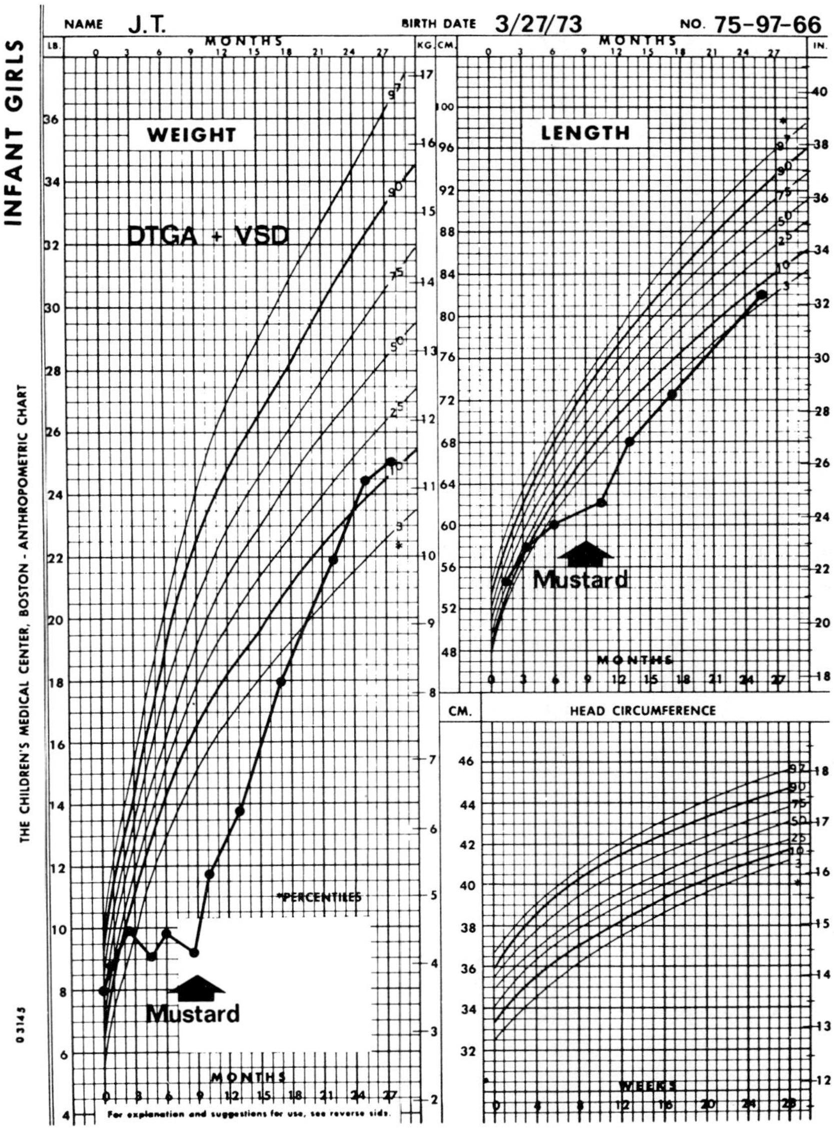

Fig. 3. Growth curves in an infant with D-transposition of the great arteries (DTGA) and ventricular-septal defect (VSD) prior to and following Mustard procedure and VSD closure. Progressive cardiac failure and hypoxemia resulted in marked growth retardation. Following repair, catch-up growth is demonstrated with a return to the expected growth curve.

surgery occurs in patients operated upon at an early age. This has been documented for patients with patent ductus arteriosus division,[21] coarctation repair,[21] and Blalock-Taussig shunt.[21] Weight gain is usually more impressive than linear growth.[10,19] The benefit of surgery on growth is greater in girls with patent ductus arteriosus or coarctation than in boys with similar lesions.[21] It is interesting that girls are not only more resistant to outside influences interfering with growth than boys, but after the influence has ceased to operate, they catch up with their normal curve more rapidly than boys.[1]

Improvement in growth may occur within months after operation[13,16,17] and is observed in most patients within 1-2 yr.[5,21] Significant growth spurts, however, may still occur at a later time,[5] and the surgical effect on growth cannot be considered final until after growth of the individual is completed (Fig. 2). Acceleration of weight is usually evident within months after surgery, while catch-up in height sometimes requires years.

When cardiac corrective operations have been performed in infants with large left-to-right shunts[16] or tetralogy of Fallot,[13] great improvement in weight has been noted approximately 6

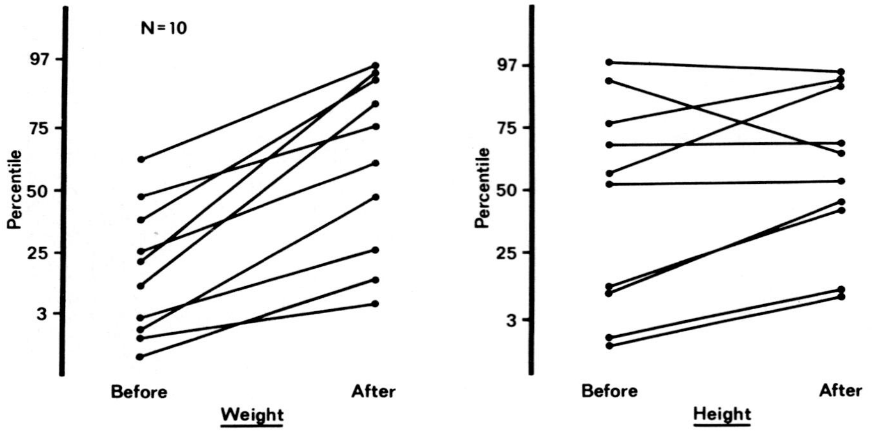

Fig. 4. Change in weight and height percentiles after Mustard operation in ten patients with D-transposition of the great arteries and intact ventricular septum.

mo postoperatively. Head circumference abnormalities at the time of operation came to lie in the normal range, but there was little change in linear growth over a 1-yr follow-up period.[16]

In judging the effects of surgery, one must consider the overall longitudinal growth pattern associated with a particular malformation. It has been suggested that growth in some children with congenital heart disease approaches closer to normal growth in the postadolescent years, whether or not the children are operated upon.[10] This phenomena could probably be observed in patients with initially large left-to-right shunt and subsequent spontaneous closure (e.g., ventricular-septal defect) or development of pulmonary-vascular obstructive disease (e.g., patent ductus arteriosus).

The effects of surgery on growth may be variable. While significant improvement occurs in most patients, there is no improvement in some and dramatic growth spurts in others (Fig. 4). The variability in response to surgery may be related to one or more of the following (Table 2): (A) The difficulty in separating the effects of the illness from that of genetic endowment. The growth inhibition in children with congenital heart disease may be secondary to associated genetic or other constitutional factors with the cardiovascular abnormality a noncontributory or aggravating cause. Normally, the heights of mothers and children are positively correlated.[43] (B) Children with congenital heart disease have reduced cell number when this parameter is related to chronological age or height.[28,44] The mitotic rate, set by intrinsic genetic control, supply of nutrients, oxygen, and so forth, controls cell number which then relates to the total size of the individual. Despite clinical improvement after surgery, too much time has been lost in some patients, at a time when growth by multiplication is so important. Hence, muscle or other tissue mass may never reach expected levels.[31] (C) Growth failure could result from simultaneous teratogenic effects on the developing heart and other tissues. This may be the result of a mutant gene or fetal infection, such as maternal rubella. Growth failure in patients with congenital heart disease is, by and large, secondary to the postnatal effect of the cardiac disease. There is an increased incidence, however, of prenatal or intrauterine growth retardation in infants with a variety of malformations, including ventricular-septal defect[18,25,45] and patent ductus arteriosus. (D) A variety of syndromes are characterized by failure to thrive which may occur with and without the presence of congenital heart disease (e.g., Noonan syndrome). Sex chromosomal abnormality (e.g., Turner syndrome) or somatic chromosomal abnormality (e.g., Down syndrome) are commonly associated with growth retardation. (E) Additional congenital defects, cardiac or extracardiac, by their own pathologic actions during the postnatal period may produce a greater degree of stunting.[40]

Table 2. Factors Which May Be Responsible for Persistent Growth Retardation in Postoperative Patients

1. Hereditary or genetic constitution
2. Hemodynamically significant residual lesions
3. Sequelae or complications of surgery
4. Associated cardiac or extracardiac anomalies
5. Age at operation
6. Chromosome abnormality and/or other hereditary and nonhereditary syndromes or recognizable patterns of malformations
7. Intrauterine growth retardation

(F) Children with normal growth preoperatively, or those that have reached the end of growth potential, cannot be expected to have accelerated linear growth. (G) Significant residual hemodynamic abnormalities, complications, or sequelae of a surgical procedure may produce continued inhibitory effects on growth.

SPECIFIC MALFORMATIONS

Patent Ductus Arteriosus

Significant retardation of growth occurs in 22%–50% of children with patent ductus arteriosus.[5,6,19,46] The lag from standards is usually greater with respect to weight than height and more evident in males than females.[21] Patients with additional anomalies,[5,6] maternal rubella,[6] and prematurity[6] are more prevalent among the group of patients with retarded height than in the group of patients without such abnormality. Irrespective of age, stature is not affected by heart size, but weight is.[5] Following division or ligation of the patent ductus arteriosus, there is acceleration of growth.[5,17,21] Thirty per cent (15/50) of patients with isolated patent ductus arteriosus and growth impairment (height and weight below the 10th percentile) were within normal limits within 6 mo after surgery.[46] In another study, 90% of patients who exhibited satisfactory weight gain did so within 2 yr postoperatively.[6] The younger the age at operation, generally under 3–7 yr, the greater the degree of improvement in growth.[4,21,47] In some studies, height and weight maturation were not depressed by increasing age at operation,[5,6] and final growth distribution of patients was the same.[19]

Height acceleration is largely uninfluenced by preoperative weight but linked to preoperative height. Children who are short and who have tall mothers are more apt to accelerate in height and weight.[5] Studies on the influence of pulmonary-artery hypertension on pre- and postoperative growth are inconclusive.[6,21] Mean height and weight in patients with pulmonary-artery hypertension 1 yr postoperatively is statistically significantly below normal.[21] The degree of retardation and its response to surgery may depend on factors other than the patent ductus arteriosus, such as the presence of associated anomalies, intrauterine growth failure,[5] congenital rubella,[6] maternal height,[5] or other associated syndromes.

Simple Coarctation of the Aorta

Growth in children with simple coarctation of the aorta is usually normal,[9] but may be impaired.[17,19,21] In 100 consecutive patients with coarctation, preoperative mean height and weight were below normal for Finnish standards.[21] One year postoperatively, the mean height and weight no longer differed from normal. Similar improvement has been noted in other studies.[17,19]

Ventricular-Septal Defect

Infants and children with large ventricular-septal defect are very stunted in growth, particularly with respect to weight. The more severe the hemodynamic disturbance,[25] congestive heart failure,[17] or pulmonary artery hypertension,[19,48,49] the greater the clinical and skeletal[25] growth retardation. Some improvement in percentile rank is evident in childhood[25] and adolescence,[15] possibly as the result of spontaneous diminution in the size of the defect. Pulmonary-vascular obstructive disease in older children with ventricular-septal defect does not aggravate the growth retardation.[17]

Improvement in growth is observed after palliative[12,50,51] or corrective[17] surgery. An effective pulmonary-artery band results in accelerated growth, especially with respect to weight.[12,50,51] Resumption of growth actually provides a good index for an effective pulmonary-artery band even in the absence of catch-up growth and return to normal channels.[18] The greatest degree of postoperative improvement is often observed in the most severely affected infants. Among 35 of 40 patients with ventricular-septal defect who were below the third percentile, only ten failed to advance above it after pulmonary-artery banding (average follow-up, 3½ yr).[12] In one study, however, with a shorter follow-up period (mean 25 mo, range 1–63 mo), 20 of 27 infants initially below the third percentile remained there.[52] Failure to accelerate or resume normal growth with hemodynamic control may be due to intrauterine growth retardation[18] or the presence of associated malformations. Following ventricular-septal defect repair in older children, growth may not accelerate.[19] The largest increase in weight and height postoperatively is seen in those with congestive heart failure in infancy.[17]

Tetralogy of Fallot

Moderate growth disturbance is present in most patients with tetralogy of Fallot.[19,53] The delay in weight maturation may be more pronounced than height[8,21,33] and growth more impaired in boys than girls.[8,21] Weight in children with tetralogy of Fallot often begins to lag at about the age of 6 mo, but the height usually not before 3 yr.[54] The retardation and growth has been shown in some studies, but not others,[17,21] to be more severe in patients with marked hypoxemia[8] or secondary polycythemia.[33]

Palliative surgery has been demonstrated to have a beneficial effect on weight and linear growth in all[15,17,19,21,55] but a few studies.[13] Of 95 cases with Blalock-Taussig shunt (mean follow-up period of 8 yr), 33% were below the third percentile for height and weight preoperatively and only 17% postoperatively.[19] The greatest postoperative acceleration in growth in 100 consecutive cases occurred when surgery was performed under 7 yr of age.[21] Growth rate is likely to be greater following Blalock-Taussig shunt than after an ascending aorta to pulmonary-artery anastomosis (Waterston) because the latter is often associated with excessive pulmonary flow and congestive heart failure.

As would be expected, the increase in linear growth is considerably greater after repair of tetralogy than palliative surgery with Blalock-Taussig shunt[17] with a similar response in patients with or without a prior shunt.[17] In infants and young children, the favorable effect on growth of repair in contrast to palliation may be striking[13] within 6 mo after surgery. Figure 2 illustrates the beneficial effect of surgical repair on growth in an older child with tetralogy of Fallot.

D-transposition of the Great Arteries

Growth retardation is common in infants and children with D-transposition of the great arteries, particularly when congestive heart failure is present. From 32% to 45% of children are more than two standard deviations below the normal mean for height and weight.[17,19]

Growth in infants with D-transposition of the great arteries and intact ventricular septum after early and adequate atrial-septal defect creation is often normal. Weight gain is observed even in older children with D-transposition of the great arteries and pulmonary-vascular obstructive disease after atrial septectomy.[57] Following corrective operation by Mustard procedure, there is an acceleration of height and weight, but many children, nevertheless, remain smaller than normal.[17,20] The greatest increase in growth occurs in patients operated on when relatively young.[20] Improvement in growth is dramatic in some (Fig. 3), yet others fail to improve. The effect of the Mustard operation on growth in ten children with D-transposition and intact ventricular septum is shown in Figure 3. All but one of the children had an atrial septectomy prior to the Mustard procedure. Mean age at repair was $2\frac{8}{12}$ yr (range $\frac{11}{12}$–$5\frac{10}{12}$) and at last follow-up visit, $5\frac{10}{12}$ yr (range $4\frac{4}{12}$–$9\frac{6}{12}$). Postoperative cardiac catheterization performed in 7/10 children revealed no significant hemodynamic abnormality.

Pulmonary Stenosis

Children with pulmonary stenosis have a normal growth pattern. Delay in height and weight maturation, greater than two standard deviations from normal, has, however, been reported in 15% of patients[19] and said to be in part related to the hemodynamic severity of the lesion.[17]

Improvement in height and weight maturation has been reported postoperatively.[17] The percentile distribution for patients after valvotomy is normal.[19] Failure to thrive after surgery may be due to the common association of this lesion with a number of syndromes which are known to independently inhibit growth, (for example, Noonan, Leopard, and congenital rubella syndromes).

Aortic Stenosis

Infants with critical aortic stenosis and congestive heart failure may have a lag in growth, but this is infrequently observed in older children. Retardation of growth below the third percentile has been described in 16% of patients with aortic stenosis[19] and an acceleration of both height and weight noted postoperatively.[17] Growth retardation may be expected to persist in children with supravalvar aortic stenosis associated with hypercalcemia and those with subvalvar stenosis and Turner syndrome.

Atrial-septal Defect Secundum

A significant lag in height and weight maturation may occur in infants with atrial-septal defect and congestive heart failure. Only a mild growth disturbance is present in older children.[17] Thirteen per cent of patients are said to be below the third percentile with no relationship between the degree of growth retardation and pulmonary-artery pres-

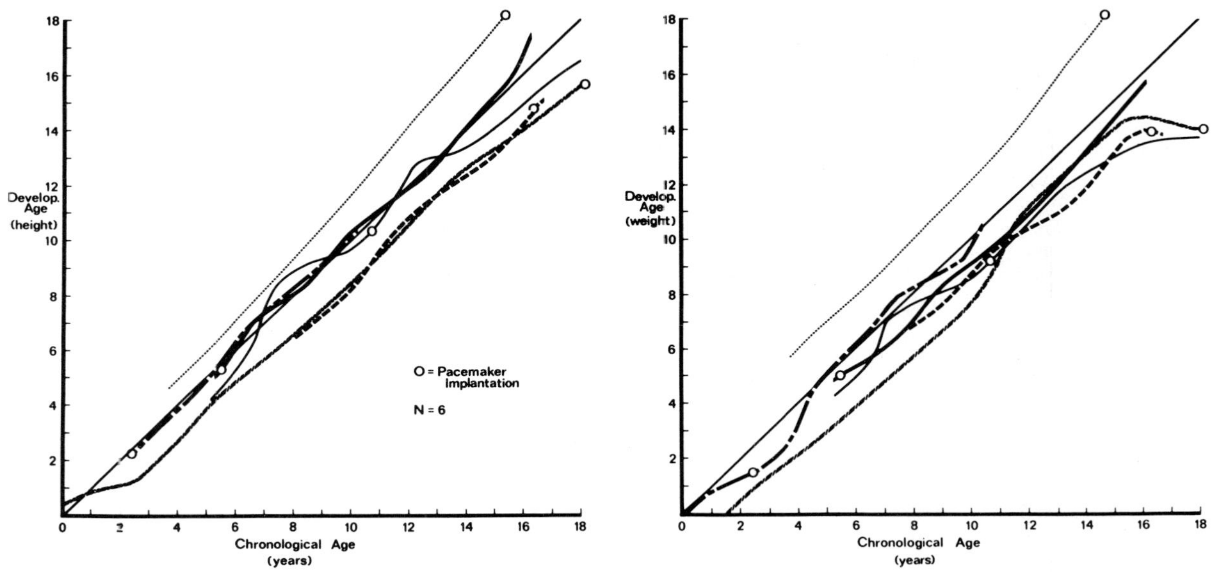

Fig. 5. Growth curves (weight and height) in six children with congenital complete heart block and no associated cardiac malformations. Weight age is usually below average for chronologic age, and height age may also lag. Pacemaker implantation in three of the patients during early childhood had no significant effect on height but improved weight maturation in one child.

sure.[19] Surgical closure of the atrial-septal defect in children does not significantly affect the patient's height or weight percentile.[17,19]

Tricuspid Atresia

Forty per cent of all patients with tricuspid atresia have marked retardation in height and weight.[19] A superior vena cava to pulmonary-artery anastomosis (Glenn shunt) results in an increased weight gain which may, however, be only transient.[14]

Congenital Heart Block

Little information is available on the growth pattern of children with congenital complete heart block before or after implantation of a pacemaker. The height and weight maturation of six children followed at our institution is shown in Fig. 5. In each case, the indication for inserting a pacemaker was an Adams-Stokes episode. Placement of a pacemaker during early childhood in three of the patients did not alter height maturation. Weight gain, however, was demonstrated in one patient.

REFERENCES

1. Sinclair D: Human growth after birth. Oxford Medical Publications, 1973
2. Israelsohn WJ: Description and modes of analysis of human growth. In: Tanner JM (ed): Human Growth: Symposium of the Society of Human Biology, vol. 3. London, Pergamon, 1960
3. A Guide to Screening. EPSDT. Medicaid. U.S. Department of Health Education and Welfare, Social and Rehabilitation Service, In conjunction with the American Academy of Pediatrics. 1974
4. Engle MA, Holswade GR, Goldberg HP, et al: Persistent problems pertaining to patency of the ductus arteriosus. I. Persistence of growth retardation after successful surgery. Pediatrics 1:70, 1958
5. Umansky R, Hauk AJ: Factors in the growth of children with patent ductus arteriosus. Pediatrics 30:540, 1962
6. Krovetz LJ: Weight gain in children with patent ductus arteriosus. Dis Chest 44:274, 1963
7. Ekstrom G: The surgical treatment of patent ductus arteriosus. A clinical study of 290 cases. Acta Chir Scand (Suppl 169) 1952
8. Linde LM, Dunn OJ, Schrireson R, et al: Growth in children with congenital heart disease. J Pediatr 70:413, 1967
9. Adams FH, Lund GW, Disenhouse RB: Observations on the physique and growth of children with congenital heart disease. J Pediatr 44:674, 1954
10. Robinson SJ, Bayer LM: Growth history of children with congenital heart defects. I. Effects of operative intervention. Child Dev 40:315, 1969
11. Reed RB, Stuart HC: Patterns of growth in height and weight from birth to eighteen years of age. Pediatrics 24:904, 1959

12. Subramanian S, Wagner HR: Pulmonary artery banding and debanding in patients with ventricular septal defect, in Barratt-Boyes BG (ed): Heart Disease in Infancy. London, Livingstone, 1973, p 127

13. Starr A, Bonchek LJ, Sunderland CO: Total correction of tetralogy of Fallot in infancy. J Thorac Cardiovasc Surg 65:45, 1973

14. Willman VL, Barner HB, Mudd JG, et al: Superior vena cava-pulmonary artery anastomosis. J Thorac Cardiovasc Surg 67:380, 1974

15. Bayer LM, Robinson SJ: Growth history of children with congenital heart defects. Am J Dis Child 117: 564, 1969

16. Clarkson PM: Growth following corrective cardiac operation in early infancy, in Barrett-Boyes BG (ed): Heart Disease in Infancy. London, Livingstone, 1973, p 75

17. Feldt RH, Strickler GB, Weidman WH: Growth of children with congenital heart disease. Am J Dis Child 117:573, 1969

18. Menahem S, Venables AW: Pulmonary artery banding in isolated or complicated ventricular septal defects. Results and effects on growth. Br Heart J 34:87, 1972

19. Mehrizi A, Drash A: Growth disturbance in congenital heart disease. J Pediatr 61:418, 1962

20. Mair DD, Danielson GK, Wallace RB, et al: Long-term follow-up of Mustard operation survivors. Circulation 50:46 (Suppl II), 1973

21. Suoninen P: Physical growth of children with congenital heart disease. Acta Paediatr Scand (Suppl) 225:1, 1971

22. Allen CM: Infant mortality from congenital cardiac malformations in California, 1957–1960. Am J Pub Health, 58:1368, 1968

23. Greulich WW, Crimson CS, Turner ML: The physical growth and development of children who survived the atomic bombing of Hiroshima or Nagasaki. J Pediatr 43: 121–145, 1953

24. Danilowicz DA: Delay in bone age in children with cyanotic congenital heart disease. Radiology 108:655, 1973

25. Menahem S: The clinical growth of infants and children with ventricular septal defect. Aust Paediatr J 8:1, 1972

26. Krieger I: Growth failure and congenital heart disease. Am J Dis Child 120:497, 1970

27. Iber FL, Cheek DB, Wolf KP: Nitrogen metabolism in children with congenital cardiac defects and severe growth retardation. Am J Clin Nutr 20:1166, 1967

28. Naeye RL: Organ and cellular development in congenital heart disease and in alimentary malnutrition. J Pediatr 67:447, 1965

29. Lees MH, et al: Relative hypermetabolism in infants with congenital heart disease and undernutrition. Pediatrics 36:183, 1965

30. Rook GD, Lopez R, Shimizu N, et al: Folic acid deficiency in infants and children with heart disease. Br Heart J 35:87, 1973

31. Cheek DB: Human Growth, Body Composition, Cell Growth Energy and Intelligence. Philadelphia, Lea and Febiger, 1968

32. Cooke RE, Boyden DG, Haller E: The relationship of acidosis and growth retardation. J Pediatr 57:326, 1960

33. Campbell M, Reynolds G: The physical and mental development of children with congenital heart disease. Arch Dis Child 24:294, 1949

34. White RI Jr, Jordan CE, Fischer KC, et al: Delayed skeletal growth and maturation in adolescent congenital heart disease. Invest Radiol 6:326, 1971

35. Elliot DA, Cheek DB: Muscle cell growth in rats with exposure to hypoxia and food. Soc Pediatr 1966

36. Cheek DB, Grastone JE, Rowe RD: Hypoxia and malnutrition in newborn rats: Effects on RNA, DNA and protein in tissues. Am J Physiol 217:642, 1969

37. D'elaqueiviere-Richardson L, Forbes S, Valdivia E: Effects of simulated high altitude on the growth rate of albino guinea pigs. J Apply Physiol 20:1022, 1965

38. Frisancho AR, Thomas RB, Baker PT: Growth patterns of a highland Peruvian population: A preliminary analysis. Dept. of Sociology and Anthropology, Pennsylvania State University, 1965

39. Fyler DC, Rosenthal A: Neonatal heart disease, in Avery GB (ed): Neonatology. Philadelphia, Lippincott (in press)

40. Greenwood R, Rosenthal A, Parisi L, et al: Extracardiac anomalies in infants with congenital heart disease. Pediatrics (in press)

41. Krieger I, Good MH: Adrenocortical and thyroid function in the deprivation syndrome. Am J Dis Child 120:95, 1970

42. Eid EE: A follow-up study of physical growth following failure to thrive with special reference to a critical period in the first year of life. Acta Paediatr Scand 60: 39, 1971

43. Pearson K, Lee A: On the laws of inheritance in man. Biometrica 2:357, 1903

44. Cheek DB, Graystone JE, Mehrizi A: The importance of muscle cell number in children with congenital heart disease. Bull Johns Hopkins Hosp 118:160, 1966

45. Hoffman JIE: Natural history of congenital heart disease: Problems in its assessment with special reference to ventricular septal defects. Circulation 37:97, 1968

46. Lynxwiler CP, Wells CRE: Patent ductus arteriosus: A report of 180 operations. South Med J 43:61, 1950

47. Adams FH, Forsyth WB: The effect of surgery on the growth of patients with patent ductus arteriosus. J Pediatr 39:330, 1951

48. Miller RH, Schiebler GL, Grumbar P, et al: Relation of hemodynamics to height and weight precentiles in children with ventricular septal defects. Am Heart J 78: 523, 1969

49. Maxwell GM, Wurfel L, Burnell RH: A study of growth in congenital heart disease with a note on the effect of surgery. Aust Paediatr J 2:188, 1966

50. Goldblatt A, Bernhard WF, Nadas AS, et al: Pulmonary artery banding: Indications and results in infants and children. Circulation 32:172, 1965

51. Idriss FS, Riker WL, Paul MH: Banding of the pulmonary artery: A palliative surgical procedure. J Pediatr Surg 3:465, 1968

52. Girod DA, Hurwitz RA, King H, et al: Recent re-

sults of two stage surgical treatment of large ventricular septal defect. Circulation 50:9 (Suppl II), 1973

53. Nadas AS, Fyler DC: Pediatric Cardiology (ed 3). Philadelphia, Saunders, 1973

54. Bakhtina GG, Lensky GB, Prilepko LP: The physical development of young children suffering from Fallot tetralogy. Kardiologiia 9:26, 1968

55. Banik NDD, Westland R, Falkner F: Growth retardation in cyanotic congenital heart disease. J Indian Med Assoc 48:282, 1967

56. Hakkila J, Makela TE, Halonen P: Absorbtion of ^{131}I triolein in congestive heart failure. Am J Cardiol 5: 295, 1960

57. Rosenthal A, Freed MD, Litwin SB et al: Atrial septectomy in patients with D-transposition of the great arteries, ventricular septal defect and severe pulmonary vascular obstructive disease. Circulation 50:35 (Suppl II), 1973

58. Powell GF, Brasel JA, Blizzard RM: Emotional deprivation and growth retardation simulating idiopathic hypopituitarism. N Engl J Med 276:1279, 1967

Prosthetic Valve Replacement in Children

Michael D. Freed and William F. Bernhard

SINCE THE SUCCESSFUL INSERTION of a caged ball valve prosthesis in the aortic position by Harken[1] and mitral position by Starr,[2] valve replacement for the treatment of acquired disease in adults has become widely accepted. In comparison with the adult experience, where more than 100,000 prostheses of one model alone have been implanted,[3] similar operations in children have been infrequent with fewer than 300 cases reported in the literature. The reluctance to replace valves in young children is readily understandable. In addition to the usual prosthetic related complications such as thromboembolism, infection, ball variance, and red cell hemolysis, fears have been expressed regarding the anticoagulation management of children whose activity level may predispose them to trauma and possibly a fatal hemorrhage.

The durability of prosthetic valves has also been questioned, since the required valve life for children may be extended to 50–60 yr. This exceeds the usual period of simulated function in an accelerated pulse duplicator used to test prostheses for adults. A final consideration involves the possibility of repeated valve replacements as a consequence of normal growth in children undergoing initial valve replacement in infancy or early childhood.

Despite these difficulties, there are children with congenital and rheumatic heart disease in whom severe incapacitation has required the implantation of a prosthesis. At the Children's Hospital Medical Center (CHMC) Boston, 54 children and young adults have undergone valve replacement in the last decade (1964–1974). This report will summarize our experience in this area as well as that of others, in an attempt to update the current status of prosthetic valve replacement in children. Included in our series are all patients with rheumatic heart disease whose valve replacement was done under 16 yr of age, and those with congenital defects who underwent cardiac surgery for the first time when < 16 yr old. An example of the latter category is a patient with ventricular septal defect (VSD) and prolapsed aortic cusp with regurgitation who underwent VSD closure at 12 yr of age followed by aortic valve replacement at age 18. We have not included replacement of the pulmonary outflow tract with a xenograft valve conduit since the problems encountered are quite different.

There were a total of 28 patients with mitral valve replacement, 21 with aortic replacement, one with tricuspid replacement, and four double (mitral and aortic) valve replacement. All patients had preoperative cardiac catheterizations and several underwent postoperative studies.

CARDIAC LESIONS REQUIRING VALVE REPLACEMENT

Aortic Valve Replacement

Isolated aortic valve replacement (AVR) was performed in 21 children at CHMC, and 20 of these had congenital abnormalities of the aortic valve. They ranged in age from 2 to 26 yr with a median of 14 yr. Two-thirds (14/21) were males.

The most common anomaly, present in seven patients, was ventricular septal defect (VSD) with aortic regurgitation (AR), (Table 1). The association of AR with VSD is not rare. It was present in 25 out of 327 children with VSD (8%) catheterized at our institution between 1959 and 1969. In six of the seven patients the valve replacement was performed at the time of the VSD closure, but in one child progressive AR developed 6-yr after VSD closure during an episode of bacterial endocarditis (BE).

Six other patients had congenital aortic stenosis (AS) secondary to a bicuspid aortic valve. In each case, a prior open aortic valvulotomy had afforded some relief, but inadequate initial operation or restenosis 11–15 yr later (4/6), or associated aortic

From the Departments of Cardiology and Cardiovascular Surgery, Children's Hospital Medical Center and the Departments of Pediatrics and Surgery, Harvard Medical School, Boston, Mass.

Supported by a grant from the John A. Hartford Foundation, and National Heart and Lung Institute, U.S. Department of Health, Education, and Welfare, Bethesda, Md.

Reprint requests should be addressed to Michael D. Freed, M.D., Department of Cardiology, Children's Hospital Medical Center, 300 Longwood Ave., Boston, Mass. 02115.

Table 1. Cardiac Diagnosis in Patients Requiring Valve Prosthesis*

Aortic			21
Congenital		20	
Ventricular septal defect and aortic regurgitation	7		
Aortic stenosis postvalvulotomy	6		
Bicuspid aortic valve and bacterial endocarditis	4		
Sinus of valsalva aneurysm	1		
Truncus arteriosus	1		
Cystic medial necrosis of the aorta	1		
Rheumatic heart disease		1	
Mitral			28
Congenital		21	
Endocardial cushion defect and mitral regurgitation	10		
Congenital mitral stenosis	6		
Coarctation of the aorta and mitral regurgitation	2		
Endocardial fibroelastosis and mitral regurgitation	1		
Corrected transposition of great arteries	1		
Iatrogenic mitral regurgitation	1		
Rheumatic heart disease		7	
Tricuspid			1
Status post-Mustard repair of D-transposition of the great arteries	1		
Multiple			4
Rheumatic heart disease	2		
Marfan syndrome	1		
Congenital aortic regurgitation and mitral regurgitation	1		

*Children's Hospital Medical Center, Boston, Mass. 1964–1974.

regurgitation (2/6) required reoperation. These patients tended to be older than the rest and, except for one 2-yr old, all were over 21 at the time of their reoperation for valve replacement. No child under 16 with AS required aortic valve replacement as a primary operation.

In four children with mild AS secondary to a bicuspid aortic valve, severe AR developed after bacterial endocarditis. Here, a valve replacement was necessary 6 mo–8 yr later because of progressive cardiac enlargement. In all four cases the organism isolated from blood culture was strep viridans.

The diagnosis in single cases requiring valve replacement included AR associated with sinus of valsalva aneurysm, cystic medial necrosis with dilatation of the aortic root, rheumatic heart disease, and truncal regurgitation in a patient with truncus arteriosus.

Previous published reports indicate that congenital abnormalities of the aortic valve are more often responsible for valve replacement in children than acquired disease. In reports by Bleiden[4] (13 cases), Taguchi[5] (eight cases) and van de Water[6] (five cases), congenital defects, with or without superimposed endocarditis, were responsible for at least 60% of the valve replacements. In a review of the American Literature by Klint,[7] 60% (21/35) of all aortic valve replacements in children were for congenital defects. The majority of patients with aortic valve replacements had VSD with AR, with bicuspid aortic valves and ruptured sinus of valsalva aneurysms the next most common lesions.

Mitral Valve Replacement

Mitral valve replacement was performed in 28 children at the CHMC. Seventy-five percent of these had congenital heart disease (Table 1). The age of the patients ranged from 9 mo to 30 yr, with a median of 10 yr. Seventeen were girls and 11 were boys.

The most common reason for mitral valve replacement in the congenital group was mitral regurgitation (MR) secondary to an endocardial cushion defect (ECD). Of ten children in this category, five had an atrial septal defect (ASD) primum closed 1–10 yr earlier, while five others had mitral valve replacement as a primary operation along with patch closure of the ASD. The youngest patient was 9 mo of age and the oldest 26 yr.

Six patients had mitral valve replacement for congenital mitral stenosis and one of these had had two previous mitral commissurotomies.

Two children undergoing mitral valve replacement had congenital MR associated with coarctation of the aorta. Both patients had their coarctation resected as infants (2 and 3 mo of age) but subsequently developed progressive cardiac enlargement necessitating valve replacement at 4 and 5 yr of age, respectively. Diagnosis in other patients with congenital heart disease included one child each with endocardial fibroelastosis and MR, severe left atrioventricular valve regurgitation in association with corrected transposition of the great arteries, and regurgitation developing after iatrogenic injury to the mitral valve at the time of resection of an obstructing subaortic membrane. Seven children with severe rheumatic mitral regurgitation, one acute and six chronic, required valve replacement.

On a review of the pertinent literature it is apparent that rheumatic heart disease accounts for about half the mitral valve replacements.[7] Large series of cases from other countries including Mexico,[8] Israel[9,10] and South Africa,[11] attest to the prevalence of this problem elsewhere, but even in the United States,[12-14] progressive rheumatic mitral regurgitation necessitated mitral valve replacement in a significant group of pediatric patients.

Other cardiac lesions associated with MR that have required replacement include cardiomyopathy,[4] Marfan syndrome,[4,15-17] subaortic stenosis,[4] sickle cell anemia,[18] and complete atrioventricular canal.[4,17]

Tricuspid Valve Replacement

We have had little experience with tricuspid valve replacement at the CHMC. It was used in one child with D-transposition of the great arteries who developed severe tricuspid regurgitation (TR) 6-mo following a Mustard procedure.[19] This problem has previously been described by Tynan.[20]

Bleiden[4] reported seven patients undergoing tricuspid valve replacement, five with Ebstein's disease and two others for congenital tricuspid valve abnormalities producing regurgitation. Tricuspid valve replacement following trauma,[7] bacterial endocarditis,[8,14] repair of tetrology of Fallot[14] and in endocardial fibroelastosis have also been reported.

Multiple Valve Replacement

Four patients in our institution have required double valve replacements (aortic and mitral): two girls with rheumatic heart disease, a boy with Marfan syndrome, and a girl with a bicuspid aortic valve, AR and MR of unknown etiology. Other authors have reported multiple valve replacements for rheumatic heart disease[4,5,9,10,21,22] and in patients with complete atrioventricular canal.[5] Two cases of a triple valve replacement (aortic, mitral, and tricuspid) for rheumatic heart disease have also been described.[7,10]

OPERATION

Choice of Valves

Aortic prosthesis. Although five different prostheses have been used for replacement in the aortic position in our series, the majority of patients have received either a Starr-Edwards valve 10 or a Bjork-Shiley prosthesis 7 (Table 2).

Table 2. Types of Prosthetic Valves Used in Children*

Aortic position		21
Starr-Edwards	10	
Bjork-Shiley	7	
McGovern	2	
Cutter	1	
Braunwald-Cutter	1	
Mitral position		28
Kay-Shiley	10	
Starr-Edwards	6	
Bjork-Shiley	3	
Gott-Daggett	3	
Porcine xenograft	3	
Cutter	2	
Beall	1	
Tricuspid		1
Bjork-Shiley	1	
Multiple		4
Starr-Edwards (aortic and mitral)	4	
Repeat valve replacement (mitral)		2
Porcine xenograft	2	

*Children's Hospital Medical Center, Boston, Mass. 1964-1974.

The dimensions of the aortic valve annulus and ascending aorta are the dominant factors in determining the most appropriate prosthesis in the pediatric age group. Accordingly, a low profile, centrally opening device would seem to be the most appropriate for use today (Bjork-Shiley), although much of the early experience was gained with the Starr-Edwards ball valve. This latter prosthesis is associated with marked turbulence and eddying during ventricular systole, and has a further disadvantage in the form of a protruding cage which makes insertion difficult in patients with a small ascending aorta.

The Braunwald-Cutter prosthesis is of limited usefulness in children because of problems similar to those associated with the Starr-Edwards valve. In addition, the Dacron cloth-covered prosthesis may be associated with hazards of excessive fabric wear and buildup of connective tissue in the orifice area which may obstruct movement of the poppet. Limited early experience was obtained with the McGovern and Cutter valves, but they are not currently being used as the valve of choice. However, the youngest patient to undergo successful aortic valve replacement at this hospital (21 mo of age) had a modified Cutter ball implanted 6-yr ago.

Use of either an aortic valve homograft or gluteraldehyde preserved xenograft valve is precluded in many pediatric patients because of the reduction in valve area produced by the intraluminal mass of valve tissue, along with the supportive stent. However, in patients with an adult sized aortic root, tissue valves are an important alternative to all current prostheses, and do not require long-term postoperative anticoagulation.

Mitral prosthesis. A low-profile valve is also appropriate for mitral valve replacement in most children, since the left ventricular cavity size is often limited in young patients. Although the Kay-Shiley disc valve was employed early in our experience, (ten children), a high incidence of thromboembolic complications has led to adoption of the centrally opening Bjork-Shiley valve (three patients). Starr-Edwards mitral valves have been used successfully, (six children) but are of value only in those older patients in whom the cage will not obstruct the left ventricular outflow tract.

The Gott-Daggett valve employed in our initial search for a suitable low-profile prosthesis (three children) has not been utilized since 1966, because of concern that the flexing monocusp leaflet might fatigue fracture. However, one anticoagulated patient with this valve is doing well 10 yr after replacement for congenital mitral stenosis (parachute valve).

Use of tissue valves on a stent in the mitral area have also been employed recently in three patients as a primary operation and in two others for repeat valve replacement. This device is limited in usefulness because of the size of the tissue mass on the valve stent which encroaches upon the effective valve area. One xenograft* was employed in a child from abroad where anticoagulation management at home would have been difficult. Two additional patients received xenograft valves because of thromboembolic complications of Starr-Edwards and Kay-Shiley valves inserted 9 and 3 yr previously.

In older patients with an adequate sized mitral annulus and as a repeat valve replacement in children who received a small prosthetic valve early in life, use of the porcine xenograft may become the procedure of choice.

Operative Technique

Valve replacements were performed during cardiopulmonary bypass using standard surgical methods. Technical details varied somewhat since the operations were performed by four different surgeons over a period of 10 yr. Left coronary perfusion or local myocardial hypothermia was used to protect the heart during aortic valve replacement and intermittent aortic cross clamping provided improved visability for mitral valve replacement.

Multiple interrupted stitches were used for fixation of the prosthesis to the excised valve remnants employing fine silk or Tevdec suture material. A Kay-Cross disc-oxygenator was employed initially in our experience and was replaced in 1972 by a disposable Bently bubble-oxygenator. During perfusion body temperature was reduced to 30°C and flow rates were maintained between 2000-2200 ml/min/m.^{2}

RESULTS OF SURGERY

Aortic Valve Replacement

Of 21 children and adolescents undergoing aortic valve replacements in our series, there were three operative deaths (mortality of 14%). These three patients had a similar postoperative course characterized by difficulty in weaning from cardiopulmonary bypass, and a low output state progressing to death within 72 hr. They were among the youngest operated upon ($1\frac{1}{2}$, 4, and 10 yr of age). Figure 1 depicts the relationship

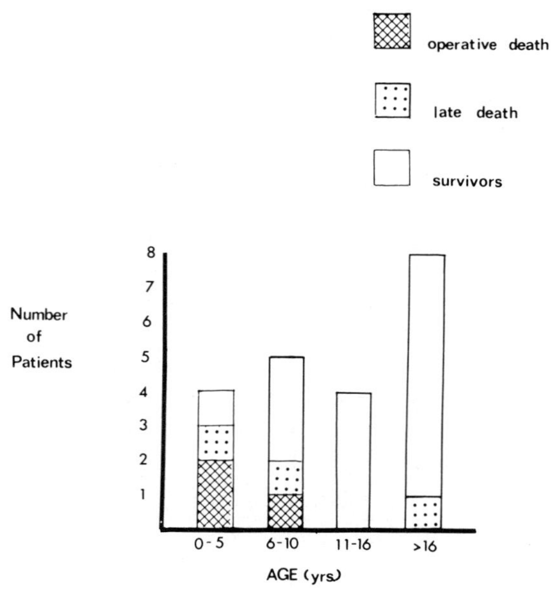

Fig. 1. Operative and late mortality following isolated aortic valve replacement related to age at operation. Note an operative mortality of 50% (2/4) in children under 6 yr compared to a mortality of 6% (1/17) in older patients.

*Hancock Laboratories, Anaheim, Calif.

between operative mortality and age at time of operation. Two of four children operated upon under 5 yr of age died, but only one operative death occurred among 17 patients over 5 yr of age (mortality 6%). The youngest individual in our series to undergo aortic valve replacement, an 18-mo old with truncus arteriosus, died as a consequence of pulmonary vascular obstructive disease (grade 4 changes noted in the pulmonary arterioles at postmortem examination).

There were three late deaths among the 18 survivors, 2 mo, 8 mo, and 3 yr postoperatively (late mortality of 14% and total mortality 28%). These patients died suddenly at home. One child early in the series (1964) died after an episode of prolonged vomiting. Postmortem examination was unrevealing, and it was postulated that an arrhythmia occurred secondary to digitalis toxicity. A second child, operated upon in 1965, had a stormy course with mediastinitis and dehiscence of his sternum and died 8 mo postoperatively. Postmortem examination disclosed constrictive pericarditis and paravalvular leak. The third late death involved a 6-yr old girl with cystic medial necrosis of the aorta. She died at home 3 yr after operation, and no postmortem examination was carried out.

The total mortality was also related to the year in which the operation was performed, (Fig. 2) with deaths in three of four children operated on prior to 1967, compared to three of 17 operations since that time. Operative mortality since 1967 has been 12% (2/17). Figure 3 depicts the overall survival statistics by the actuarial method of life tables.[23] After an initial drop representing operative mortality, the curve levels off at a 65 ± 12% survival at 9 yr. This value is comparable to the adult experience.

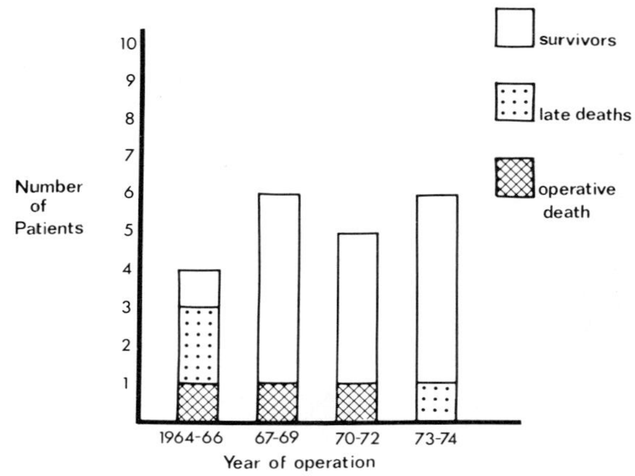

Fig. 2. Operative and late mortality following isolated aortic valve replacement related to year of operation. Prior to 1967 overall mortality was 75% (3/4). Since 1967 it has been reduced to 18% (3/17).

The 15 survivors have been followed for periods of 6 mo–9 yr, (median 3 yr) and all are asymptomatic (class I New York Heart Association) in school or working.

One patient developed complete heart block postoperatively and had a fixed rate pacemaker implanted.

Klint[7] in a review of the American Literature in 1972 noted a total operative mortality similar to ours (14.3%), among 35 children reported with

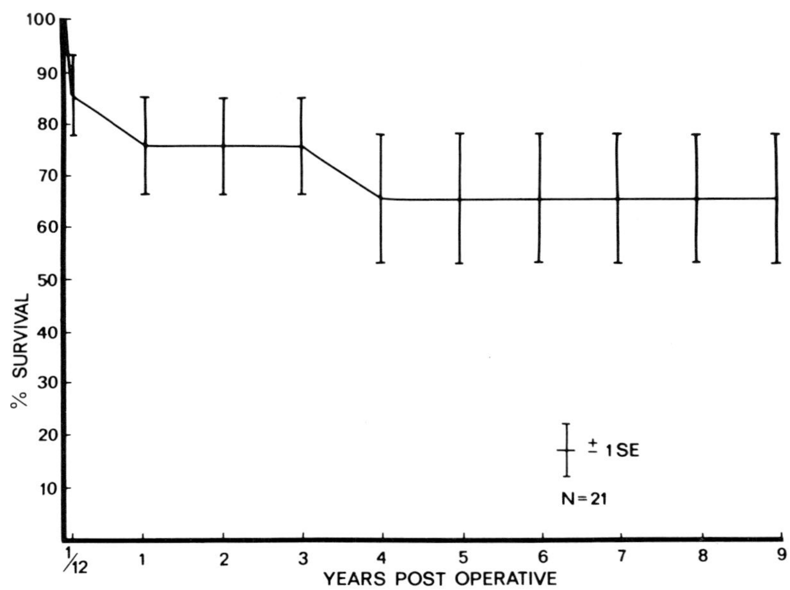

Fig. 3. Survival curves in patients with isolated aortic valve replacement. After a large initial drop representing operative mortality, curve levels off at 65± (12%).

aortic valve replacement. More recently Bleiden et al.[4] described an early mortality of 38% (5/13), but indicated that four of these were very early in their series with an operative mortality of 14% (1/7) since 1966. All reported series including our own involve patients operated upon over at least a 6–10-yr period. Obviously surgical results in the 1970s will be better than those recorded during early period of valve replacement (1960s).

We believe that elective, aortic valve replacement in children who are over 5 yr of age can now be performed at a risk similar to that of the adult population (approxmately 4%).[24,25]

Mitral Valve Replacement

Among 28 patients who underwent surgery, there were seven operative deaths (25%). Four of these occurred in our initial experience (Fig. 4), with a decrease in mortality to 7% (1/14) since 1970. In the group of mitral valve replacements deaths were also related to age at time of operation (Fig. 5). Four of six patients (66%) under 5 yr of age expired early in the postoperative period in a low-output state. Postmortem examination in two of these indicated that the valve cage obstructed the left ventricular outflow tract. There were also three operative deaths among 22 children (14%) over 5 yr of age.

Four late deaths occurred for a combined mortality of 39% (11/28). One patient with congenital mitral stenosis, bilateral hydronephrosis, and a ureteroileostomy (ileal bladder), died 2 yr after valve replacement from recurrent bacterial endo-

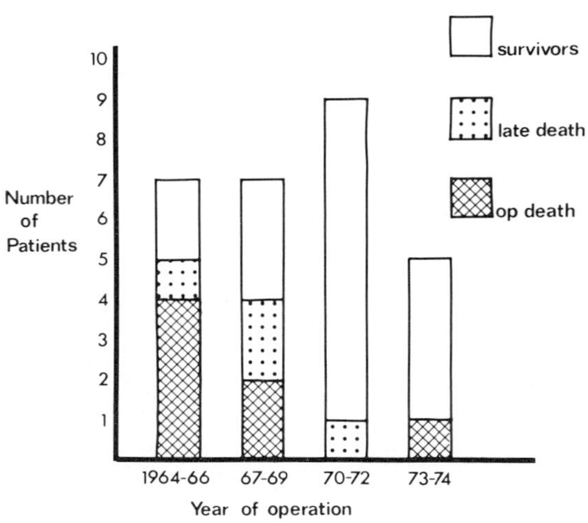

Fig. 4. Operative and late mortality of isolated mitral valve replacement related to year of operation. Since 1967 the operative mortality has been 14%.

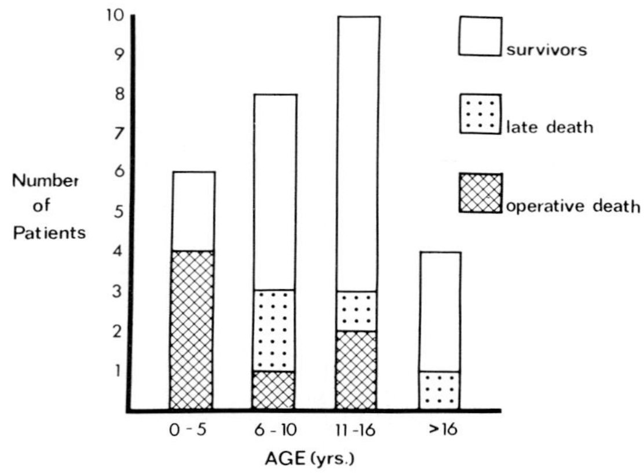

Fig. 5. Operative and late mortality following isolated mitral valve replacement related to age at operation. Operative mortality was 66% (4/6) among children under 6 yr and 14% among the older patients.

carditis involving the prosthesis. A second patient, a 9-yr old girl operated on in 1965, died 1 yr later with staphylococcus aureus septicemia and disseminated intravascular coagulation. A third child anticoagulated with Coumadin, developed a CNS hemorrhage (prothrombin time 31.9 sec, control 12 sec) and expired several days later. At postmortem he was found to have ruptured an aneurysm involving one of several congenital cerebral arteirovenous malformations. The fourth late death, a 24-yr old man, died 3 mo following surgery with pneumonia. Fig. 6 presents an actuarial life table of isolated mitral valve replacements. The projected 10 yr survival is 58%.

Two patients have required a cardiac pacemaker because of surgically induced complete atrioventricular block. In one, block was transient and a sinus rhythm with first degree atrioventricular block, left anterior hemiblock and right bundle branch block was observed on the tenth postoperative day. However, a demand pacemaker was inserted because of fear that patients with surgically created bifasicular block who have complete heart block transiently in the postoperative period may develop fatal arrhythmias.[26] Two patients have required a second valve replacement because of recurrent, life threatening emboli (9 yr and 3 yr after insertion of a Starr-Edwards and Kay-Shiley prosthesis, respectively). Both were reoperated upon uneventfully and received porcine xenograft valves.

The clinical improvement in children after mitral valve replacement has been dramatic. Small, frail, severely incapacitated children have had an impres-

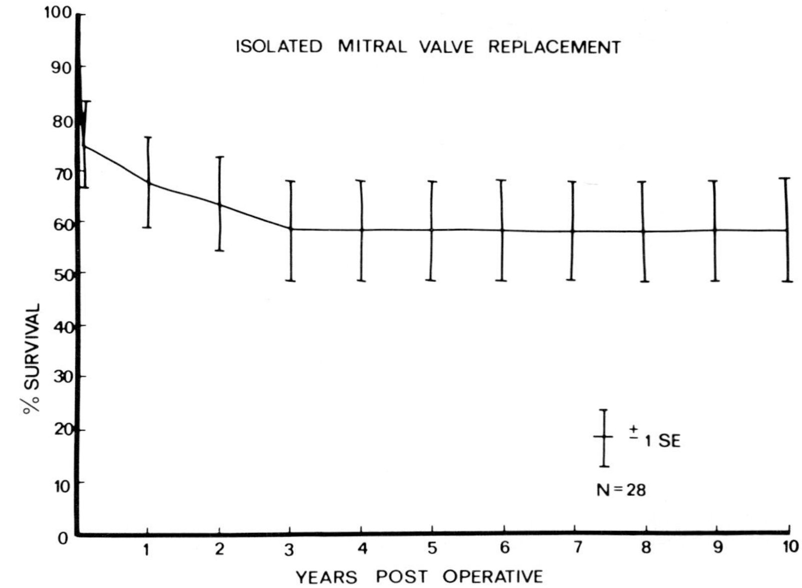

Fig. 6. Survival curve in patients with isolated mitral valve replacements. After a large initial drop representing operative mortality, curve levels off at 58 ± (10%).

sive spurt in both height and weight maturation and have returned to normal full activities for age. Congestive heart failure has improved and cardiomegaly has dimished (Fig. 7). Hemodynamic confirmation of improvement following mitral valve replacement has recently been obtained[27] and suggests that children have a quicker postoperative reversion to normal cardiac performance, than do adults with comparable hemodynamics.

The reported early and late mortality for mitral valve replacement in the pediatric group is slightly higher than that for aortic valve replacement. The overall mortality as calculated by Klint[7] was 17% (19/111), but many of the accumulated cases were single case reports of survivors. Among the larger reported series the early operative mortality was 14%[11,17] and total mortality 24%–42%. In Bleiden's study of mitral valve replacements,[4] yearly improvement in the results was similar to those observed with aortic valve replacement. They found a combined (early and late) mortality of 75% (6/8) among patients operated upon before 1966, and only 18% (2/11) since.

Although mitral valve replacement continues to be more hazardous than aortic valve replacement, we currently feel that elective operation in children over 5 yr of age should carry an operative mortality of less than 10%.

Tricuspid

We have performed only one tricuspid valve replacement in a child with tricuspid incompetence following Mustard repair of transposition of the great arteries. He died early in the postoperative period. Although few tricuspid valve replacements have been performed in children, others[4,7] have reported a mortality of 36%–43%.

Multiple Valve Replacement

These procedures have also carried a high risk in the past. Three of four patients in our series have died, two early in the postoperative period secondary to a low-output syndrome, and another 5-mo later with mediastinitis and dehiscence of the aortic suture line. The remaining patient is doing well 2 yr after operation.

Of 13 children undergoing double valve replacement, reported in the literature prior to 1972,[4,7] six have died (mortality of 46%). More recently the group from South Africa[22] has reported a mortality of only 14% (1/7) among children operated upon for rheumatic heart disease between 1968 and 1971.

The recipients of the triple valve replacements were alive 4 and 7 mo after operation.[7,10]

MANAGEMENT

At the initial medical postoperative evaluation, usually 6 weeks after surgery, a series of laboratory tests are obtained as base line values. These usually include a chest x-ray in the anteroposterior and lateral projection and a standard 12 lead electrocardiogram. A complete blood count including reticulocyte count, hematocrit, hemoglobin con-

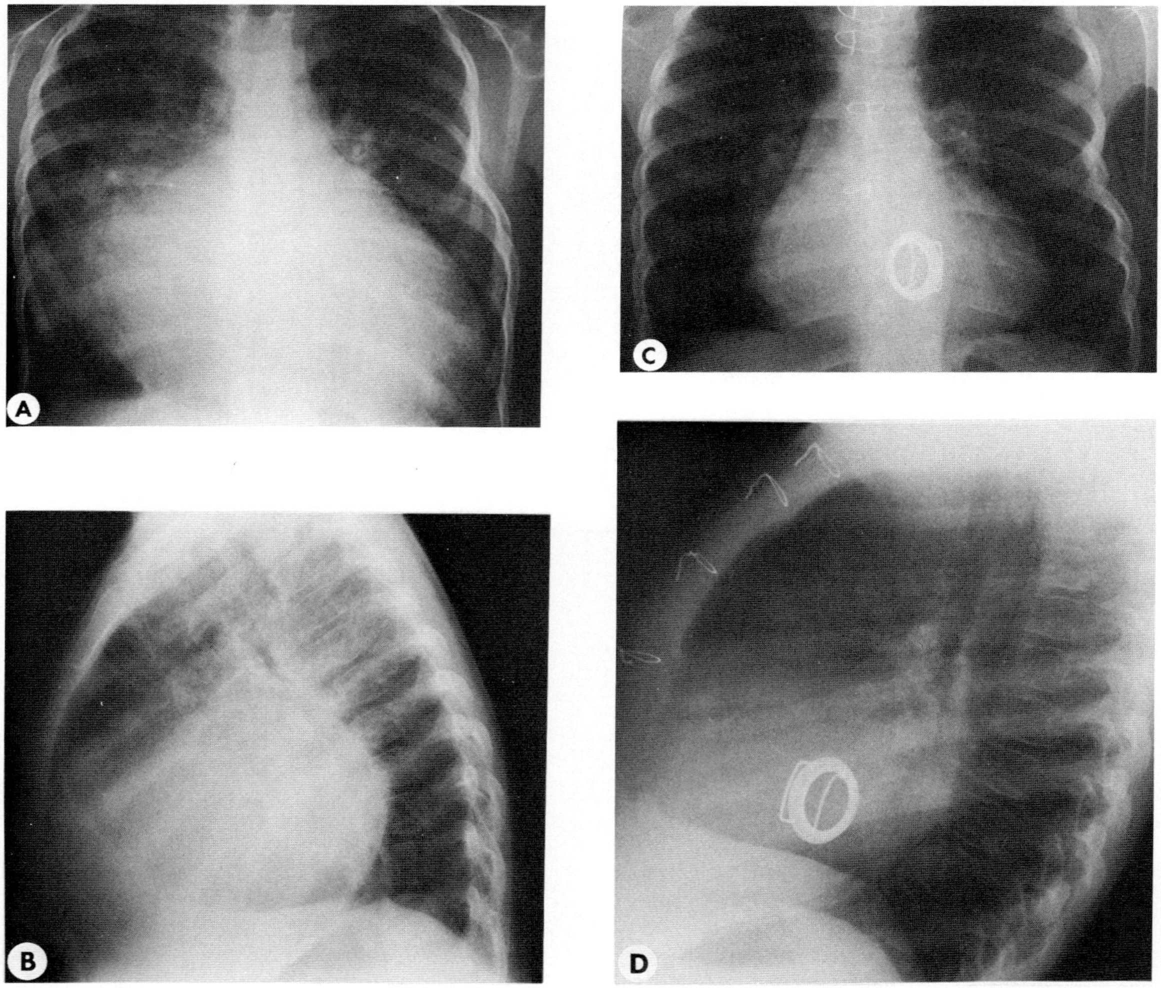

Fig. 7. Chest roentgenograms of a 4-yr old girl with mitral regurgitation. Successful resection of coarctation of the aorta was performed at 3 mo of age. (A) Anteroposterior, (B) Left lateral x-ray on the day prior to surgery, (C) Anteroposterior, and (D) Left lateral x-ray 2 yr later. Note significant reduction of left atrial and left ventricular size and the improvement of pulmonary venous engorgement.

centration; serum haptoglobin, lactic dehydrogenase, and bilirubin are obtained to evaluate possible hemolysis. A phonocardiogram is obtained for evaluation of opening and closing clicks. Changes in these sounds may be of use in evaluation of ball variance or thrombus on the struts. A prothrombin time is obtained to assess the adequacy of anticoagulation. Prothrombin times are obtained frequently until levels stabilize and thereafter approximately monthly. Dosage of Coumadin varies widely and has to be individualized. The problems in regulation of dosage do not appear to be more difficult in the younger age groups than in adolescents or adults.

After stabilization in the postoperative period the children are seen approximately every 6 mo. At each visit a hematocrit, hemoglobin, and reticulocyte count are obtained. Chest x-rays and electrocardiogram are obtained annually. Other tests are obtained upon specific indication. Repeat cardiac catheterizations in the past have only been for specific indications.

COMPLICATIONS

Valve replacement in adults has been well documented to be associated with a variety of postoperative complications. These include thromboembolism, bleeding secondary to anticoagulation

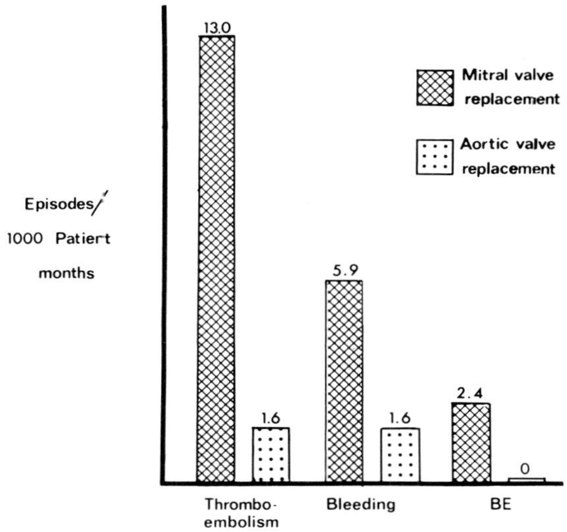

Fig. 8. The incidence of complications after valve replacement in children (number of episodes/1000 patient months). Thromboembolism, bleeding, and bacterial endocarditis (BE) are more common following mitral valve replacement.

therapy, infection, red cell hemolysis, and ball variance. Our experience and that of others, suggests that these problems occur in the pediatric age group with approximately the same incidence as in adults (Fig. 8).

Thromboembolism

Thromboembolism has been the most frequently reported complication of prosthetic valve replacement in adults. The incidence has varied widely depending upon the type, location, and particular model of the device employed, ranging from 55% with the early Starr–Edwards mitral valves[28] to <1% with certain tissue valve prostheses.

Valve replacement in children is so unusual and the types of valves employed so varied, that it is hard to obtain meaningful statistics from our clinical experience. All of our patients, with the exception of three who received porcine xenograft mitral valves and one other with a Braunwald–Cutter prosthesis in the aortic position, have been anticoagulated with Coumadin.

Among 18 survivors of mitral replacement using a cage or disc valve anticoagulated and followed for 844 mo, five (28%) have had a total of 11 symptomatic embolic episodes or an average of 13.0/1000 patient mo. This rather high incidence may reflect the fact that almost half the mitral valves were replaced with Kay–Shiley prostheses now known to be associated with a high incidence of embolization.[29] Two patients, one receiving an early model Starr–Edwards valve and the other a Kay–Shiley device, have undergone a second valve replacement because of recurrent cerebral and coronary emboli. Both had porcine xenografts implanted. Two other patients have residual hemiplegias.

Our experience with aortic valve replacements is considerably better with only one cerebral embolus among 18 (6%) survivors followed for 624 mo, an embolic incidence of 1.6/1000 patient mo. Others have noted a 15% incidence of thromboembolic complications in children,[4,9,17] although a few have quoted a lower incidence.[5,7,11,14] An occasional death has been reported[8,10,11,13,14] due to emboli or clot restricting valve function.

Hopefully, with an increased use of newer, less thrombogenic prosthetic valves, and the adaptation of preserved homograft and xenograft valves, the occurrence of thromboembolic complications can be further reduced.

Bleeding

In an attempt to reduce the thrombogenicity of prosthetic valves most surgeons have anticoagulated adult patients with sodium Warfarin. This regimen has added a new problem to patient management; that of hemorrhage. The incidence of severe bleeding among a large group of adults followed by Friedl et al.[30] was 10%, with another 39% of 170 patients noted to have soft tissue bleeding or epistaxis after minor trauma.

A fear that children might be more prone to accidents and serious hemorrhage had convinced some physicians not to use anticoagulants at all in the management of young valve recipients.[11] Others have instituted and maintained anticoagulation indefinitely.[6–10,13,14] Since 1965, it has been our policy to anticoagulate all patients except those receiving xenograft valves, and the cloth covered Braunwald–Cutter aortic prosthesis.

Among 17 of our patients surviving aortic valve replacement who were anticoagulated there has been one potentially serious hemorrhage and two minor bleeding episodes. A 22-yr old man developed flank pain and hematuria associated with a prolonged prothrombin time 3 mo following surgery. One of the minor hemorrhages was a prolonged nosebleed, and the other a hematoma secondary to a soft tissue laceration. None of the cases required hospitalization and no transfusions were necessary.

Eighteen of our patients who survived mitral valve replacement and were anticoagulated sustained five episodes of hemorrhage requiring hospitalization, with one death. Three young women had menorrhagia requiring transfusion and one eventually underwent hysterectomy to control severe pelvic hemorrhage. Another case involved a 10-yr old boy with recurrent headaches who was found to have a subdural hematoma with no antecedent history of trauma. A final patient, a 16-yr old boy, presented 6 wk postoperatively with a severe cerebral hemorrhage secondary to a ruptured cerebral arteriovenous communication. The prothrombin time on admission was 31.9 sec with a control of 12.5 sec. This child later died.

In summary, only one patient undergoing aortic valve replacement has had a serious hemorrhagic episode, but five patients with mitral valve replacement have required hospitalization, an incidence of 5.9/1000 patients mo. Our initial fears concerning a possible high incidence of hemorrhagic disorders in the youngest children due to unavoidable trauma has not been realized. No serious bleeding was noted in any child under 10 yr (10 children followed for 312 mo). This experience is similar to that reported in Klint's[7] review where bleeding was encountered in only eight children among 118 anticoagulated. One death, however, has been reported in a 13-yr old girl who had central nervous system hemorrhage 1 mo following mitral valve replacement.[8]

Infection

Bacterial endocarditis (BE) acquired at cardiac surgery is a well documented complication in both adults and children. Although the results of carefully controlled, double blind studies are not conclusive on the subject, we have used prophylactic antibiotics prior to, during, and after all valve replacements. Nevertheless, we have one patient, the first in this series, who developed a sternal infection and dehiscence after antibiotic coverage during surgery with penicillin and streptomycin. He responded to mediastinal drainage and massive doses of antibiotics.

Two patients, among 40 operative survivors, developed BE 2 mo and 3 mo following mitral valve replacement. One child had congenital bilateral hydronephrosis, and prior to cardiac surgery, had undergone a nephrectomy and a right uretero-ileostomy (ileal bladder). He developed two episodes of bacterial endocarditis on the basis of bacteremia from his infected kidney, and died at home 1 mo after a second course of antibiotics. The other patient developed BE due to candida 3 mo after repeat valve replacement with a porcine xenograft in the mitral position. This patient is currently under treatment with amphotericin B.

It is interesting to note that among all of our patients (54), there were seven episodes of BE preoperatively and only two following surgery. The incidence of BE after prosthetic valve replacement in our institution is similar to that observed in adults (approximately 4%).[31] Others have reported BE following valve replacement in children[4,9,17] usually terminating fatally.

Intravascular Hemolysis

Intravascular hemolysis following valve replacement was first reported by DeCesare[32] and has been found to be accelerated by prosthetic valve malfunction or paravalvular leak.[33] In our experience, virtually all children had evidence of chronic hemolysis with decreased serum haptoglobin, increased lactic dehydrogenase values, and mild reticulocytosis. However, none of our patients has had symptoms secondary to hemolysis, nor have transfusions been necessary. Two young women have developed cholelithiasis 3–4 yr postmitral valve replacement, but thus far, neither has been operated upon. The association between gallstones and hemolysis from prosthetic valves has recently been reported in adults.[34] Some authors[6,7,14,35] have suggested that hemolysis may be a problem in children, but it appears to be no more common than that noted in the adult experience.

Ball Valve Variance

Ball variance has been reported in some adults with prosthetic valve replacement and attributed to shrinkage or swelling of the silastic (Dow Corning Trademark) ball secondary to lipid uptake. The Starr–Edwards model No. 1000 appears to have been the worst offender in this regard.[36]

We have not experienced this problem, but a 9-yr old boy, reported by Miller,[35] presented with severe hemolytic anemia secondary to a crevice in a silastic ball that developed 2 yr after implantation of a model No. 1000 Starr–Edwards valve. Both Bleiden[4] and Stanton[14] have reported deaths in children in whom the ball shrunk and dislodged from the cage. With new Starr valve models employing hollow Stellite balls, this problem seems to have been eliminated.

Growth

One of major reasons for the reluctance to carry out valve replacements in children has been the fear that repeated operations might be necessary due to stenosis produced by normal growth. These concerns were reinforced by an early report (1966) of a reoperation on a 2-yr old child to replace a valve that had been inserted only 1 yr previously.[37] Our experience suggests that this is the exceptional case rather than the rule. None of 40 operative survivors at our institution has required reoperation so far for this reason. A review of the literature disclosed only one other case[4] where this was necessary.

It has been estimated that in an adult a mitral valve area of greater than 1.5 cm^2 would not cause significant obstruction with virtually unlimited physical exertion.[38] Similarly an aortic valve area of greater than 1.0 cm^2 is also probably compatible with a near normal existence.[39] In our series of 54 patients only two had smaller valves implanted. A 9-mo old with severe mitral regurgitation after an atrial septal defect (primum) repair had a mitral valve replacement with a 17 mm Bjork–Shiley (valve area 1.0 cm^2) and a 18-mo old with truncus arteriosus with stenosis and regurgitation has had the same size valve inserted in the "aortic" position. Only three other children were within 50% of these levels—a 3-yr old with congenital mitral stenosis who had a No. 1 Kay–Shiley inserted (valve area 1.5 cm^2),[41] a 4-yr old with congenital mitral stenosis who had a O M Starr–Edwards valve inserted (valve area 1.54 cm^2),[41] and a 2-yr old with congenital aortic stenosis who had a Smeloff–Cutter A-1 placed in the aortic position (valve area 1.19 cm^2).[41] The vast majority of the children with aortic and mitral valve replacements had "adult" sized devices inserted that were probably adequate for full growth even though the effective valve area in prosthetic valves in a group of children in vivo has been found to be only 75%–90% of the predicted orifice area.[27] Since most children undergoing valve replacement have regurgitant lesions with cardiomegaly and dilatation of the valve ring, they can accommodate large valves. The five patients in our series receiving valves of marginal size all were under 5 yr of age and had stenotic lesions. In this small group repeat valve replacements may be necessary in the future.

Our findings confirm previous reports in the literature. Although some authors have anticipated problems in a few of the smaller children,[4,5,11,15,27] all patients over 6 yr of age have received adult sized valves.[6–8,12,13,16,17,27] Finally, as Taguchi points out, "the possibility of reoperation in certain infants or small children . . . . . would not seem to be an inordinate price to pay for survival into adulthood."[27]

SUMMARY AND CONCLUSIONS

Valve replacement has been necessary in childhood for a variety of congenital and acquired forms of heart disease. At the Children's Hospital most of the aortic valve replacements have been for congenital abnormalities, with ventricular septal defect and aortic regurgitation being the most common lesion followed by valvar aortic stenosis. In the group of patients undergoing mitral valve replacement, the most common congenital defect was endocardial cushion defect with mitral regurgitation. However, rheumatic heart disease also accounted for a significant proportion of cases. Tricuspid and multiple valve replacements have been rarely required in our institution.

Although a wide variety of valve models have been used in the past, a low-profile, centrally opening device would seem to be the most appropriate today. Tissue valves have many potential advantages, but their long-term durability has not yet been proven and their size makes them currently not applicable in small children.

Aortic valve replacement has been associated with an overall mortality of 28% in the last decade (14% operative and 14% late death), but since 1967 operative mortality has been reduced to 6% and late mortality to 12%. Operative mortality in patients over 5 yr of age has been 6% since 1964. Actuarial life tables indicate an expected 9 yr survival rate of 65 ± 12%.

Mitral valve replacement continues to be more hazardous, with an operative mortality of 25% and an overall mortality of 39%. Operative mortality since 1967 has been 14%. Life tables estimate a 10-yr survival rate of 58 ± 10%. Age at the time of operation and date of procedure influenced the results. Tricuspid and double valve replacements were infrequent and associated with a high risk.

The complications identified with valve replacements in the adult population also affect children. Thromboembolism, spontaneous bleeding secondary to Warfarin anticoagulation, and bacterial endocarditis have occurred in our cases with an incidence similar to the adult experience. Concern about an increased risk of bleeding in anticoagulated children because of the high activity level has not been observed. Hemolytic anemia and ball variance, while not observed in our series has been reported by others in children. Initial fears about the need for repeated valve replacements with normal growth have not been realized, although this may be necessary in a small group of children operated upon before 5 yr of age.

While valve replacement in children is far from a panacea, it has been life saving in many young patients. The sight of a previously thin, frail, irritable apprehensive child bounding into clinic, and the reports of parents proudly discussing their discovery of a "child they have to hold down" reinforces the belief that valve replacement has a definite place in pediatric cardiovascular surgery. With continued improvements in the prostheses, valve replacement will undoubtably be performed with less trepidation in the future.

REFERENCES

1. Harken DE, Soroff HS, Taylor WJ, et al: Partial and complete prostheses in aortic insufficiency. J Thorac Cardiovasc Surg 40:744, 1960

2. Starr A, Edwards ML: Mitral replacement: Clinical experience with a ball-valve Prosthesis. Ann Surg 154:726, 1961

3. Bonchek LI, Dobbs JL, Matar AF, et al: Roentgenographic identification of Starr–Edwards prosthesis. Circulation 47:154, 1973

4. Bleiden LC, Castaneda AR, Nicoloff DM, et al: Prosthetic valve replacement in children: Results in 44 patients. Ann Thorac Surg 14:545, 1972

5. Taguchi K, Total prosthetic valve replacement in children under 10 years of age. Can Med Assoc J 98:765, 1968

6. Van De Water JM, Wolfe RR, Mulder DG: Total heart-valve replacement in the pediatric age group. J Thorac Cardiovasc Surg 53:515, 1967

7. Klint R, Hernandez A, Weldon C, et al: Replacement of cardiac valves in children. J Pediatr 80:980, 1972

8. Pérez-Alvarez JJ, Perez-Treviño C, Reta-Villalobos A, et al: Valvular prosthesis in children. Surgery 65:668, 1969

9. Vidne B, Levy MJ: Heart valve replacement in children. Thorax 25:57, 1970

10. Borman JB, Appelbaum A, Freund U: Results with cardiac valve protheses in children with rheumatic heart disease. J Thorac (Torino) Surg 13:272, 1972

11. van der Horst RL, le Roux BT, Rogers NMA, et al: Mitral valve replacement in childhood. A report of 51 patients. Am Heart J 85:624, 1973

12. Collins HA, Daniel RA Jr, Scott HW Jr, et al: Surgery for mitral valvular disease during childhood and adolescence. J Thorac Cardiovasc Surg 51:639, 1966

13. Ainger LE, Pate JW, Lawyer NG, et al: Prosthetic mitral valve replacement in children. J Pediatr 70:577, 1967

14. Stanton RE, Gallaher ME, Meyer BW, et al: Replacement of cardiac valves in children. Am J Dis Child 120:503, 1970

15. Shahin W, Eshkol D, Levy MJ: Valve replacement for mitral insufficiency in an infant with Marfan's syndrome J Pediatr Surg 4:350, 1969

16. Pifarre R, Caralps JM, Sinha SN: Mitral valve replacement for regurgitation in an infant with Marfan's syndrome. J Thorac Cardiovasc Surg 67:233, 1974

17. Bloodwell RD, Hallman GL, McNamara DG, et al: Cardiac valve replacement for congenital mitral valvular disease in children. J Pediatr Surg 4:9, 1969

18. Craenen J, Kilman J, Hosier DM, et al: Mitral valve replacement in a child with sickle cell anemia. J. Thorac Cardiovasc Surg 63:797, 1972

19. Mustard WT: Successful two-stage correction of transposition of the great vessels. Surgery 55:469, 1964

20. Tynan MJ, Aberdeen E, Stark J: Tricuspid incompetence after the Mustard operation for transposition of the great arteries. Circulation 45–46 (Suppl):111, 1972

21. Windsor HM, Shananhan MX: Cardiac valve replacement in the child. Med J Aust 1:649, 1968

22. van der Horst RL, le Roux BT, Rogers NMA, et al: Prosthetic valve replacement in children. Singapore Med J 14:420, 1973

23. Anderson RP, Bonchek LI, Grunkemeier GL, et al: The analysis and presentation of surgical results by actuarial methods. J Surg Res 16:224, 1974

24. Isom OW, Dembrow JM, Glassman E, et al: Factors influencing long-term survival after isolated aortic valve replacement. Circulation 49–50 (Suppl II):154, 1974

25. Karp RB, Kirklin JW, Kouchoukos NT, et al: Comparison of three devices to replace the aortic valve. Circulation 49–50 (Suppl II): 163, 1974

26. Wolff GS, Rowland TW, Ellison RC: Surgically induced right bundle branch block with left anterior hemiblock: An ominous sign in the postoperative tetralogy of Fallot: Circulation 46:587, 1972

27. Taguchi K: Hemodynamic evaluation of the prosthetic valve replacement among children under 10 years of age. Hiroshima J Med Sci 21:1, 1972

28. Results of Dr. Starr, As of September 1973. (Supplied by courtesy of Edwards Laboratory).

29. Vogel JHK, Paton BC, Overy HR, et al: Abnormal hemodynamic function after disc myral valve replacement. Circulation 39–40 (Suppl):141, 1969

30. Friedli B, Aerichide N, Grondin P, et al: Thromboembolic complications of heart valve prostheses. Am Heart J 81:702, 1971

31. Slaughter L, Morris JE, Starr, A: Prosthetic valvular endocarditis: A 12 year review. Circulation 47:1319, 1973

32. DeCesare W, Rath C, Hufnagel C: Hemolytic anemia of mechanical origin with aortic valve prosthesis. N Engl J Med 272:1045, 1965

33. Kastor JA, Akbarian M, Buckley MJ, et al: Paravalvular leaks and hemolytic anemia following insertion of Starr–Edwards aortic and mitral valves. J Thorac Cardiovasc Surg 56:279, 1968

34. Merendino KA, Manhas DR: Man-made gallstones: A new entity following cardiac valve replacement. Ann Surg 177:694, 1973

35. Miller BL, Pearson HA, Wheat MW, et al: Delayed onset of hemolytic anemia in a child: An indicator of ball variance of aortic valve prosthesis. Circulation 40:55, 1969

36. Hylen JC: Durability of prosthetic heart valves. Am Heart J 81:299, 1971

37. Robinson G, Young D: Secondary implantation of a mitral valve prosthesis in a child. Ann Thorac Surg 2:208, 1966

38. Friedberg CK: Diseases of the Heart (ed 3). Philadelphia, Saunders, 1966, p 1033

39. Friedberg CK: Diseases of the Heart (ed 3). Philadelphia, Saunders, 1966, p 1129

40. Courtesy of Shiley Laboratories

41. Roschke EJ, Harrison EC: Size comparisons of commercial prosthetic heart valves. Med Instrum 7:277, 1973

Evaluation and Management of Patients After Surgical Repair of Congenital Heart Diseases

Welton M. Gersony and Ehud Krongrad

AN ESTIMATED 25,000 babies are born each year with congenital heart disease in the United States.[1] Until the last decade, the great majority of patients who reached adulthood had either mild abnormalities or had undergone successful surgery for a single, usually simple defect. These individuals were virtually all hemodynamically normal, and rarely developed late complications which would require further management. In the past 10 yr however, technical advances and remarkable surgical accomplishments have led to physiologic correction of a large number of patients who hitherto would not have reached maturity. Thus, among the present generation of children who have been operated upon for congenital heart disease, many will emerge into adulthood with "repaired" complex lesions, and some will present to the adult cardiologist and internist with a number of new diagnostic and therapeutic challenges.

The purpose of this review is to provide physicians with information regarding potential late complications and the management of the postoperative patient after cardiac surgery for congenital heart disease. Special problems associated with repair of specific defects will be outlined, and questions will be considered regarding the eventual clinical effects of mild residual anatomic, hemodynamic, and electrocardiographic abnormalities.

GENERAL CONSIDERATIONS

Growth

Many children with severe congenital heart disease who show growth retardation prior to surgical correction will have an accelerated period of growth immediately after surgery.[2–5] Those who do not have severe residual defects will eventually display a growth pattern equivalent to that of the general population. Improvement is especially striking in patients who displayed congestive heart failure prior to operation.[2] A persistent growth deficit in patients with successfully repaired congenital heart disease is most often the result of associated congenital anomalies (e.g., small head circumference, chromosomal aberration, or single gene anomaly).[2,6–9]

An increased incidence of scoliosis has been reported[10–13] in the young adult with congenital heart disease, particularly in the cyanotic patient. This association may be due to general impairment of cortical bone formation, cardiomegaly, or a manifestation of an associated congenital defect.[10] The incidence of scoliosis in these patients increases with age and has no relationship to specific heart disease, side of the aortic arch, or the site of thoracotomy.[10,11] Scoliosis is particularly prevalent in the young adult with heart disease and associated vertebral malformations.[13] Since a precise etiologic factor has not been determined for the development of scoliosis in the majority of patients, it is not yet clear whether early corrective surgery might reduce the incidence of this association. It is therefore important that patients with a history of congenital heart disease be observed carefully for the eventual development of scoliosis, especially in the presence of predisposing factors such as (1) cyanotic heart disease, (2) coarctation of the aorta, (3) cardiomegaly, and (4) previous open heart surgery. Recognition of deformities prior to the adolescent growth spurt allows a greater chance that orthopedic management will be successful. Therapy includes braces and surgical intervention depending on the severity of the deformity.

Physical Examination

The great majority of children and young adults with a history of correction of congenital heart disease will be acyanotic and free of cardiovascular symptoms. In the absence or following reversal of cyanosis, clubbing usually will be absent but may

From the Division of Pediatric Cardiology, Department of Pediatrics, College of Physicians and Surgeons, Columbia University, and Babies Hospital, Columbia-Presbyterian Medical Center, New York, N.Y.

Supported by NIH grants 5 TOI HE-05389-14, and HE 12738-04.

Reprint requests should be addressed to Welton M. Gersony, M.D., Director, Division of Pediatric Cardiology, College of Physicians and Surgeons, Columbia University, New York, N. Y. 10032.

Table 1. Complications Following Surgical Correction of Congenital Heart Disease

Potential Late Complication	Comment
Bacterial endocarditis	Routine antibiotic prophylaxis recommended post surgery (except isolated ASD 2° and PDA).
Pulmonary vascular obstructive disease	Progresses only when pulmonary pressure and resistance were elevated prior to surgery and correction carried out after infancy.
Persistent L ⟶ R shunt	May be present after repair of ventricular septal defect but usually hemodynamically insignificant.
Late complete heart block	More likely with acquired right bundle branch block—LAH and/or history of early postoperative heart block which spontaneously resolved.
Slow junctional pacemaker	Occasionally observed; most often after Mustard operation for transposition of the great arteries.
Sudden death	Extremely rare; associated with an arrhythmia.
Constrictive pericarditis	Rare, but has been reported.
Thromboembolization	Late embolization infrequently may occur following prosthetic valve insertion.
Hemolysis	Infrequent. Reported after valve replacement, endocardial cushion defect repair, and aortic valvuloplasty.
Residual pulmonary insufficiency	Common after tetralogy of Fallot and pulmonary stenosis correction. No apparent adverse clinical manifestations.
Residual aortic insufficiency	May occur after aortic valvotomy and may persist after repair of ventricular septal defect with prolapsed aortic cusp. Clinical course depends on severity.
Residual mitral insufficiency	Observed after repair of endocardial cushion defect, corrected transposition of the great vessels, and congenital mitral insufficiency.
Residual tricuspid insufficiency	Observed after correction of pulmonary stenosis, transposition of the great arteries, tetrology of Fallot and endocardial cushion defect.
Restenosis following aortic or pulmonic valvotomy or coarctation repair	More likely if surgical correction was done in early infancy. May require reoperation.
Myocardial or coronary heart disease	Increased likelihood when left ventricular obstruction was severe and long standing prior to surgical relief of aortic stenosis or coarctation of the aorta.
Calcification or dysfunction of right ventricle—pulmonary artery homograft or heterograft	No serious malfunctions yet described.
Obstruction of pulmonary or venous return after Mustard operation (transposition of the great arteries)	Described as an early complication, but no reports of late obstruction (beyond 3 yr postop).
Psychiatric problems	Uncommon.
Scoliosis	Not unusual during adolescence in postoperative patients.

be occasionally noted in mild form. If an unoperated patient is encountered who displays cyanosis, it can be assumed that (1) he has not had proper evaluation and treatment, (2) he has developed pulmonary vascular obstructive disease which negated the possibility of surgical correction, or (3) he has an extremely complex anatomic malformation currently not amenable to surgical repair.

Examination of children and young adults with congenital heart disease may show absent, decreased, or asymetric peripheral pulses. Patients who have undergone a Blalock-palliative shunt will reveal absence of the brachial pulse on the side of the anastomosis. Absent or diminished pulses may also result from an arteriotomy performed for left heart catheterization, or following insertion of an arterial line in the immediate postoperative period.

Scars indicating past cardiac catheterization may be noted in the inguinal, antecubital, or axillary regions. A right thoracotomy scar is usually the result of thoracotomy for repair of atrial septal defect or a previous pulmonary to systemic anastomosis such as a Waterston or a Blalock-Taussig anastomosis. A left thoracotomy scar may indicate past surgery for patent ductus arteriosus, coarctation of the aorta, or Potts anastomosis. The median sternotomy is the most commonly used route for surgical repair of intraventricular defects and valvar anomalies. Scars in the right or left inferior abdominal quadrant indicate previous iliac cardiopulmonary bypass.

The presence of cardiac murmurs in the postoperative period will vary according to the nature of the original defect. Many patients will have functional systolic ejection murmurs at the left mid sternal border. Residual harsh systolic ejection murmurs and early diastolic murmurs at the base are common following repair of pulmonic stenosis, tetralogy of Fallot, coarctation of the aorta, or aortic stenosis; and are of varying significance. Mitral or tricuspid insufficiency murmurs may be heard after repair of endocardial cushion defects, transposition of the great arteries, and coarctation of the aorta. Continuous murmurs over the axillae and back related to increased bronchial collateral blood flow may persist following surgery for coarctation of the aorta or extreme tetralogy of Fallot.[14]

The second heart sound will usually be normally split in the late postoperative period, but wide splitting is occasionally heard for some time following atrial septal defect closure, as well as in other conditions in which a right bundle branch block persists after surgery. Patients with pulmonary vascular obstructive disease will have a loud single or narrowly split S_2.

The Electrocardiogram

A right bundle branch block pattern (RBBB) following right ventriculotomy is the most frequent electrocardiographic manifestation of open heart surgery. This pattern may be due to either proximal or distal disruption of the right bundle branch.[15,18] There have been no reports concerning late clinical manifestations attributed to RBBB. However, prognostic significance of the post ventriculotomy RBBB pattern lies in the eventual observation as to whether atrioventricular conduction will be maintained in the face of an acquired left bundle branch block later in life.

The postoperative development of an RBBB pattern associated with a counterclockwise superiorly oriented frontal plane QRS axis, "left anterior hemiblock" (RBBB-LAH) has been of recent concern.[19-26] Current evidence suggests that patients with RBBB-LAH may be divided into three groups:[27] (1) patients with congenital anomalies of the specialized conduction system, such as endocardial cushion defects, display this ECG pattern as a result of asynchronous activation of the left ventricle.[28] Presumably, these individuals do not have an increased risk of late complete heart block. (2) Following surgery, RBBB-LAH may result from peripheral disruption of the right bundle branch and anterior fascicles of the left bundle branch during surgery. These patients do not exhibit atrioventricular conduction disturbances immediately after surgery, and presumably do not carry an increased risk of complete heart block during early adulthood.[27] (3) Patients who show evidence of atrioventricular conduction disturbances immediately following surgery in association with RBBB-LAH may have injured the distal part of the His bundle.[29,30] With further healing and fibrosis such patients may be prone to the development of complete heart block or sudden death. This type of injury may also involve more proximal fibers of the His bundle resulting in P–R prolongation ("trifascicular block pattern").[31]

Complete heart block following open heart surgery requires insertion of an artificial pacemaker. Patients with implanted pacemakers are protected from the risks of severe bradycardia and Adams–Stokes attacks. Long-term management of acquired surgical block has been successful despite frequent surgical procedures for battery replacement. Even small infants have sustained normal growth and development during prolonged pacemaker therapy.[32] Already an infrequent complication, heart block may be virtually eliminated by the widespread use of electrophysiologic methods for mapping of the specialized conduction system during surgery.[33,34]

Injury to the sinus node during cardiac bypass may result in postoperative dysrrhythmias including sinus arrest with subsidiary slow junctional rhythm, sinus bradycardia, and the bradycardia-tachycardia syndrome (Fig. 2).[35-41] Although most frequent in patients after correction of transposition of the great arteries,[35-40] injury to the sinus node may occasionally occur after other types of open heart surgery.[41] Most patients are asymptomatic but the clinical significance of these rhythm disturbances may become more apparent later in life. It is possible that some of the reported late sudden deaths are associated with surgical injury to the sinus node.[35,42,43]

Episodes of supraventricular tachycardia and

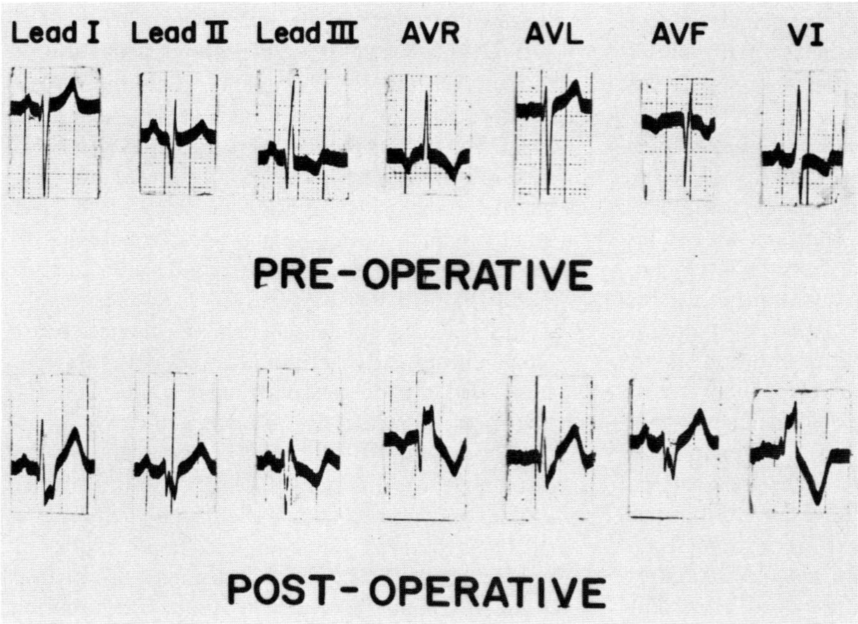

Fig. 1. Electrocardiograms prior to and after surgical repair of Tetralogy of Fallot. Preoperative electrocardiogram showing right axis deviation (QRS Â = 120°). Postoperative tracing reveals RBBB and left superior axis (QRS Â = −60°).

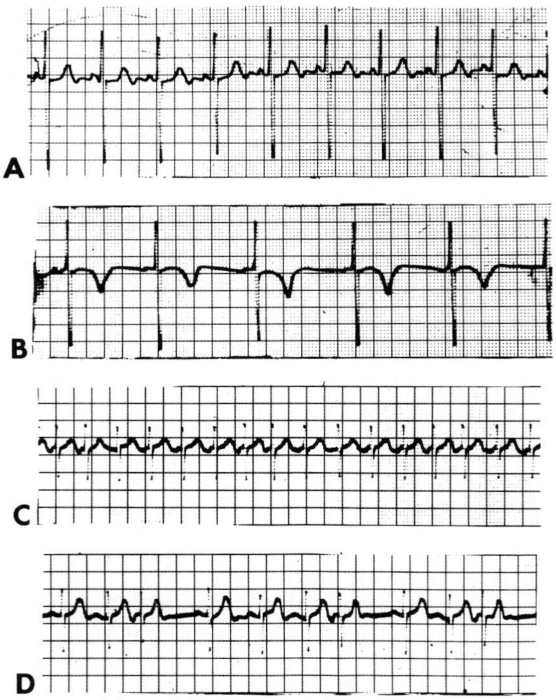

Fig. 2. Selected tracings from continuous electrocardiograms in a patient 2 yr following Mustard operation for repair of D-transposition of the great arteries. (A) At rest, regular, rhythm, heart rate = 100/min. (B) 2 hr later, during sleep, junctional rhythm, heart rate = 55/min. (C) 12 hr later, while crying, supraventricular tachycardia, heart rate = 167/min. (D) after cessation of crying, irregular rhythm as tachycardia regresses.

persistent premature ventricular contractions are other dysrhythmias which are occasionally encountered following open heart surgery but these disturbances rarely require chronic antiarrhythmic therapy. However, late tachyarrhythmias on occasion may become serious complications and can result in sudden death.[43]

Chest X-ray

Most patients with congenital heart disease will display a relatively normal chest x-ray following surgical correction, usually within 1 or 2 yr of operation. However, in some instances, preoperative cardiomegaly may persist for years, perhaps indefinitely. Mild cardiac enlargement is usually the result of the removal of pericardium and subsequent loss of pericardial tensile strength following surgery,[44] a phenomenon similar to that observed in patients with congenital absence of the pericardium.[45] Cardiomegaly may also be associated with pulmonary insufficiency such as seen following pulmonary valvotomy, insertion of a right ventricular outflow patch, or in the congenital absence of the pulmonary valve.[46–49] Residual intracardiac shunts or mitral or tricuspid regurgitation also may account for postoperative cardiac enlargement, but should be accompanied by characteristic physical findings. Patients with complete heart block and increased stroke index also will show an increase in cardiac size. Pulmonary vascular markings are normal in most young adults who

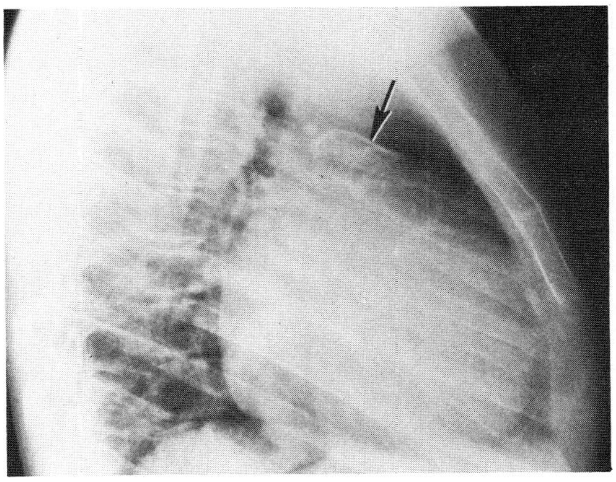

Fig. 3. Lateral view of the chest in a patient 3 yr after pulmonary homograft insertion for repair of pulmonary atresia. Arrow indicates calcification.

had surgical correction of a congenital heart lesion during childhood.

Physical Activities

Physical activity for most young adults with a history of successfully repaired congenital heart disease will be unimpaired. Women will tolerate pregnancy without difficulty.[50,51] Hemodynamic studies following corrective surgery have shown that if no residual anomalies are present, cardiovascular function during rest is usually similar to that observed in the normal population. However, patients have been reported who display subtle hemodynamic abnormalities for some time following surgery.[52–56] Furthermore, some individuals who show normal hemodynamics during the basal state at cardiac catheterization will display abnormal response to exercise.[52–54] Recent reports suggest, however, that the duration of cardiac overload prior to correction may be an important determinant in the reversability of myocardial malfunction.[57,58] For example, some patients operated upon for ventricular septal defect over 10 yr of age may show cardiovascular impairment during exercise whereas none of the patients operated upon under 2 yr of age, even those who have had congestive heart failure, will display exercise-related hemodynamic abnormalities.[57] Age related differences in response to exercise have also been demonstrated after correction of pulmonic stenosis.[58]

In general, the reported hemodynamic abnormalities following successful correction are mild and there are no indications that progression should be expected in adult life. When residual anomalies are present, physical capacity is dependent on the type and severity of the defects which remain. If cardiac abnormalities are severe, reoperation must be considered. Incomplete correction is most common in patients who have undergone procedures which involve the semilunar valves. Residual mild to moderate right ventricular outflow obstruction or pulmonary insufficiency are well tolerated and restriction of activities is not indicated. Significant postoperative aortic valvular abnormalities are of greater concern and some limitations of physical effort may be desirable. The degree of physical activity suggested for patients with residual aortic stenosis or aortic insufficiency depends upon: (1) hemodynamic severity of the lesion as measured at cardiac catheterization, (2) associated electrocardiographic changes which indicate myocardial abnormalities ("strain pattern"), and (3) evidence of ventricular irritability. Even after successful surgery, rough competitive sports should be discouraged for this group of patients.

Among patients in whom anatomic factors or pulmonary vascular disease do not currently allow for the possibility of correction, restriction of activities is in most instances self-imposed. Many of these individuals will live many years of productive lives despite severe physiologic handicaps.

A detailed summary regarding physical, recreational, and occupational guidelines for patients with congenital heart disease has been provided by the congenital heart disease study group of the American Heart Association.[59,60]

Antimicrobial Prophylaxis

Antimicrobial prophylaxis is advocated for patients with various forms of congenital heart disease in order to avoid the development of bacterial endocarditis.[61] This complication may occur following any procedure which predisposes to bacteremia, such as dental manipulation, and nasopharyngeal surgery,[62–66] genitourinary instrumentation and surgery in adults,[67–72] skin infections,[73] bronchoscopy,[74] and labor.[75]

Palliative surgery does not decrease the incidence of bacterial endocarditis. This infection is not infrequent among patients with palliative systemic-to-pulmonary artery shunts such as the Blalock-Taussig, Pott's, or Waterston anastomoses. It is therefore important that particular care in the prevention of infective endocarditis should be exercised in this group of patients.

Little data are available regarding endocarditis among patients who have undergone corrective heart surgery, but in many patients the factors which predispose to infection remain. Residual deformities of valvar cusps are common following aortic and pulmonary valvotomy. Abnormalities of the mitral and tricuspid valves also persist following correction of endocardial cushion defects or other congenital lesions. Various prosthetic materials are utilized in the repair of intracardiac shunts, the reconstruction of the right ventricular outflow tract, the widening of various pulmonary or systemic vessels, valve replacements, and valve containing conduits.

It would seem prudent to administer antimicrobial prophylaxis to most postoperative patients. Since the incidence of bacterial endocarditis following repair of patent ductus arteriosus and atrial septal defect secundum (without mitral valve abnormalities) is virtually nil, prophylaxis against bacterial endocarditis is not recommended postoperatively in these conditions.[61]

Cerebrovascular Accidents and Thromboembolism

Cerebrovascular accidents occur mainly in severely cyanotic patients with congenital heart disease who display reduced arterial oxygen tension.[76,77] Infants who develop cerebrovascular accidents will often be relatively anemic; whereas adolescents or adults will appear with marked polycythemia. Some patients will show permanent residual central nervous system damage after recovery from the original insult. Early repair of cyanotic heart disease will undoubtedly contribute to the reduction of the incidence of this severe complication during childhood.

Postoperative thromboembolism is an extremely infrequent occurrence in patients with congenital heart disease. Embolization is known to occur most often following aortic or mitral valve replacement, and in rare instances, following dislodgement of patch materials used for closure of intracardiac defects.[78] Improvements in operative techniques, prosthetic valve design, the use of cloth covered valves or tissue containing grafts, and postoperative anticoagulation have served to reduce the incidence of thromboembolism over the past decade.[79–83]

Chronic anticoagulation therapy is advisable following mitral valve replacement.[82] After aortic valve replacement with cloth covered prosthesis, anticoagulation therapy may not be necessary as additional protection from thromboembolism.[82]

Since an adolescent youth may be expected to be more active physically, anticoagulation might carry a more significant risk for hemorrhagic complications in this age group. Therefore, it is important that the patient and his family realize the potential hazard involved in anticoagulation and the threat of uncontrolled bleeding associated with physical injury.

Among the general population, an increased incidence of pulmonary thromboembolism is known to occur with the use of oral contraceptives.[84,85] This risk is related to the estrogen content of these preparations. Some patients with congenital heart disease and pulmonary vascular changes may be in particular peril from an additional insult to their pulmonary circulation. The use of oral contraceptives containing estrogen should be discouraged in any woman showing evidence of pulmonary vascular disease. These patients should be advised as to alternate methods of contraception.

Hemolytic Anemia

Hemolytic anemia may occur in some patients following corrective cardiac surgery for congenital heart disease. This syndrome has been reported most often following insertion of prosthetic valves[86–88] and rarely following correction of an endocardial cushion defect,[89–90] systemic-to-pulmonary artery shunts and aortic valvuloplasty.[91–94] A precise diagnosis is based on the demonstration of extra corpuscular hemoglobin in serum or urine, decreased or absent serum haptoglobin, and decrease of red cell survival time.[91] Hemolytic anemia following cardiovascular surgery may be either transient or chronic, and can begin months after surgery. Some patients in whom severe hemolysis is present will require reoperation in order to eliminate the mechanical basis for red cell destruction.

Genetic Considerations

For many years most congenital cardiac defects were considered to be nonhereditary, primarily because the only cardiac lesions amenable to familial and genetic studies were those associated with relative longevity and mild symptomatology.[95-101] Thus, the exclusion of more severe and lethal defects from genetic studies appears to have led to a biased impression that certain heart defects and not others are familial.[95]

The proper diagnosis and management of almost all congenital heart disease over the last two decades has resulted in the emergence of young adults with a previous history of significant heart disease capable of leading a normal family life. For this reason relatively large aggregates of offspring to parents with various and severe forms of congenital heart defects are becoming available for genetic studies of congenital heart defects. It has been established that an increased incidence occurs among probands with various forms of congenital heart disease.[102,103] The familial recurrence rate of the various forms of a congenital heart defect is estimated to be between 1%–5% for the first offspring.[95,102] The risk to offspring of patients with ventricular septal defect and atrial septal defect has been established to be 21 and 37 times higher, respectively, than the expected frequency among the general population.[104] Although limited data is available regarding the risk to offsprings of parents with other forms of congenital defects, an increased incidence has been reported.[50]

For many years some centers encouraged the interrelationship and social activities of children with congenital heart defects by establishing various clubs, social meetings, and summer camps. Emerging data regarding the genetics of congenital heart disease may cast doubts regarding the advisability of such activities, which increase the possibilities of intermarriage among these patients.[103]

SPECIFIC DEFECTS

Tetralogy of Fallot

Children who have undergone open heart correction for tetralogy of Fallot usually do not show late signs or symptoms of cardiac malfunction. Follow-up studies have revealed that for the great majority of patients, general health is excellent, child bearing is unaffected, and educational and occupational status is equivalent to that of the general population.[50] Most of these reports have concerned young adults followed into the third decade of life; later evaluation awaits the passage of time. Despite these encouraging results, residual hemodynamic and electrophysiologic abnormalities which have been observed in the postoperative period continue to raise questions as to the long-term prognosis in some patients. Indeed, in a few instances late complications have been documented. The long-term effects of surgical correction of tetralogy of Fallot must be considered in several areas.

Residual Defects

Trivial or even moderately severe residual anatomic and hemodynamic abnormalities may persist following intracardiac repair of tetralogy of Fallot but in most instances the postoperative clinical course is not seriously affected. Studies carried out 1 to 10 yr after correction have reported elevated mean systolic right ventricular pressures at rest in the range of 44–46 mm mercury, as a result of mild outflow tract obstruction.[65-107] However, right ventricular performance has been markedly abnormal during exercise, only in the presence of severe residual pulmonary stenosis.[108]

Pulmonary insufficiency is common and does not appear to influence the late postoperative status of patients with tetralogy of Fallot.[105,106,109-111] Even marked incompetence of the pulmonary valve created by insertion of a right ventricular outflow patch has not been associated with significant late morbidity.[50] On rare occasions, tricuspid valve regurgitation will be created when the insertion of the papillary muscle of the conus is injured during right ventricular infundibulectomy. When both the pulmonary and tricuspid valves are insufficient, significant limitation of right ventricular function may be observed, and a chronic syndrome of right ventricular failure associated with liver congestion may be encountered. Under these unusual circumstances, one or both valves could eventually require replacement.

Surgical correction of extreme tetralogy of Fallot with pulmonary atresia is accomplished by reconstruction of the right ventricular outflow tract using homografts or various types of heterografts.[112] These valve-containing conduits have been successful in bypassing total obstruction of the right ventricular outflow tract and in many instances have prevented massive pulmonary insufficiency. Calcifications may be recognized along the lining of homografts (Fig. 3). Long-term experience with homografts and valve-containing conduits is not available.

Persistent intraventricular communications are

not infrequently documented at hemodynamic study after correction of tetralogy of Fallot, but only in rare instances are large defects discovered among long-term survivors.[50] Reoperation is not indicated for small left-to-right shunts.

Pulmonary Artery Hypertension

Late pulmonary vascular obstructive disease has not been reported among patients with tetralogy of Fallot whose pulmonary artery pressure has been documented to be within the normal range prior to operation. However, some individuals who undergo corrective surgery will have had earlier palliative operations which have resulted in an extremely large pulmonary flow and elevated pulmonary artery pressures. Pulmonary hypertension rarely occurs after a Blalock–Taussig operation, but may occasionally be observed following Waterston or Pott's anastomoses.[113] In a report of 64 patients from this institution, two late deaths occurred, and both were among patients who fell into this category.[50]

Some patients with tetralogy of Fallot have only one functional pulmonary artery.[111] This may be due to a congenital absence of one vessel or as a result of a previous shunt procedure which resulted in thrombosis of the right or left pulmonary artery at the site of the anastomosis. Following intracardiac correction, the pulmonary artery pressure in these patients will often be higher than normal, presumably on a flow basis. At this time, no cases have been reported who have developed pulmonary vascular obstructive disease or other late clinical complications.

Electrocardiographic Abnormalities

Right bundle branch block is virtually universal on the electrocardiogram following repair of tetralogy of Fallot. It has been well shown that this pattern is usually produced at the time of right ventriculotomy rather than during the repair of the ventricular septum.[15,16] RBBB + LAH is present in 10%–20% of operated patients (Fig. 1).[27] The prognosis for individuals with this electrocardiographic pattern varies significantly.[27] (See the section on General Considerations–Electrocardiogram.) A history of transient heart block in the immediate postoperative period or the development of P-R prolongation may indicate an increased risk of late dysrythmias and sudden death among these patients.[19,24,27]

Pulmonary Stenosis

The late results of repair of valvular pulmonary stenosis have been excellent.[114–118] Mild pulmonary insufficiency or occasionally a small residual gradient may remain in the postoperative period. Two sets of circumstances should alert the physician to a significant residual pulmonary artery-right ventricular gradient (1) Despite the demonstration of significant right ventricular infundibular hypertrophy by angiography prior to surgery, an infundibulectomy still may not have been carried out. This is because valvulotomy alone will be sufficient to relieve the valvar gradient and the secondary infundibular obstruction most often will regress with time.[115] However, unrelieved infundibular stenosis may be of sufficient magnitude to eventually require reoperation. (2) A significant number of patients in whom closed pulmonary valvotomies were carried out in early infancy will require a second operation later in life.

Patients with significant residual right ventricular outflow gradient may be diagnosed rather readily by physical examination (length and intensity of murmur, behavior of the second sound) and the electrocardiogram.[116] With successful repair, the ECG will show regression of right ventricular potentials and a frontal plane axis shift towards normal. Occasionally, a mild right ventricular conduction defect will be encountered as a permanent electrocardiographic abnormality despite complete elimination of the obstruction. However, the persistence of a definite right ventricular hypertrophy pattern, suggests the presence of significant pulmonary stenosis.

Aortic Stenosis

Aortic valvotomy for valvar aortic stenosis during infancy and childhood must be considered a palliative operation. Only rarely is the left ventricular-aortic gradient completely abolished, since the surgeon must be careful not to substitute significant aortic insufficiency for aortic valve obstruction. A malformed aortic valve, subject to the abuses of a high pressure system and the likelihood of late calcification, may require replacement at some time later in life. The purpose of early valvotomy for severe obstruction is twofold: (1) protection of left ventricular myocardium from the chronic effects of severe hypertension through childhood, adolescence, and the early adult years, (2) lessening of the possibility of sudden death.[119–123]

In severe cases of aortic stenosis, myocardial fibrosis, subendocardial ischemia, and papillary muscle dysfunction have been documented.[124–126] These myocardial changes produce persistent and progressive electrocardiographic abnormalities. Little is known about regression of myocardial hypertrophy after relief of left ventricular outflow obstruction, although experimental evidence suggests that if severe afterload is removed, wall thickness will become reduced.[127] This might imply that early intervention for significant aortic stenosis may have long-term benefits. There are no clinical data which indicate that myocardial insufficiency can be expected in adolescence or early adulthood among patients in whom congenital aortic stenosis has been successfully corrected prior to the onset of left ventricular decompensation. Repeated cardiac catheterizations may be required to assess the severity of residual stenosis. Late postoperative follow-up data concerning the effects of valvotomy on myocardial function, incidence of restenosis, or the age of onset of coronary artery disease are not available.

Surgical relief of discrete subvalvar and supravalvar aortic stenosis will not result in residual aortic valve deformities, but incomplete repair of subvalvar stenosis may occasionally be documented. The prognosis for patients in whom complete elimination of obstruction has been achieved appears to be excellent.

Coarctation of the Aorta

Coarctation of the aorta was one of the earliest defects amenable to surgical correction. However, until recently, little information has been available as to the long-term outlook for postoperative patients. The incidence of "recoarctation" is age related and infants are more likely to require a second operation. Improved techniques have lowered the necessity for a second procedure, even when repair is done in the neonatal period.[128]

Late narrowing at the anastomosis is usually due to scarring rather than as a result of a fixed orifice at the repair site which does not maintain the circumferential growth rate of the immediate proximal and distal aortic segments.[129] The true incidence of residual coarctation may be greater than recognized by differential arm and leg blood pressure determination at rest.

Maron and his associates reported a high incidence of early cardiovascular disease in a retrospective analysis of postoperative cases.[130] Two hundred and forty-eight patients were evaluated 11–25 yr after surgery. Only 12% had died. The mean age at operation was 20 yr. In a hospital examination of 59 patients, 78% had evidence of cardiovascular disease and 40% had hypertension at least as high as had been recorded prior to surgery. Premature mortality appeared to be related to the duration of preoperative hypertension, but whether corrective surgery earlier in childhood will be protective remains to be determined.

The physician must be aware that a significant number of patients with coarctation of the aorta also have bicuspid aortic valves and some will have mitral valve abnormalities.[131] Although significant aortic valve gradients are uncommon in childhood, calcification may lead to significant stenosis later in life. Auscultation for the murmurs of aortic stenosis or mitral insufficiency must be emphasized during routine physical examination of these patients.

Ventricular Septal Defect

The great majority of patients who have undergone successful repair of ventricular septal defect can be expected to live a normal life following surgery. A low intensity left sternal border ejection systolic murmur may be present, the electrocardiogram will show RBBB, and a mild to moderate increase in heart size may be noted on the chest x-ray; but none of these observations have been linked to late complications. However, the physician should be aware of possible exceptions to this optimistic outlook.

Residual Defects

Small residual left-to-right shunts are present after correction of ventricular septal defects in some patients.[132–134] Large defects which remain after inadequate repair will most often require reoperation in the early postoperative period, but an occasional patient may be seen many years after the initial procedure in whom a large residual defect persists. Decision as to reoperation depends upon clinical evaluation of the patient, the presence of pulmonary artery hypertension, and the size of the shunt.

Patients with pulmonary hypertension at the time of closure of ventricular septal defect should be observed closely in order to assess the state of the pulmonary vascular bed. Since the electrocardiogram usually exhibits a right bundle branch block pattern following surgery, the ECG may not be helpful in the evaluation of progressive right ventricular overload. In estimating the severity of pulmonary vascular obstructive disease in these patients therefore, one must rely on clinical status, physical examination (right ventricular impulse, loud S_2), radiologic evidence of large proximal pulmonary arteries, and hemodynamic evaluation by means of repeat cardiac catheterization.

Patients with severe pulmonary vascular obstruction should be encouraged to avoid vigorous physical activity and travel to high altitudes. They may be adversely affected by excessive exercise, anesthesia, external heat, fever, or the injection of hyperosmotic contrast material. Patients with severe pulmonary vascular obstructive disease have little cardiac reserve and any acute changes in pulmonary or systemic hemodynamics carry the risk of sudden death.[135–137] Although life expectancy is shortened for these patients, many will survive and enjoy useful lives for many years.[138]

Aortic Insufficiency

Certain high ventricular septal defects will be associated with prolapse of an aortic valve cusp into the defect, resulting in aortic insufficiency and/or rupture of the sinus of Valsalva into the right ventricle.[139–142] Since, under these circumstances, the ventricular septal defect tends to be small or even closed by the aortic cusp, the major clinical and hemodynamic findings relate almost entirely to the severity of aortic insufficiency. Most of the patients with ventricular septal defect and aortic insufficiency are recognized in the first decade of life, but this association must be considered if aortic insufficiency is discovered in an adult with a history of ventricular septal defect. Early closure of the ventricular septal defect may not eliminate aortic insufficiency since inherent abnormalities of the aortic valve are present in some cases. Surgical correction requires aortic valvuloplasty as well as ventricular septal defect closure but aortic valve replacement is hardly necessary.[140,141,143] Early operation is recommended in order to prevent long term effects of aortic insufficiency on the left ventricular myocardium. Long-term results of surgery have been encouraging. However, observation for residual aortic regurgitation must be maintained postoperatively.

Complete Heart Block

Complete heart block is an infrequent result of surgery for ventricular septal defect; at present, the incidence is almost nil. However, when this complication occurs, insertion of an artificial pacemaker is mandatory. When junctional pacemaker, characterized by narrow QRS duration and heart rate in the range of 60–80, is present, pacemaker implantation may not be necessary. Late onset of heart block has been extremely rare among patients who have had sinus rhythm postoperatively.

Atrial Septal Defect (Secundum)

Following surgical correction of atrial septal defect, children with growth retardation will improve in a striking fashion.[144,145] Furthermore, even patients who are considered to be asymptomatic prior to surgery will show a subjective improvement in functional capacity following correction.[145] Cardiac examination of postoperative patients will often reveal residual left sternal border systolic murmurs, but diastolic murmurs of tricuspid flow will invariably disappear following successful repair.[146] A widely split second sound may persist indefinitely despite elimination of the intracardiac shunt.[146] This may be due in part to persistent right ventricular conduction delay after operation.

Most patients will display a gradual reduction of cardiac size by x-ray postoperatively. However, occasionally, cardiomegaly may persist for a prolonged period of time.[144] Within the first 2 yr following surgery, mild to moderate cardiac enlargement, a large pulmonary artery segment, and an increased pulmonary vascular pattern do not necessarily indicate that a residual cardiac shunt is present.[144]

Arrhythmias consisting of junctional rhythm and ectopic atrial activity are common in the immediate postoperative period, but are usually self-limiting. Persistent arrhythmias and complete heart block are uncommon. The electrocardiogram improves following surgery, and the preoperative rightward oriented QRS axis will shift to the left.[144,145] The electrocardiograph pattern of right ventricular conduction delay improves, with a decrease in R or R′ voltage in V_1, but the pattern of right ventricular conduction delay will persist in most patients.[147]

It has been suggested that minimal right ventricular dysfunction is more likely to persist when atrial septal defects are closed at an older age, since these patients were subject to more prolonged cardiac overload.[52,148,149]

Endocardial Cushion Defects

Atrial Septal Defect Primum, Atrioventricular Canal

Factors affecting the surgical results of patients with endocardial cushion defect are more complex than for atrial septal defect of the secundum type.[150–153] (1) The complete closure of an endocardial cushion defect may be technically difficult since the precise demarcation of the lower part of the lesion is not always immediately apparent. Residual shunts may be more common. (2) The defect may be in close proximity to the specialized conduction system of the heart, increasing the risk of postoperative complete heart block. (3) Mitral valve clefts are almost invariably present. Mitral valvuloplasties may well be imperfect, and if residual insufficiency is severe, left atrial hypertension may be greater than when the atrial septal defect was open and served to decompress the left atrium. In some cases with severe mitral incompetence, valve replacement may be necessary.[152] (4) Preoperative pulmonary hypertension is present with endocardial cushion defects when there is an associated ventricular septal defect (partial or complete atrioventricular canal). If pulmonary resistance is elevated, progressive pulmonary vascular obstructive disease may occur, even after surgical correction.

Postoperatively, right ventricular forces on the ECG gradually diminish over the years. The typical counterclockwise superiorly oriented frontal plane QRS axis does not change following surgical correction of an endocardial cushion defect. This pattern is most probably the result of inhomogenous activation of the left ventricle and is not affected by the elimination of the intracardiac shunt. Late development of complete heart block in these patients[154] is probably due to latent injury to the specialized conduction system during surgery, rather than late manifestations of the intrinsic properties of the conduction system.

Following surgery, a considerable decrease in heart size and pulmonary vascular markings on chest x-ray will usually occur. However, similar to postoperative patients with other types of left-to-right shunts, an enlarged heart and increased pulmonary vascular markings may be present for some time. Residual mitral insufficiency may also affect the appearance of the cardiac silhouette.

D-Transposition of the Great Arteries

The grave prognosis for patients with transposition of the great arteries has been reversed during the last decade. This has occurred largely as a result of a vigorous approach to management including: (1) the introduction of the balloon atrial septostomy, performed immediately during the neonatal period at the initial cardiac catheterization.[155,156] This results in improved mixing of pulmonary and systemic venous blood and marked reduction of lethal hypoxemia. (2) The success of a second stage operation which rechannels atrial blood flow to opposite ventricles (Mustard procedure). This operation is usually carried out between 1 and 2 yr of age.

More than half of the patients with transposition of the great arteries will have additional cardiac lesions. Infants who have an associated ventricular septal defect may require pulmonary artery banding after atrial septostomy during the first year of life prior to complete correction. Others, with ventricular septal defect and severe pulmonic stenosis, may need an early systemic-pulmonary arterial shunt. Thus, early palliative operations for transposition of the great arteries will attempt to either increase or decrease pulmonary blood flow, depending on the associated defects.[159,160] Correction of patients with ventricular septal defect and severe pulmonic stenosis is usually accomplished after 5 yr of age by creation of a right ventricular to pulmonary artery communication using an aortic hemograft or a synthetic conduit. The ventricular septal defect is utilized as an outflow from the left ventricle to the aorta, thus avoiding the necessity for the Mustard operation.[112,162]

Residual Defects

Following correction of transposition of the great arteries, the patients become acyanotic, improve their growth and developmental pattern, and are able to lead active and unrestricted lives. However, persistent abnormalities following surgery have been recognized in a number of patients. These include (1) residual intraatrial shunts, (2) superior and/or inferior vena cava obstruction, (3) pulmonary venous obstruction, (4) tricuspid regurgitation, (5) cardiac dysrhythmias, and (6) pulmonary vascular obstructive disease. The question as to how long the right ventricle will be able to adequately maintain systemic circulation is unresolved.

Residual intraatrial shunts usually occur at the superior vena cava-right atrial junction and favor the streaming of systemic venous blood into the systemic circulation.[162-165] This results in arterial oxygen desaturation to a degree dependent on the magnitude of the right-to-left shunt. In most patients, these shunts are small resulting in a decrease of systemic oxygen saturation to about 90%. This is not clinically recognized as cyanosis and may be detected only by special techniques such as dye dilution curves at the time of a postoperative catheterization. Mild arterial desaturation may also be the result of incorporation of the coronary sinus into the newly created "left atrium." Small intraatrial shunts are of no clinical significance and do not require further treatment. However, when intraatrial shunts are large, reoperation may be required to repair the residual defect.

Systemic venous obstruction may occur postoperatively at the site of the intraatrial baffle.[42,162,166,167] Mild obstruction is well tolerated and does not require treatment. When venous obstruction is severe, signs and symptoms will appear. Intermittent periorbital edema is noted initially after periods of lying flat and this may progress to persistent facial edema. An enlarged liver, ascites, and dependent edema may also be recognized. Medical treatment emphasizing an upright position during rest and judicious use of the diuretics may relieve symptoms to some degree, but surgical relief of the obstruction is eventually required.

Injury to the tricuspid apparatus causing tricuspid regurgitation or obstruction to pulmonary venous return by the atrial baffle may result in elevated pulmonary venous pressure and chronic pulmonary congestion.[42,162,167,168] Some patients with postoperative tricuspid incompetence have been reported, who have required insertion of an artificial valve to control massive regurgitation.[42]

Arrhythmias

Particular concern as to the long-term effects of present surgical treatment of patients with transposition of the great arteries stems from the frequent occurrence of cardiac arrhythmias following the Mustard operation. Most rhythm disturbances observed among these patients are supraventricular in origin and are due to sinus node injury and apparent interruption of atrial tracts (Fig. 2).[35,36,38-40] Many patients display an intermittent or permanent slow subsidiary junctional pacemaker. Some individuals have developed complete heart block following surgery.[164,169] Late sudden death has been reported.[35,42,43]

Right Ventricular Function

Although the great majority of patients operated upon for transposition of the great arteries are clinically well, decrease in right ventricular contractility,[167] depressed cardiac index,[170] and ejection fraction[171] have been reported. Concern as to long term cardiac function in these patients underscores the need for close followup of cardiac performance over the years.

Truncus Arteriosus

Correction of truncus arteriosus is currently accomplished by closure of the ventricular septal defect and insertion of a right ventricle to pulmonary artery conduit.[112] Most of the patients successfully repaired have been over 6 yr of age, and had preoperative hemodynamic studies which revealed that pulmonary resistance was not elevated to a severe degree. Nevertheless, long-term results will undoubtedly depend on whether pulmonary vascular obstructive disease is present. No long-term data are available as to the effect of surgical correction on the possible arrest or regression of mild to moderate pulmonary vascular disease. When unilateral absence of a pulmonary artery is present, prognosis may be more guarded because pulmonary vascular obstructive disease tends to progress more rapidly in these patients.[172] The long-term prognosis also depends on the proper function of the prosthetic conduit and competence of the truncal valve. Postoperative right ventricular failure in patients might be due to potentially correctable right ventricular to pulmonary artery obstruction at the conduit level rather than to progressive pulmonary vascular obstructive disease.[112] Truncal valve insufficiency is present prior to surgery in some patients and when severe requires replacement with a prosthetic valve in addition to the right ventricular-pulmonary artery conduit.

L-Transposition of the Great Arteries (Corrected Transposition)

The long-term outlook for patients with L-transposition is affected by the presence of various associated intracardiac defects and an increased incidence of atrioventricular block.[173] Until recently, total correction of this defect was associated with a prohibitive incidence of surgical complete heart block. Recent advances in the intraoperative delineation of the cardiac conduction system may decrease the risk of this complication.[174] Some patients with L-transposition have Ebstein type deformities of the left sided AV valve[174,175] which may require insertion of a prosthesis. Although the threat of spontaneous complete heart block remains, patients who have undergone successful correction of the associated defects are expected to be active and asymptomatic.

Patent Ductus Arteriosus

Division of a patent ductus arteriosus eliminates the possibility of recurrence. Rechannelization has been reported when a patent ductus arteriosus has been ligated but not divided.[176] However, with the exception of small infants, ligation has not been utilized over the past decade. The risk of pulmonary artery hypertension and elevated pulmonary resistance parallels that of ventricular septal defect. In the absence of pulmonary vascular disease, the cardiac status can be considered to be normal in postoperative patients.

Total Anomalous Pulmonary Venous Drainage

Surgical repair of total anomalous pulmonary venous drainage associated with pulmonary artery hypertension in infancy can be accomplished with virtually normal postoperative hemodynamics.[177] Similarly, nonobstructive total anomalous pulmonary venous drainage corrected later in childhood has not been associated with late complications.[178]

Tricuspid Atresia

Most patients with tricuspid atresia and decreased pulmonary blood flow benefit from superior vena cava to pulmonary artery anastomosis (Glenn procedure).[179,180] However, the development of venous collaterals several years after surgery may decrease the efficiency of the shunt.

Physiologic correction of tricuspid atresia has been carried out by means of direct right atrial to main pulmonary artery (or right ventricle) conduit following the earlier palliative Glenn operation.[181,182] Significant follow-up information is not yet available regarding this recent innovative operation.

Pulmonary Atresia With Intact Ventricular Septum

A number of patients with pulmonary atresia and intact ventricular septum with under-sized right ventricles have survived early pulmonary valvotomy and/or systemic to pulmonary arterial shunt.[183–186] Later angiographic studies have documented adequate growth of the right ventricular chamber,[187] and a few children have undergone subsequent open heart correction utilizing a valve containing conduit bypass from the right ventricle to the pulmonary artery.[161]

REFERENCES

1. National Center for Health Statistics. Heart facts reference sheets. USPHS, 1974.

2. Feldt RH, Stickler GB, Weidman WH: Growth of children with congenital heart disease. Am J Dis Child 117:573, 1969

3. Krovetz LJ: Weight gain in children with patent ductus arteriosus. Dis Chest 44:274–283, 1963

4. Ritter DG, Wallace RB, Weidman WH: Immediate and late results of the complete repair of severe tetralogy of Fallot. Heart Bull 14:92–94, 1965

5. Robinson SJ, Bayer LM: Growth history of children with congenital heart defects. I. Effect of operative intervention. Child Dev 307–314, 1969

6. Okada R, Johnson D, Lev M: Extracardial malformations associated with congenital disease. Arch Pathol 85: 649, 1968

7. Engle MA, Ehlers KH: Cardiovascular malformations in association with chromosomal aberrations, in Watson H (ed): Pediatric Cardiology. St. Louis, Mosby, 1968, p 688

8. Ehlers KH, Engle MA: Heart disease in hereditary syndromes, in Watson H (ed): Pediatric Cardiology. St. Louis, Mosby, 1968, p 676

9. Bayer LM, Robinson SJ: Growth history of children with congenital heart defects. Am J Dis Child 117:564, 1969

10. Roth A, Rosenthal A, Hall JE, et al: Scoliosis and congenital heart disease. Clin Orthop 93:95, 1973

11. Luke MJ, McDonnell EJ: Congenital heart disease and scoliosis. J Pediatr 73:725, 1968

12. White RI, Jr, Jordan CE, Fischer KC, et al: Skeletal changes associated with adolescent congenital heart disease. Am J Roentgenol Radium Ther Nucl Med 116:531, 1972

13. Marisaki N: Spinal scoliosis associated with congenital heart disease. J Jap Orthop Assoc 38:699, 1964

14. Moss AJ, Marcano B, Ruttenberg HD, et al: Intrapulmonary shunts in cyanotic congenital heart disease after surgical correction. Am J Cardiol 23:818, 1969

15. Gelband H, Waldo AL, Kaiser GA, et al: Etiology of right bundle branch block in patients undergoing total correction of tetralogy of Fallot. Circulation 44:1022, 1971

16. Krongrad E, Hefler SE, Bowman FO, Jr, et al: Further observations on the etiology of the right bundle branch block pattern following right ventriculotomy. Circulation 50:1105, 1974

17. Titus JL, Daugherty GW, Kirklin JW, et al: Lesions of the atrioventricular conduction system after repair of ventricular septal defect: Relation to heart block. Circulation 28:82, 1963

18. Okoroma EO, Guller B, Maloney JD, et al: Etiology of right bundle branch block following closure of ventricular septal defect. Pediatr Res 8(4):74, 1974

19. Wolff GS, Roland TW, Ellison RC: Surgically induced right bundle branch block with left anterior hemiblock. An ominous sign in postoperative tetralogy of Fallot. Circulation 46:587, 1972

20. Kulbertus HE, Coyne JJ, Hallidie-Smith KA: Conduction disturbance before and after surgical closure of ventricular septal defect. Am Heart J 77:123, 1969

21. Rosenbaum MD, Corrado G, Oliveri R, et al: Right bundle branch block with left anterior hemiblock surgically induced in tetralogy of Fallot. Relation to the mechanism of electrocardiographic changes in endocardial cushion defect. Am J Cardiol 26:12, 1970

22. Chesler E, Beck W, Schrire V: Left anterior hemiblock and right bundle branch block before and after surgical repair of tetralogy of Fallot. Am Heart J 84:45, 1972

23. Cairns JA, Dobell ARC, Gibbons J, et al: Benign prognosis of right bundle branch block and left anterior hemiblock after intracardiac repair of tetralogy of Fallot. (Abstr) Am J Cardiol 33:129, 1973

24. Godman MJ, Roberts NK, Izukawa T: Late postoperative conduction disturbances after repair of ventricular septal defect and tetralogy of Fallot. Analysis of His bundle branch recordings. Circulation 49:214, 1974

25. Downing JW, Kaplan S, Bore KE: Post surgical left anterior hemiblock and right bundle branch block. Br Heart J 34:263, 1972

26. Bocala RR, Guller B, Danielson GK, et al: Left anterior hemiblock and complete repair of tetralogy of Fallot. (Abstr) Pediatr Res 8:347, 1974

27. Steeg CN, Krongrad E, Davachi F, et al: Post surgical left anterior hemiblock pattern in tetralogy of Fallot. Circulation 51:1026–1029, 1975

28. Boineau JP, Moore NE, Patterson DF: Relationship between the ECG, ventricular activation and ventricular conduction system in ostium primum ASD. Circulation 48:556, 1973

29. Krongrad E, Rosen MR, Merker C, et al: Creation of counterclockwise superiorly oriented frontal plane loops in isolated blood perfused canine hearts. Pediatr Res 7:300/72, 1973

30. Watt TB, Pruitt RD: Focal lesions in the canine bundle of His Their effects on ventricular excitation. Circulation Res 31:531, 1972

31. Krongrad E, Rosen MR, Merker C, et al: Creation of trifascicular block in isolated blood perfused canine hearts. Circulation (Abstr)IV–21, 1973

32. Griffiths SP, Hayes CJ, Bowman FO, Jr, et al: Long term follow-up of two infants with implanted cardiac pacemakers. (submitted for publication)

33. Krongrad E, Malm JR, Bowman FO, Jr, et al: Electrophysiological delineation of the specialized A-V conduction system in patients with congenital heart disease. I. Delineation of the His bundle proximal to the membraneous septum. J Thorac Cardiovasc Surg 67:875, 1974

34. Krongrad E, Malm JR, Bowman FO, Jr, et al: Electrophysiological delineation of the specialized A-V conduction system in patients with congenital heart disease. II. Delineation of the distal His bundle and the right bundle branch. Circulation 49:1232, 1974

35. El-Said G, Rosenberg HS, Mullins CE, et al: Dysrhythmias after Mustard's operation for transposition of the great arteries. Am J Cardiol 30:526, 1972

36. Gillette PC, El-Said GM, Sivarajan N, et al: Electrophysiological abnormalities after Mustard's operation for transposition of the great arteries. Br Heart J 36:186, 1974

37. Waldo AL, Krongrad E, Bowman FO, Jr, et al: Electrophysiological considerations during total repair of transposition of the great vessels. Circulation 46(II):34, 1972 (Abstr)

38. Rodriguez-Fernandez HL, Kelley PT, Collado A, et al: Hemodynamic data and angiographic findings after Mustard repair for complete transposition of the great arteries. Circulation 46:799, 1972

39. Stanton RE, Lindesmith GG, Meyer BW: Arrhythmias following the Mustard operation for transposition of the great vessels. Circulation 45, 46(Supp. II):225, 1972 (Abstr)

40. Issacson R, Titus JL, Meredith J, et al: Apparent interruption of arterial conduction pathways after surgical repair of transposition of the great arteries. Am J Cardiol 30:533, 1972

41. Nugent EW, Varghese PJ, Row RD: "Sluggish" sinus node syndrome in children after open heart surgery for acyanotic congenital heart disease. Pediatr Res 7:298/70, 1973

42. Mair DD, Danielson GK, Wallace RB, et al: Late follow-up of Mustard operation survivors. Circulation (Suppl II), 49, 50:46, 1974

43. Lambert EC, Memon VA, Wagner HR, et al: Sudden unexpected death from cardiovascular disease in children. Am J Cardiol 34:89, 1974

44. Marshall RJ, Shepherd JT: Cardiac function in

health and disease, in Pericardial Disease. Philadelphia, Saunders, 1968, p 339 (Chap 14)

45. Morgan JR, Rogers AK, Forkner AD: Congenital absence of the left pericardium. Ann Intern Med 74:370, 1971

46. Blount SG: Follow-up of five patients with pulmonic valve insufficiency as a result of pulmonic valvuloplasty in 1953, in Kidd BSL, Keith JD (eds): The Natural History and Progress in Treatment of Congenital Heart Defects. Springfield, Ill, Thomas, 1971.

47. Kaplan S, Helmsworth JA, McKinivan CE, et al: The fate of reconstruction of the right ventricular outflow tract. J Thorac Cardiovasc Surg 66:361, 1973

48. Stafford EG, Mair DD, McGoon DC, et al: Tetralogy of Fallot with absent pulmonary valve: Surgical considerations and results. Circulation (Suppl III) 47–48:24, 1973

49. Ellis K: Postoperative roentgen evaluation of total correction of tetralogy of Fallot. Circulation 47:1335, 1973

50. Gersony WM, Malm JR: Late results of repair of tetralogy of Fallot, in Kirklin JW, (ed): Advances in Cardiovascular Surgery. New York, Grune & Stratton, 1973, p 17

51. Copeland WE, Wooley CF, Ryan JM, et al: Pregnancy and congenital heart disease. Am J Obstet Gynecol 86:107, 1963

52. Epstein SE, Beiser GD, Goldstein RE, et al: Hemodynamic abnormalities in response to mild and intense upright exercise following operative correction of an atrial septal defect or tetralogy of Fallot. Circulation 47:1065, 1973

53. Johnson AM: Impaired exercise response and other residua of pulmonary stenosis after valvulotomy. Br Heart J 24:375, 1962

54. Jonsson B, Lee SJK: Haemodynamic effects of exercise in isolated pulmonary stenosis before and after surgery. Br Heart J 30:60, 1968

55. Graham TP: Ventricular performance in patients following corrective surgery for congenital heart disease, in: A perspective on new techniques in congenital and acquired heart disease. Adv Cardiol, vol II. Brasel, Karger, 1974, pp 81–106

56. Maron BJ, Redwood DR, Hirshfeld JW, Jr, et al: Postoperative assesment of patients with ventricular septal defect and pulmonary hypertension, response to intense upright exercise. Circulation 48,864, 1973

57. Krongrad E, Ritter DG, Weidman WH, et al: Long term prognosis for infants with total correction of ventricular septal defect. Circulation 46(Suppl II):178, 1972, (Abstr)

58. Stone MF, Bessinger B, Lucas RV, et al: Pre and post operative rest and exercise hemodynamics in children with pulmonary stenosis. Circulation 49:1102, 1974

59. Engle MA, Adams FH, Betson C, et al: Resources for optimal long term care of congenital heart disease. Circulation 44A:205, 1971

60. Committee report of the American Heart Association Ad Hoc Committee on Rehabilitation of the Young Cardiac (Chairman, Weidman WH): Recreational activity and career choice recommendations for use by physicians counseling physical education directors, vocational counselors, parents and young patients with heart disease. Circulation 43:459, 1971

61. Committee Report: Prevention of Bacterial Endocarditis. Circulation 46:459, 1971

62. Round H, Kirkpatrick H, Hails B: Further investigation of bacterial infection of the mouth. Proc Roy Soc Med 29:1552, 1936

63. Okell C, Elliott S: Bacteremia and oral sepsis with special reference to the etiology of subacute endocarditis. Lancet 2:869, 1935

64. Harvey W, Capone M: Bacterial endocarditis related to cleaning and filling teeth. Am J Cardiol 7:793, 1961

65. Glaser K, Dankner A, Mathes S, et al: Effect of penicillin on bacteremia following dental extraction. Am J Med 4:55, 1948

66. Roads P, Sibley J, Billings C: Bacteremia following tonsillectomy. JAMA 157:877, 1955

67. Sullivan NM, Sutter VL, Mims MM, et al: Clinical aspects of bacteremia after manipulation of the genitourinary tract. J Infect Dis 127:49, 1973

68. Last PM, Harolison PA, Marsh JA: Bacteremia after urological instrumentation. Lancet 2:74, 1966

69. Slade N: Bacteremia and septicemia after urological operations. Proc Roy Soc Med 51:331, 1958

70. Miller A, Gillespie WA, Linton KB, et al: Post operative infection in urology. Lancet 2:608, 1958

71. Merrit W: Bacterial endocarditis as a complication of transurethral prostatic resection. J Urol 65:100, 1951

72. Speck WT, Dresdale SS, Krongrad E, et al: Absence of bacteremia after mistrumentation of the genitourinary tract in children. J Pediatr 85:224, 1974

73. McCauley D: Acute endocarditis in infancy and early childhood. Am J Dis Child 88:715, 1954

74. Burman SO, Bronchoscopy and bacteremia. J Thorac Cardiovasc Surg 40:635, 1960

75. Redleaf P, Fadell E: Bacteremia during parturition. JAMA 169:1284, 1959

76. Phornphutkul C, Rosenthal A, Nadas AS, et al: Cerebrovascular accidents in infants and children with cyanotic congenital heart disease. Am J Cardiol 32:329, 1973

77. Tyler RH, Clark DB: Cerebrovascular accidents in patients with congenital heart disease. Arch Neurol Psychiat 77:483, 1957

78. Gersony WM, White NR: Patch embolization following repair of ventricular septal defect. A complication of bacterial endocarditis. Am J Cardiol 26:315, 1970

79. Isom WO, Dembrow JM, Glassman E, et al: Factors influencing long term survival after isolated aortic valve replacement. Circulation (Suppl II) 49–50:163, 1974

80. Karp RB, Kirklin JW, Kouchoukos NT, et al: Comparison of three devices to replace the aortic valve. Circulation (Suppl II) 49–50:163, 1974

81. Isom OW, Williams CD, Spencer FC, et al: Evaluation of anticoagulant therapy in cloth covered prosthetic valves. Circulation (Suppl II)45–46:93, 1972

82. Paton BP: Artificial cardiac valves current status and future developments, in: A perspective on new techniques in congenital and acquired heart disease. Adv Cardiol II:192–197. Basel, Karger, 1974

83. Davies H, Roberts I: Homograft valves ten years later: The physicians' viewpoint, in: A perspective on new

techniques in congenital and acquired heart disease. Adv Cardiol II:198–210. Basel, Karger, 1974

84. Inman WHW, Vessey MP, Westerholm B, et al: Thromboembolic disease and the steroidal content of oral contraceptives. A report to the committee on Safety of Drugs. Br Med J 2:203, 1970

85. Sartwell PE, Masi AT, Arthes FG, et al: Thromboembolism and oral contraceptives: An epidemiological case control study. Am J Epidem 90:365, 1969

86. Stevenson TD, Baker HJ: Haemolytic anemia following the insertion of a lucite ball valve prosthesis into the cardiovascular system. Circulation 13:586, 1964

87. Reed WA, Dunn M: Fatal hemolysis following ball valve replacement of the aortic valve. J Thorac Cardiovasc Surg 48:436, 1964

88. Kloster FE, Bristow JD, Griswold HE: Medical problems in mitral and multiple valve replacement. Prog Cardiovasc Dis 7:504, 1965

89. Neill CA: Postoperative hemolytic anemia in endocardial cushion defects. Circulation 30:801, 1964

90. Verdon TA, Jr, Forrester RH, Crosley WH: Hemolytic anemia after open heart repair of ostium primum defects. N Engl J Med 269:444, 1963

91. Marsh GW, Lewis SM: Cardiac hemolytic anemia. Sem Hematol 6:133, 1969

92. Westring DW: Aortic valve disease and hemolytic anemia. Ann Intern Med 65:203, 1966

93. Gersony WM, Willerson WD, Johnson AF, et al: Aortic valvuloplasty during acute rheumatic fever. J Thorac Cardiovasc Surg 55:598, 1968

94. Eyster E, Mayer K, McKenzie S: Traumatic hemolysis with iron deficiency anemia in patients with aortic valve lesions. Ann Intern Med 68:995, 1968

95. Neill CA: Genetics of congenital heart disease. Ann Rev Med 24:61, 1973

96. Zetternist P: Multiple occurrence of atrial septal defect in a family. Acta Paediatr 49:741, 1960

97. Campbell M, Polani PE: Factors in the aetiology of atrial septal defect. Br Heart J 23:477, 1961

98. Johnsson BW, Sievers J: Inheritance of atrial septal defect. Lancet 1:1224, 1967

99. Williamson EM: A family study of atrial septal defects. J Med Genetics 6:255, 1969

100. Bizzaro RO, Callahan JA, Feldt RH, et al: Familial atrial septal defect with prolonged atrioventricular conduction. Circulation 41:677, 1970

101. Nora JJ, Meyer TC: Familial nature of congenital heart diseases. Pediatr 37:329, 1966

102. Nora JJ: Etologic factors in congenital heart disease. Pediatr Clin N Am 18:1059, 1971

103. Nora JJ: Genetic counseling in congenital heart disease, in A perspective on new techniques in congenital and acquired disease. Advances in Cardiology vol II. Brasel, Karger, 1974, pp 56–66

104. Nora JJ, Dodd PF, McNamara DG, et al: Risk of offspring of parents with congenital heart disease. JAMA 209:2052, 1969

105. Bristow JD, Kloster FE, Lees MH, et al: Serial cardiac catheterization and exercise hemodynamics after correction of tetralogy of Fallot. Circulation 41:1057, 1970

106. Olley PM: Follow-up of children treated with intracardiac repair for tetralogy of Fallot, in Kidd BSL, Keith JD (eds): The Natural History and Progress in Treatment of Congenital Heart Defects. Springfield, Ill, Thomas, 1971

107. Bjernulf A, Cullhed I, Hallein A, et al: Primary and late results of open correction of Fallot's disease. Acta Med Scand 184:89, 1968

108. Joransen JA, Moller JH: Postoperative hemodynamics studies in tetralogy of Fallot. Circulation 45–46(Suppl II):98, 1972 (Abstr)

109. Gotesman MS, Beck W, Barnard CN, et al: Results of repair of Fallot's tetralogy. Circulation 40:803, 1969

110. Kirklin JW, Karp RB: The tetralogy of Fallot from a surgical viewpoint. Philadelphia, Saunders, 1970

111. Malm JR, Blumenthal S, Bowman FO, Jr, et al: Factors that modify hemodynamic results in total correction of tetralogy of Fallot. J Thorac Cardiovasc Surg 52:502, 1966

112. Wallace RB, McGoon DC, Danielson GK: Complete correction of truncus arteriosus, pulmonary atresia, and transposition of the great arteries with ventricular septal defect and pulmonary stenosis, in: A Perspective on New Techniques in Congenital and Acquired Heart Disease. Advanced Cardiology vol II. Basel, Karger, 1974, pp 11–17

113. Kimsley RH, McGoon DC, Danielson GK, et al: Pulmonary arterial hypertension after repair of tetralogy of Fallot. J Thorac Cardiovasc Surg 67:110, 1974

114. Lillehei CW, Simmons RL, Todd DB: Late hemodynamic response to isolated pulmonary stenosis by open operation during pulmonary bypass. Circulation 37:258, 1965

115. Engle MA, Holswade GR, Goldberg HP, et al: Regression after open valvulotomy of infundibular stenosis accompanying severe valvular pulmonic stenosis. Circulation 17:862, 1958

116. Tandon R, Nadas AS, Gross RE: Results of open heart surgery in patients with pulmonic stenosis and intact ventricular septum. Circulation 31:190, 1965

117. Braimbridge MV, Oakley CM, Bentall HH, et al: Pulmonary valve stenosis without ventricular septal defect: results of surgery. Thorax 21:164, 1966

118. Engle MA, Ito T, Goldberg HP: The fate of the patient with pulmonic stenosis. Circulation 30:554, 1964

119. Conkle DM, Jones M, Morrow AG: Treatment of congenital aortic stenosis. Arch Surg 107:649, 1973

120. McGoon DC, Geha AS, Scofield EL, et al: Surgical treatment of congenital aortic stenosis. Dis Chest 55: 388, 1969

121. Campbell M: The natural history of congenital aortic stenosis. Br Heart J 30:514, 1968

122. Doyle EF, Arumugham P, Lara E, et al: Sudden death in young patients with congenital aortic stenosis. Pediatrics 53:481, 1974

123. Schwartz LS, Goldfisher J, Sprague OJ, et al: Syncope and sudden death in aortic stenosis. Am J Cardiol 23:647, 1969

124. Vincent WR, Buckberg GD, Hoffman JIE: Left ventricular subendocardial ischemia in severe valvar and supravalvar aortic stenosis. Circulation 49:326, 1974

125. Lewis AB, Heyman MA, Stranger P, et al: Evaluation of subendocardial ischemia in valvar aortic stenosis in children. Circulation 49:978, 1974

126. Moller JH, Nakib A, Edwards JE: Infarction of papillary muscles and mitral insufficiency associated with congenital aortic stenosis. Circulation 34:87, 1966

127. Cutilletta AF, Rudnik MM, Dowell RT, et al: Regression of myocardial hypertrophy. Pediatr Res 4:348/74, 1974 (Abstr)

128. Hartmann AF, Goldring D, Hernandez A, et al: Recurrent coarctation of the aorta after successful repair in infancy. Am J Cardiol 25:405, 1970

129. Ibarra-Perez C, Casteneda AR, Varco RL, et al: Recoarctation of the aorta. Ninteen year clinical experience. Am J Cardiol 23:778, 1969

130. Maron BJ, Humphries JO, Rowe RD, et al: Prognosis of surgically corrected coarctation of the aorta. A 20-year postoperative appraisal. Circulation 47:119, 1973

131. Freed MD, Keane JF, Van-Praah R, et al: Coarctation of the aorta with congenital mitral regurgitation. Circulation 49:1175, 1974

132. Lueker RD, Vogel JHK, Blount SG: Cardiovascular abnormalities following surgery for left to right shunts. Circulation 40:785, 1969

133. Cartmill TB, DuShane JW, McGoon DC, et al: Results of repair of ventricular septal defect. J Thorac Cardiovasc Surg 52:486, 1966

134. Allen HD, Anderson RC, Noren GR, et al: Postoperative follow-up of patients with ventricular septal defect. Circulation 50:465, 1974

135. Young D, Mark H: Fate of the patient with the Eisenmenger syndrome. Am J Cardiol 28:658, 1971

136. Brammell HL, Vogel JHK, Pryor R, et al: The Eisenmenger syndrome, a clinical and physiological reappraisal. Am. J. Card. 28:679, 1971.

137. Krongrad E, Helmholz HF, Jr, Ritter DG: Effect of breathing Oxygen on patients with severe pulmonary vascular obstructive disease. Circulation 47:94, 1973

138. Clarkson PM, Frye RL, DuShane JW, et al: Prognosis for patients with ventricular septal defect and severe pulmonary vascular obstructive disease. Circulation 38:129, 1968

139. Tatsuno K, Konno S, Ando M, et al: Pathogenetic mechanisms of prolapsing aortic valve and aortic regurgitation associated with ventricular septal defect. Circulation 49:1028, 1973

140. Kawashima Y, Danno M, Shimizu Y, et al: Ventricular septal defect associated with aortic insufficiency. Circulation 47:1057, 1973

141. Bonfils-Roberts EA, DuShane JW, McGoon DC, et al: Aortic sinus fistula: Surgical considerations and results of operation. Ann Thorac Surg 12:492, 1971

142. Glasser SP, Cheitlin MD, McCarty RJ, et al: Thirty-two cases of interventricular septal defect and aortic insufficiency. Am J Med 53:473, 1972

143. Spencer FC, Doyle EF, Danilowicz DA, et al: Long term evaluation of aortic valvuloplasty for aortic insufficiency and ventricular septal defect. J Thorac Cardiovasc Surg 65:15, 1973

144. Young D: Late results of closure of secundum atrial septal defect in children. Am J Cardiol 31:14, 1973

145. Petersson PO: Atrial septal defect of secundum type. Acta Paediatr Scand (Suppl)174, 1967

146. Hoffman LE, Krovetz LJ, VanMierop LHS, et al: Secundum atrial septal defects in children. Ann Thorac Surg 7:104, 1969

147. Davies DH, Pryor R, Blount SG, Jr: Electrocardiographic changes in atrial septal defect following surgical correction. Br Heart J 22:274, 1960

148. Nadas AS: The role of the physician in the management of patients with atrial septal defect. Prog Cardiovasc Dis 8:1, 1965

149. Tikoff G, Schmidt AM, Kuida H, et al: Heart failure in atrial septal defect. Am J Med 39:533, 1965

150. Griffiths SP, Ellis K, Burris JO, et al: Postoperative evaluation of mitral valve function in ostium primum defect with cleft mitral valve (partial form of atrioventricular canal) Circulation 40:21, 1969

151. Rastelli GC, Weidman WH, Kirklin JW: Surgical repair of the partial form of persistent common atrioventricular canal, with special reference to the problem of mitral valve incompetence. Circulation 39–40(Suppl I): I-31, 1965

152. McMullen MH, McGoon DC, Wallace RB, et al: Surgical treatment of partial atrioventricular canal. Arch Surg 107:705, 1973

153. Wallace RB, McGoon DC, Danielson GK: Complete atrioventricular canal, in: Perspective on New Techniques in Congenital and Acquired Heart Disease. Advanced Cardiology II: Basel, Karger, 1974, pp 26–35

154. Moss AJ, Klyman G, Emmanouilides GC: Late onset of complete heart block. Newly recognized sequela of cardiac surgery. Am J Cardiol 30:884, 1972

155. Rashkind WJ, Miller WW: Creation of an atrial septal defect without thoracotomy. JAMA 196:173, 1966

156. Rashkind WJ, Miller WM: Transposition of the great arteries. Results of palliation by balloon atrioseptostomy in 31 infants. Circulation 38:453, 1968

157. Mustard WT: Successful two-stage correction of transposition of the great vessels. Pediatr Surg 55:469, 1964

158. Mustard WT, Keith JD, Trusler GA, et al: The surgical management of transposition of the great vessels. J Thorac Cardiovasc Surg 48:953, 1964

159. Clarkson RM, Barratt-Boyes BG, Neutze JM, et al: Results over a ten-year period of palliation followed by corrective surgery for complete transposition of the great arteries. Circulation 45:1251, 1972

160. Danielson GK, Mair PP, Ongley PA, et al: Repair of transposition of the great arteries by transposition of venous return. J Thorac Cardiovasc Surg 61:96, 1971

161. McGoon DC, Wallace RB, Danielson GK: Homografts in reconstruction of congenital cardiac anomalies. Mayo Clinic Proc. 47:101, 1972

162. Stark J, Tynan MJ, Ashcraft KW, et al: Obstruction of pulmonary veins and superior vena cava after the Mustard operation for transposition of the great arteries. Circulation 45&46(Suppl I):116, 1972

163. Morgan JR, Miller BL, Daicoff GR, et al: Hemodynamic and angiographic evaluation after Mustard procedure for transposition of the great arteries. J Thorac Cardiovasc Surg 64:878, 1972

164. Rodriguez-Fernandez HL, Kelly DT, Collado A, et al: Hemodynamic data and angiographic findings after Mustard repair for complete transposition of the great arteries. Circulation 46:799, 1972

165. Friedli B, Godman MJ, Kidd L, et al: Late results of the baffle repair for transposition of the great arteries. Am J Cardiol 33:137, 1974 (Abstr)

166. Rizk G, Moller JH, Amplatz K: The angiographic appearance of the heart following the Mustard procedure. Diagn Radiology 106:269, 1973

167. El-Said G, Mullins CE, Nihill MR, et al: Hemodynamic changes after Mustard's operation for transposition of the great arteries. Am J Cardiol 31:129, 1973 (Abst)

168. Tynan M, Aberdeen E, Stark J: Tricuspid incompetence after the Mustard operation for transposition of the great arteries. Circulation 45&46(Suppl I):I–III, 1972

169. Champsaur GL, Sokol DM, Trusler GA, et al: Repair of transposition of the great arteries on 123 pediatric patients: Early and long term results. Circulation 47:1032, 1973

170. Parr GVS, Blackstone E, Kirklin JW, et al: Cardiac performance after Mustard procedure. Circulation 47&48 (Suppl IV):3, 1973 (Abstr)

171. Jarmakani JMM, Canent RV: Pre and post-operative right ventricular function in children with transposition of the great vessels. Circulation 47&48(Suppl IV): 34, 1973 (Abstr)

172. Mair DD, Ritter DG, Davis GD, et al: Selection of patients with truncus arteriosus for surgical correction. Anatomic and hemodynamic considerations. Circulation, 49:144, 1974

173. Freidberg DZ, Nadas AS: Clinical profile of patients with congenital corrected transposition of the great arteries. N Engl J Med 282:1053, 1970

174. Kupersmith J, Krongrad E, Gersony WM, et al: Electrophysiologic identification of the specialized conduction system in corrected transposition of the great vessels. Circulation 50:795, 1974

175. Schiefler GL, Edwards JE, Burchell HB, et al: Congenital corrected transposition of the great vessels: A study of 33 cases. Pediatrics 27:(Suppl II)851, 1961

176. Gross RE, Longino LA: The patent ductus arteriosus: Observations from 412 surgically treated cases. Circulation 3:125, 1951

177. Hordof AJ, Hayes CJ, Bowman FO, Jr, et al: Hemodynamic assessment of total anomalous pulmonary venous connection following correction during infancy. Am J Cardiol 33:144, 1974 (Abstr)

178. Gomes MMR, Feldt RH, McGoon DC, et al: Total anomalous pulmonary venous connection, J Thorac Cardiovasc Surg 60:116, 1972

179. Glenn WWL, Ordway NK, Talner NS, et al: Circulatory bypass of the right side of the heart: IV shunt between superior vena cava and distal right pulmonary artery: Report of clinical application in thirty-eight cases. Circulation 31:172, 1965

180. Glenn WL, Gardner TH, Jr, Talner NS, et al: Rational approach to the surgical management of tricuspid atresia. Circulation (Suppl II)37&38:62, 1967

181. Fontan F, Baudet E: Surgical repair of tricuspid atresia. Thorax 26:240, 1971

182. Ross DN, Somerville J: Surgical correction of tricuspid atresia. Lancet 1:845, 4/21/73

183. Somerville J: Management of pulmonary atresia. Br Heart J 32:641, 1970

184. Bowman FO, Jr, Malm JR, Hayes CJ, et al: Pulmonary atresia with intact ventricular septum. J Thorac Cardiovasc Surg 61:85, 1971

185. Dhanavaravibul S, Nora JJ, McNamara DG: Pulmonary valvular atresia with intact ventricular septum. Problems in diagnosis and results of treatment. J Pediatr 77:1010, 1970

186. Luckstead EF, Mattioli L, Crosby IK, et al: Two stage palliative surgical approach for pulmonary atresia with intact ventricular septum (Type I). Am J Cardiol 29:490, 1972

187. Graham TP, Bender HW, Atwood GF, et al: Increase in right ventricular volume following valvulotomy for pulmonary atresia or stenosis with intact ventricular septum. Circulation 49–50(Suppl II):69, 1974

INDEX

a b 5 c 6 d 7 e 8 f 9 g 0 h 1 i 8 2 j